# THE OFFICIAL PATIENT'S SOURCEBOOK

## *on*

# KIDNEY FAILURE

AND P                    ITORS

ICON Health Publications
ICON Group International, Inc.
4370 La Jolla Village Drive, 4th Floor
San Diego, CA 92122 USA

Printed in the United States of America.

Last digit indicates print number: 10 9 8 7 6 4 5 3 2 1

Publisher, Health Care: Philip Parker, Ph.D.
Editor(s): James Parker, M.D., Philip Parker, Ph.D.

**Publisher's note:** The ideas, procedures, and suggestions contained in this book are not intended as a substitute for consultation with your physician. All matters regarding your health require medical supervision. As new medical or scientific information becomes available from academic and clinical research, recommended treatments and drug therapies may undergo changes. The authors, editors, and publisher have attempted to make the information in this book up to date and accurate in accord with accepted standards at the time of publication. The authors, editors, and publisher are not responsible for errors or omissions or for consequences from application of the book, and make no warranty, expressed or implied, in regard to the contents of this book. Any practice described in this book should be applied by the reader in accordance with professional standards of care used in regard to the unique circumstances that may apply in each situation, in close consultation with a qualified physician. The reader is advised to always check product information (package inserts) for changes and new information regarding dose and contraindications before taking any drug or pharmacological product. Caution is especially urged when using new or infrequently ordered drugs, herbal remedies, vitamins and supplements, alternative therapies, complementary therapies and medicines, and integrative medical treatments.

Cataloging-in-Publication Data

Parker, James N., 1961-
Parker, Philip M., 1960-

    The Official Patient's Sourcebook on Kidney Failure: A Revised and Updated Directory for the Internet Age/James N. Parker and Philip M. Parker, editors
            p.          cm.
    Includes bibliographical references, glossary and index.
    ISBN: 0-497-00989-7
    1. Kidney Failure-Popular works.        I. Title.

# Disclaimer

This publication is not intended to be used for the diagnosis or treatment of a health problem or as a substitute for consultation with licensed medical professionals. It is sold with the understanding that the publisher, editors, and authors are not engaging in the rendering of medical, psychological, financial, legal, or other professional services.

References to any entity, product, service, or source of information that may be contained in this publication should not be considered an endorsement, either direct or implied, by the publisher, editors or authors. ICON Group International, Inc., the editors, or the authors are not responsible for the content of any Web pages nor publications referenced in this publication.

# Copyright Notice

# Dedication

To the healthcare professionals dedicating their time and efforts to the study of kidney failure.

# Acknowledgements

The collective knowledge generated from academic and applied research summarized in various references has been critical in the creation of this sourcebook which is best viewed as a comprehensive compilation and collection of information prepared by various official agencies which directly or indirectly are dedicated to kidney failure. All of the *Official Patient's Sourcebooks* draw from various agencies and institutions associated with the United States Department of Health and Human Services, and in particular, the Office of the Secretary of Health and Human Services (OS), the Administration for Children and Families (ACF), the Administration on Aging (AOA), the Agency for Healthcare Research and Quality (AHRQ), the Agency for Toxic Substances and Disease Registry (ATSDR), the Centers for Disease Control and Prevention (CDC), the Food and Drug Administration (FDA), the Healthcare Financing Administration (HCFA), the Health Resources and Services Administration (HRSA), the Indian Health Service (IHS), the institutions of the National Institutes of Health (NIH), the Program Support Center (PSC), and the Substance Abuse and Mental Health Services Administration (SAMHSA). In addition to these sources, information gathered from the National Library of Medicine, the United States Patent Office, the European Union, and their related organizations has been invaluable in the creation of this sourcebook. Some of the work represented was financially supported by the Research and Development Committee at INSEAD. This support is gratefully acknowledged. Finally, special thanks are owed to Tiffany Freeman for her excellent editorial support.

# About the Editors

**James N. Parker, M.D.**

Dr. James N. Parker received his Bachelor of Science degree in Psychobiology from the University of California, Riverside and his M.D. from the University of California, San Diego. In addition to authoring numerous research publications, he has lectured at various academic institutions. Dr. Parker is the medical editor for the *Official Patient's Sourcebook* series published by ICON Health Publications.

**Philip M. Parker, Ph.D.**

Philip M. Parker is the Eli Lilly Chair Professor of Innovation, Business and Society at INSEAD (Fontainebleau, France and Singapore). Dr. Parker has also been Professor at the University of California, San Diego and has taught courses at Harvard University, the Hong Kong University of Science and Technology, the Massachusetts Institute of Technology, Stanford University, and UCLA. Dr. Parker is the associate editor for the *Official Patient's Sourcebook* series published by ICON Health Publications.

# About ICON Health Publications

In addition to kidney failure, *Official Patient's Sourcebooks* are available for the following related topics:

- The Official Patient's Sourcebook on Childhood Nephrotic Syndrome
- The Official Patient's Sourcebook on Cystocele
- The Official Patient's Sourcebook on Glomerular Disease
- The Official Patient's Sourcebook on Goodpasture Syndrome
- The Official Patient's Sourcebook on Hematuria
- The Official Patient's Sourcebook on Hemochromatosis
- The Official Patient's Sourcebook on Immune Thrombocytopenic Purpura
- The Official Patient's Sourcebook on Impotence
- The Official Patient's Sourcebook on Interstitial Cystitis
- The Official Patient's Sourcebook on Kidney Stones
- The Official Patient's Sourcebook on Lupus Nephritis
- The Official Patient's Sourcebook on Nephrotic Syndrome
- The Official Patient's Sourcebook on Peyronie
- The Official Patient's Sourcebook on Polycystic Kidney Disease
- The Official Patient's Sourcebook on Prostate Enlargement
- The Official Patient's Sourcebook on Prostatitis
- The Official Patient's Sourcebook on Proteinuria
- The Official Patient's Sourcebook on Pyelonephritis
- The Official Patient's Sourcebook on Renal Osteodystrophy
- The Official Patient's Sourcebook on Renal Tubular Acidosis
- The Official Patient's Sourcebook on Simple Kidney Cysts
- The Official Patient's Sourcebook on Urinary Incontinence
- The Official Patient's Sourcebook on Urinary Incontinence for Women
- The Official Patient's Sourcebook on Urinary Incontinence with Children
- The Official Patient's Sourcebook on Urinary Tract Infection in Children
- The Official Patient's Sourcebook on Urinary Tract Infections in Adults
- The Official Patient's Sourcebook on Vasectomy
- The Official Patient's Sourcebook on Vesicoureteral Reflux

To discover more about ICON Health Publications, simply check with your preferred online booksellers, including Barnes&Noble.com and Amazon.com which currently carry all of our titles. Or, feel free to contact us directly for bulk purchases or institutional discounts:

ICON Group International, Inc.
4370 La Jolla Village Drive, Fourth Floor
San Diego, CA 92122 USA
Fax: 858-546-4341
Web site: **www.icongrouponline.com/health**

# Table of Contents

# INTRODUCTION

## Overview

Dr. C. Everett Koop, former U.S. Surgeon General, once said, "The best prescription is knowledge."[1] The Agency for Healthcare Research and Quality (AHRQ) of the National Institutes of Health (NIH) echoes this view and recommends that every patient incorporate education into the treatment process. According to the AHRQ:

> Finding out more about your condition is a good place to start. By contacting groups that support your condition, visiting your local library, and searching on the Internet, you can find good information to help guide your treatment decisions. Some information may be hard to find—especially if you don't know where to look.[2]

As the AHRQ mentions, finding the right information is not an obvious task. Though many physicians and public officials had thought that the emergence of the Internet would do much to assist patients in obtaining reliable information, in March 2001 the National Institutes of Health issued the following warning:

> The number of Web sites offering health-related resources grows every day. Many sites provide valuable information, while others may have information that is unreliable or misleading.[3]

---

[1] Quotation from **http://www.drkoop.com**.
[2] The Agency for Healthcare Research and Quality (AHRQ):
**http://www.ahcpr.gov/consumer/diaginfo.htm**.
[3] From the NIH, National Cancer Institute (NCI):
**http://cancertrials.nci.nih.gov/beyond/evaluating.html**.

Since the late 1990s, physicians have seen a general increase in patient Internet usage rates. Patients frequently enter their doctor's offices with printed Web pages of home remedies in the guise of latest medical research. This scenario is so common that doctors often spend more time dispelling misleading information than guiding patients through sound therapies. *The Official Patient's Sourcebook on Kidney Failure* has been created for patients who have decided to make education and research an integral part of the treatment process. The pages that follow will tell you where and how to look for information covering virtually all topics related to kidney failure, from the essentials to the most advanced areas of research.

The title of this book includes the word "official." This reflects the fact that the sourcebook draws from public, academic, government, and peer-reviewed research. Selected readings from various agencies are reproduced to give you some of the latest official information available to date on kidney failure.

Given patients' increasing sophistication in using the Internet, abundant references to reliable Internet-based resources are provided throughout this sourcebook. Where possible, guidance is provided on how to obtain free-of-charge, primary research results as well as more detailed information via the Internet. E-book and electronic versions of this sourcebook are fully interactive with each of the Internet sites mentioned (clicking on a hyperlink automatically opens your browser to the site indicated). Hard copy users of this sourcebook can type cited Web addresses directly into their browsers to obtain access to the corresponding sites. Since we are working with ICON Health Publications, hard copy *Sourcebooks* are frequently updated and printed on demand to ensure that the information provided is current.

In addition to extensive references accessible via the Internet, every chapter presents a "Vocabulary Builder." Many health guides offer glossaries of technical or uncommon terms in an appendix. In editing this sourcebook, we have decided to place a smaller glossary within each chapter that covers terms used in that chapter. Given the technical nature of some chapters, you may need to revisit many sections. Building one's vocabulary of medical terms in such a gradual manner has been shown to improve the learning process.

We must emphasize that no sourcebook on kidney failure should affirm that a specific diagnostic procedure or treatment discussed in a research study, patent, or doctoral dissertation is "correct" or your best option. This sourcebook is no exception. Each patient is unique. Deciding on appropriate options is always up to the patient in consultation with their physician and healthcare providers.

## Organization

This sourcebook is organized into three parts. Part I explores basic techniques to researching kidney failure (e.g. finding guidelines on diagnosis, treatments, and prognosis), followed by a number of topics, including information on how to get in touch with organizations, associations, or other patient networks dedicated to kidney failure. It also gives you sources of information that can help you find a doctor in your local area specializing in treating kidney failure. Collectively, the material presented in Part I is a complete primer on basic research topics for patients with kidney failure.

Part II moves on to advanced research dedicated to kidney failure. Part II is intended for those willing to invest many hours of hard work and study. It is here that we direct you to the latest scientific and applied research on kidney failure. When possible, contact names, links via the Internet, and summaries are provided. It is in Part II where the vocabulary process becomes important as authors publishing advanced research frequently use highly specialized language. In general, every attempt is made to recommend "free-to-use" options.

Part III provides appendices of useful background reading for all patients with kidney failure or related disorders. The appendices are dedicated to more pragmatic issues faced by many patients with kidney failure. Accessing materials via medical libraries may be the only option for some readers, so a guide is provided for finding local medical libraries which are open to the public. Part III, therefore, focuses on advice that goes beyond the biological and scientific issues facing patients with kidney failure.

## Scope

While this sourcebook covers kidney failure, your doctor, research publications, and specialists may refer to your condition using a variety of terms. Therefore, you should understand that kidney failure is often considered a synonym or a condition closely related to the following:

- Acute Kidney Failure
- Chronic Kidney Failure

- Chronic Renal Insufficiency
- End Stage Renal Disease
- End-stage Renal Disease
- Functional Renal Failure of Cirrhosis
- Hemodynamic Renal Failure of Cirrhosis
- Hepatic Nephropathy
- Hepato-renal Syndrome
- Heyd's Syndrome
- Kidney Failure
- Kidney Failure - Acute
- Kidney Failure - Chronic
- Kidney Failure - End Stage
- Myoglobinuria with Renal Failure
- Oliguric Renal Failure of Cirrhosis
- Renal Failure
- Renal Failure - Acute
- Renal Failure - Chronic
- Renal Failure - End Stage
- Renal Failure of Cirrhosis
- Uremia

In addition to synonyms and related conditions, physicians may refer to kidney failure using certain coding systems. The International Classification of Diseases, 9th Revision, Clinical Modification (ICD-9-CM) is the most commonly used system of classification for the world's illnesses. Your physician may use this coding system as an administrative or tracking tool. The following classification is commonly used for kidney failure:[4]

- 572.4 hepatorenal syndrome
- 584.9 acute renal failure unspecified
- 584.9 acute renal failure, unspecified

---

[4] This list is based on the official version of the World Health Organization's 9th Revision, International Classification of Diseases (ICD-9). According to the National Technical Information Service, "ICD-9CM extensions, interpretations, modifications, addenda, or errata other than those approved by the U.S. Public Health Service and the Health Care Financing Administration are not to be considered official and should not be utilized. Continuous maintenance of the ICD-9-CM is the responsibility of the federal government."

- 585 chronic renal failure
- 728.89 idiopathic rhabdomyolysis
- 728.89 rhabdomyolysis
- 997.4 hepatorenal syndrome, resulting from a procedure

For the purposes of this sourcebook, we have attempted to be as inclusive as possible, looking for official information for all of the synonyms relevant to kidney failure. You may find it useful to refer to synonyms when accessing databases or interacting with healthcare professionals and medical librarians.

## Moving Forward

Since the 1980s, the world has seen a proliferation of healthcare guides covering most illnesses. Some are written by patients or their family members. These generally take a layperson's approach to understanding and coping with an illness or disorder. They can be uplifting, encouraging, and highly supportive. Other guides are authored by physicians or other healthcare providers who have a more clinical outlook. Each of these two styles of guide has its purpose and can be quite useful.

As editors, we have chosen a third route. We have chosen to expose you to as many sources of official and peer-reviewed information as practical, for the purpose of educating you about basic and advanced knowledge as recognized by medical science today. You can think of this sourcebook as your personal Internet age reference librarian.

Why "Internet age"? All too often, patients diagnosed with kidney failure will log on to the Internet, type words into a search engine, and receive several Web site listings which are mostly irrelevant or redundant. These patients are left to wonder where the relevant information is, and how to obtain it. Since only the smallest fraction of information dealing with kidney failure is even indexed in search engines, a non-systematic approach often leads to frustration and disappointment. With this sourcebook, we hope to direct you to the information you need that you would not likely find using popular Web directories. Beyond Web listings, in many cases we will reproduce brief summaries or abstracts of available reference materials. These abstracts often contain distilled information on topics of discussion.

While we focus on the more scientific aspects of kidney failure, there is, of course, the emotional side to consider. Later in the sourcebook, we provide a chapter dedicated to helping you find peer groups and associations that can provide additional support beyond research produced by medical science. We hope that the choices we have made give you the most options available in moving forward. In this way, we wish you the best in your efforts to incorporate this educational approach into your treatment plan.

*The Editors*

# PART I: THE ESSENTIALS

## ABOUT PART I

Part I has been edited to give you access to what we feel are "the essentials" on kidney failure. The essentials of a disease typically include the definition or description of the disease, a discussion of who it affects, the signs or symptoms associated with the disease, tests or diagnostic procedures that might be specific to the disease, and treatments for the disease. Your doctor or healthcare provider may have already explained the essentials of kidney failure to you or even given you a pamphlet or brochure describing kidney failure. Now you are searching for more in-depth information. As editors, we have decided, nevertheless, to include a discussion on where to find essential information that can complement what your doctor has already told you. In this section we recommend a process, not a particular Web site or reference book. The process ensures that, as you search the Web, you gain background information in such a way as to maximize your understanding.

# CHAPTER 1. THE ESSENTIALS ON KIDNEY FAILURE: GUIDELINES

## Overview

Official agencies, as well as federally funded institutions supported by national grants, frequently publish a variety of guidelines on kidney failure. These are typically called "Fact Sheets" or "Guidelines." They can take the form of a brochure, information kit, pamphlet, or flyer. Often they are only a few pages in length. The great advantage of guidelines over other sources is that they are often written with the patient in mind. Since new guidelines on kidney failure can appear at any moment and be published by a number of sources, the best approach to finding guidelines is to systematically scan the Internet-based services that post them.

### The National Institutes of Health (NIH)[5]

The National Institutes of Health (NIH) is the first place to search for relatively current patient guidelines and fact sheets on kidney failure. Originally founded in 1887, the NIH is one of the world's foremost medical research centers and the federal focal point for medical research in the United States. At any given time, the NIH supports some 35,000 research grants at universities, medical schools, and other research and training institutions, both nationally and internationally. The rosters of those who have conducted research or who have received NIH support over the years include the world's most illustrious scientists and physicians. Among them are 97 scientists who have won the Nobel Prize for achievement in medicine.

---

[5] Adapted from the NIH: **http://www.nih.gov/about/NIHoverview.html**.

There is no guarantee that any one Institute will have a guideline on a specific disease, though the National Institutes of Health collectively publish over 600 guidelines for both common and rare diseases. The best way to access NIH guidelines is via the Internet. Although the NIH is organized into many different Institutes and Offices, the following is a list of key Web sites where you are most likely to find NIH clinical guidelines and publications dealing with kidney failure and associated conditions:

- Office of the Director (OD); guidelines consolidated across agencies available at **http://www.nih.gov/health/consumer/conkey.htm**

- National Library of Medicine (NLM); extensive encyclopedia (A.D.A.M., Inc.) with guidelines available at **http://www.nlm.nih.gov/medlineplus/healthtopics.html**

- National Institute of Diabetes and Digestive and Kidney Diseases (NIDDK); guidelines available at **http://www.niddk.nih.gov/health/health.htm**

Among these, the National Institute of Diabetes and Digestive and Kidney Diseases (NIDDK) is particularly noteworthy. The NIDDK's mission is to conduct and support research on many of the most serious diseases affecting public health.[6] The Institute supports much of the clinical research on the diseases of internal medicine and related subspecialty fields as well as many basic science disciplines. The NIDDK's Division of Intramural Research encompasses the broad spectrum of metabolic diseases such as diabetes, inborn errors of metabolism, endocrine disorders, mineral metabolism, digestive diseases, nutrition, urology and renal disease, and hematology. Basic research studies include biochemistry, nutrition, pathology, histochemistry, chemistry, physical, chemical, and molecular biology, pharmacology, and toxicology. NIDDK extramural research is organized into divisions of program areas:

- Division of Diabetes, Endocrinology, and Metabolic Diseases

- Division of Digestive Diseases and Nutrition

- Division of Kidney, Urologic, and Hematologic Diseases

The Division of Extramural Activities provides administrative support and overall coordination. A fifth division, the Division of Nutrition Research Coordination, coordinates government nutrition research efforts. The Institute supports basic and clinical research through investigator-initiated

---

[6] This paragraph has been adapted from the NIDDK: **http://www.niddk.nih.gov/welcome/mission.htm**. "Adapted" signifies that a passage is reproduced exactly or slightly edited for this book.

grants, program project and center grants, and career development and training awards. The Institute also supports research and development projects and large-scale clinical trials through contracts. The following patient guideline was recently published by the NIDDK on kidney failure.

## What Is Kidney Failure?[7]

Your kidneys filter wastes from your blood and regulate other functions of your body. When your kidneys fail, you need treatment to replace the work of healthy kidneys to survive.

Developing kidney failure means that you have some decisions to make about your treatment. If you choose to receive treatment, your choices are hemodialysis, peritoneal dialysis, and kidney transplantation. Each of them has advantages and disadvantages. You may also choose to forgo treatment. By learning about your choices, you can work with your doctor to decide what's best for you. No matter which treatment you choose, you'll need to make some changes in your life, including how you eat and plan your activities. But with the help of your health care team, family, and friends, you can lead a full, active life.

## When Your Kidneys Fail

Healthy kidneys clean your blood by removing excess fluid, minerals, and wastes. They also make hormones that keep your bones strong and your blood healthy. When your kidneys fail, harmful wastes build up in your body, your blood pressure may rise, and your body may retain excess fluid and not make enough red blood cells. When this happens, you need treatment to replace the work of your failed kidneys.

## Treatment Choice: Hemodialysis

### Purpose

Hemodialysis cleans and filters your blood using a machine to temporarily rid your body of harmful wastes, extra salt, and extra water. Hemodialysis

---

[7] Adapted from the National Institute of Diabetes and Digestive and Kidney Diseases (NIDDK): **http://kidney.niddk.nih.gov/kudiseases/pubs/choosingtreatment/index.htm**.

helps control blood pressure and helps your body keep the proper balance of important chemicals such as potassium, sodium, calcium, and bicarbonate.

### How It Works

Hemodialysis uses a special filter called a dialyzer that functions as an artificial kidney to clean your blood. During treatment, your blood travels through tubes into the dialyzer, which filters out wastes and extra water. Then the cleaned blood flows through another set of tubes back into your body. The dialyzer is connected to a machine that monitors blood flow and removes wastes from the blood.

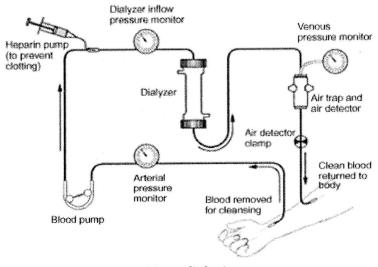

*Hemodialysis*

Hemodialysis is usually needed three times a week. Each treatment lasts from 3 to 5 or more hours. During treatment, you can read, write, sleep, talk, or watch TV.

### Getting Ready

If you choose hemodialysis, several months before your first treatment, an access to your bloodstream will need to be created. You may need to stay overnight in the hospital, but many patients have their access placed on an outpatient basis. This access provides an efficient way for blood to be carried from your body to the dialysis machine and back without causing discomfort. The two main types of access are a fistula and a graft.

- A surgeon makes a fistula by using your own blood vessels; an artery is connected directly to a vein, usually in your forearm. The increased blood flow makes the vein grow larger and stronger so that it can be used for repeated needle insertions. This is the preferred type of access. It may take several weeks to be ready for use.

- A graft connects an artery to a vein by using a synthetic tube. It doesn't need to develop as a fistula does, so it can be used sooner after placement. But a graft is more likely to have problems with infection and clotting.

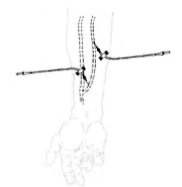

*Arteriovenous Fistula*

Needles are placed into the access to draw out the blood. You'll be given a local anesthetic to minimize any pain during dialysis.

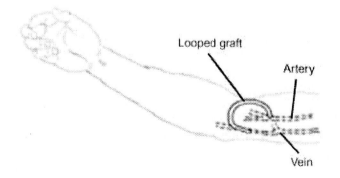

Looped graft
Artery
Vein

*Graft*

If your kidney disease has progressed quickly, you may not have time to get a permanent vascular access before you start hemodialysis treatments. You may need to use a catheter, a tube inserted into a vein in your neck, chest, or leg near the groin, as a temporary access. Some people use a catheter for long-term access as well. Catheters that will be needed for more than about 3 weeks are designed to be placed under the skin to increase comfort and reduce complications.

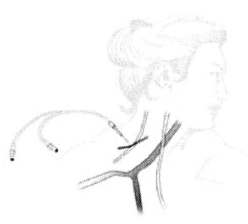

*Catheter for temporary access.*

### Who Performs It

Hemodialysis is usually done in a dialysis center by nurses and trained technicians. In some parts of the country, it can be done at home with the help of a partner, usually a family member or friend. If you decide to do home dialysis, you and your partner will receive special training.

### Possible Complications

Vascular access problems are the most common reason for hospitalization among people on hemodialysis. Common problems include infection, blockage from clotting, and poor blood flow. These problems can keep your treatments from working. You may need to undergo repeated surgeries in order to get a properly functioning access.

Other problems can be caused by rapid changes in your body's water and chemical balance during treatment. Muscle cramps and hypotension, or a sudden drop in blood pressure, are two common side effects. Low blood pressure or hypotension can make you feel weak, dizzy, or sick to your stomach.

You'll probably need a few months to adjust to hemodialysis. Side effects can often be treated quickly and easily, so you should always report them to your doctor and dialysis staff. You can avoid many side effects if you follow a proper diet, limit your liquid intake, and take your medicines as directed.

### Diet for Hemodialysis

Hemodialysis and a proper diet help reduce the wastes that build up in your blood. A dietitian is available at all dialysis centers to help you plan meals according to your doctor's orders. When choosing foods, you should remember to

- Eat balanced amounts of high-protein foods such as meat, chicken, and fish.

- Control the amount of potassium you eat. Potassium is a mineral found in salt substitutes, some fruits (bananas, oranges), vegetables, chocolate, and nuts. Too much potassium can be dangerous.

- Limit how much you drink. When your kidneys aren't working, water builds up quickly in your body. Too much liquid makes your tissues swell and can lead to high blood pressure, heart trouble, and cramps and low blood pressure during dialysis.

- Avoid salt. Salty foods make you thirsty and make your body hold water.

- Limit foods such as milk, cheese, nuts, dried beans, and dark colas. These foods contain large amounts of the mineral phosphorus. Too much phosphorus in your blood causes calcium to be pulled from your bones, which makes them weak and brittle and can cause arthritis. To prevent bone problems, your doctor may give you special medicines, which you must take with meals every day as directed.

Each person responds differently to similar situations. What may be a negative factor for one person may be positive for another. See a list of the general advantages and disadvantages of in-center and home hemodialysis below.

### In-Center Hemodialysis

Pros:

- Facilities are widely available.
- You have trained professionals with you at all times
- You can get to know other patients.

Cons:

- Treatments are scheduled by the center and are relatively fixed.
- You must travel to the center for treatment.

### Home Hemodialysis

Pros:

- You can do it at the times you choose (but you still must do it as often as your doctor orders).
- You don't have to travel to a center.
- You gain a sense of independence and control over your treatment.

Cons:

- You must have a helper.
- Helping with treatments may be stressful to your family.
- You and your helper need training.
- You need space for storing the machine and supplies at home.

### Working with Your Health Care Team

Questions you may want to ask:

- Is hemodialysis the best treatment choice for me? Why?
- If I'm treated at a center, can I go to the center of my choice?
- What should I look for in a dialysis center?
- Will my kidney doctor see me at dialysis?
- What does hemodialysis feel like?

- What is self-care dialysis?

- Is home hemodialysis available in my area? How long does it take to learn? Who will train my partner and me?

- What kind of blood access is best for me?

- As a hemodialysis patient, will I be able to keep working? Can I have treatments at night?

- How much should I exercise?

- Who will be on my health care team? How can these people help me?

- Whom can I talk with about finances, sexuality, or family concerns?

- How/where can I talk to other people who have faced this decision?


## Treatment Choice: Peritoneal Dialysis

### Purpose

Peritoneal dialysis is another procedure that removes extra water, wastes, and chemicals from your body. This type of dialysis uses the lining of your abdomen to filter your blood. This lining is called the peritoneal membrane and acts as the artificial kidney.


### How It Works

A mixture of minerals and sugar dissolved in water, called dialysis solution, travels through a soft tube into your abdomen. The sugar, called dextrose, draws wastes, chemicals, and extra water from the tiny blood vessels in your peritoneal membrane into the dialysis solution. After several hours, the used solution is drained from your abdomen through the tube, taking the wastes from your blood with it. Then you fill your abdomen with fresh dialysis solution, and the cycle is repeated. Each cycle is called an exchange.

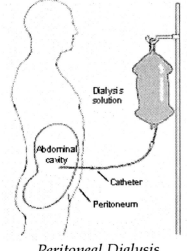

*Peritoneal Dialysis*

### Getting Ready

Before your first treatment, a surgeon places a small, soft tube called a catheter into your abdomen. The catheter tends to work better if there is adequate time--usually from 10 days to 2 or 3 weeks--for the insertion site to heal. This is another way in which planning your dialysis access can improve treatment success. This catheter stays there permanently to help transport the dialysis solution to and from your abdomen.

### Types of Peritoneal Dialysis

There are three types of peritoneal dialysis:

- Continuous Ambulatory Peritoneal Dialysis (CAPD)
- Continuous Cycler-Assisted Peritoneal Dialysis (CCPD)
- Combination of CAPD and CCPD

### Continuous Ambulatory Peritoneal Dialysis (CAPD)

CAPD is the most common type of peritoneal dialysis. It requires no machine and can be done in any clean, well-lit place. With CAPD, your blood is always being cleaned. The dialysis solution passes from a plastic bag through the catheter and into your abdomen, where it stays for several hours with the catheter sealed. The period that dialysis solution is in your abdomen is called the dwell time. Next, you drain the dialysis solution back into the bag for disposal. You then use the same catheter to refill your abdomen with fresh dialysis solution so the cleaning process can begin again. With CAPD, the dialysis solution stays in your abdomen for a dwell time of 4 to 6 hours (or more). The process of draining the used dialysis solution and replacing it with fresh solution takes about 30 to 40 minutes. Most people change the dialysis solution at least four times a day and sleep with solution in their abdomen at night. With CAPD, it's not necessary to wake up and perform dialysis tasks during the night.

## Continuous Cycler-Assisted Peritoneal Dialysis (CCPD)

CCPD uses a machine called a cycler to fill and empty your abdomen three to five times during the night while you sleep. In the morning, you begin one exchange with a dwell time that lasts the entire day. You may do an additional exchange in the middle of the afternoon without the cycler to increase the amount of waste removed and to reduce the amount of fluid left behind in your body.

## Combination of CAPD and CCPD

If you weigh more than 175 pounds or if your peritoneum filters wastes slowly, you may need a combination of CAPD and CCPD to get the right dialysis dose. For example, some people use a cycler at night but also perform one exchange during the day. Others do four exchanges during the day and use a minicycler to perform one or more exchanges during the night. You'll work with your health care team to determine the best schedule for you.

## Who Performs It

Both types of peritoneal dialysis are usually performed by the patient without help from a partner. CAPD is a form of self-treatment that needs no machine. However, with CCPD, you need a machine to drain and refill your abdomen.

## Possible Complications

The most common problem with peritoneal dialysis is peritonitis, a serious abdominal infection. This infection can occur if the opening where the catheter enters your body becomes infected or if contamination occurs as the catheter is connected or disconnected from the bags. Peritonitis requires antibiotic treatment by your doctor.

To avoid peritonitis, you must be careful to follow procedures exactly and learn to recognize the early signs of peritonitis, which include fever, unusual color or cloudiness of the used fluid, and redness or pain around the catheter. Report these signs to your doctor immediately so that peritonitis can be treated quickly to avoid serious problems.

### Diet for Peritoneal Dialysis

A peritoneal dialysis diet is slightly different from a hemodialysis diet.

- You'll still need to limit salt and liquids, but you may be able to have more of each, compared with hemodialysis.

- You must eat more protein.

- You may have different restrictions on potassium.

- You may need to cut back on the number of calories you eat because there are calories in the dialysis fluid that may cause you to gain weight.

Your doctor and a dietitian who specializes in helping people with kidney failure will be able to help you plan your meals.

### Pros and Cons

Each type of peritoneal dialysis has advantages and disadvantages. See a list below.

CAPD Pros:

- You can do it alone.

- You can do it at times you choose as long as you perform the required number of exchanges each day.

- You can do it in many locations.

- You don't need a machine.

CAPD Cons:

- It can disrupt your daily schedule.

- This is a continuous treatment, and all exchanges must be performed 7 days a week.

CCPD Pros:

- You can do it at night, mainly while you sleep.

CCPD Cons:

- You need a machine.

### Working with Your Health Care Team

Questions you may want to ask:

- Is peritoneal dialysis the best treatment choice for me? Why? If yes, which type is best?
- How long will it take me to learn how to do peritoneal dialysis?
- What does peritoneal dialysis feel like?
- How will peritoneal dialysis affect my blood pressure?
- How will I know if I have peritonitis? How is it treated?
- As a peritoneal dialysis patient, will I be able to continue working?
- How much should I exercise?
- Where do I store supplies?
- How often do I see my doctor?
- Who will be on my health care team? How can these people help me?
- Whom do I contact with problems?
- Whom can I talk with about finances, sexuality, or family concerns?
- How/where can I talk to other people who have faced this decision?

### Dialysis Is Not a Cure

Hemodialysis and peritoneal dialysis are treatments that help replace the work your kidneys did. These treatments help you feel better and live longer, but they don't cure kidney failure. Although patients with kidney failure are now living longer than ever, over the years kidney disease can cause problems such as heart disease, bone disease, arthritis, nerve damage, infertility, and malnutrition. These problems won't go away with dialysis, but doctors now have new and better ways to prevent or treat them. You should discuss these complications and treatments with your doctor.

## Treatment Choice: Kidney Transplantation

### Purpose

Kidney transplantation surgically places a healthy kidney from another person into your body. The donated kidney does the work that your two failed kidneys used to do.

### How It Works

A surgeon places the new kidney inside your lower abdomen and connects the artery and vein of the new kidney to your artery and vein. Your blood flows through the donated kidney, which makes urine, just like your own kidneys did when they were healthy. The new kidney may start working right away or may take up to a few weeks to make urine. Unless your own kidneys are causing infection or high blood pressure, they are left in place.

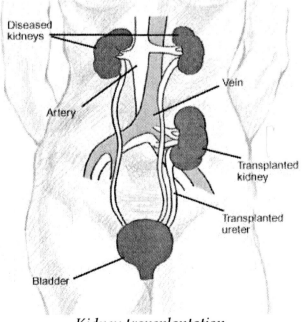

*Kidney transplantation*

## Getting Ready

The transplantation process has many steps. First, talk with your doctor, because transplantation isn't for everyone. Your doctor may tell you that you have a condition that would make transplantation dangerous or unlikely to succeed.

You may receive a kidney from a member of your family (living, related donor), from a person who has recently died (cadaveric donor), or sometimes from a spouse or a very close friend (living, unrelated donor). If you don't have a living donor, you're placed on a waiting list for a cadaveric kidney. The wait for a cadaveric donor kidney can be several years.

The transplant team considers three factors in matching kidneys with potential recipients. These factors help predict whether your body's immune system will accept the new kidney or reject it.

- Blood type. Your blood type (A, B, AB, or O) must match the donor's. This is the most important matching factor.

- Human leukocyte antigens (HLAs). Your cells carry six important HLAs, three inherited from each parent. Family members are most likely to have a complete match. You may still receive a kidney if the HLAs aren't a complete match as long as your blood type matches the organ donor's and other tests are negative.

- Cross-matching antigens. The last test before implanting an organ is the cross-match. A small sample of your blood will be mixed with a sample of the organ donor's blood in a tube to see if there's a reaction. If no reaction occurs, the result is called a negative cross-match, and the transplant operation can proceed.

## The Time It Takes

How long you'll have to wait for a kidney varies. Because there aren't enough cadaveric donors for every person who needs a transplant, you must be placed on a waiting list. However, if a voluntary donor gives you a kidney, the transplant can be scheduled as soon as you're both ready. Avoiding the long wait is a major advantage of living donation.

The surgery takes 3 to 4 hours. The usual hospital stay is about a week. After you leave the hospital, you'll have regular followup visits.

If someone has given you a kidney, the donor will probably stay in the hospital about the same amount of time. However, a new technique for removing a kidney for donation uses a smaller incision and may make it possible for the donor to leave the hospital in 2 to 3 days.

Between 85 and 90 percent of transplants from cadaveric donors are working 1 year after surgery. Transplants from living relatives often work better than transplants from cadaveric donors because they're usually a closer match.

### Possible Complications

Transplantation is the closest thing to a cure. But no matter how good the match, your body may reject your new kidney. A common cause of rejection is not taking medication as prescribed.

Your doctor will give you drugs called immunosuppressants to help prevent your body's immune system from attacking the kidney, a process called rejection. You'll need to take immunosuppressants every day for as long as the transplanted kidney is functioning. Sometimes, however, even these drugs can't stop your body from rejecting the new kidney. If this happens, you'll go back to some form of dialysis and possibly wait for another transplant.

Immunosuppressants can weaken your immune system, which can lead to infections. Some drugs may also change your appearance. Your face may get fuller; you may gain weight or develop acne or facial hair. Not all patients have these problems, though, and diet and makeup can help.

Immunosuppressants work by diminishing the ability of immune cells to function. In some patients, over long periods of time, this diminished immunity can increase the risk of developing cancer. Some immunosuppressants can cause cataracts, diabetes, extra stomach acid, high blood pressure, and bone disease. When used over time, these drugs may also cause liver or kidney damage in a few patients.

### Diet for Transplantation

Diet for transplant patients is less limited than it is for dialysis patients, although you may still have to cut back on some foods. Your diet will probably change as your medicines, blood values, weight, and blood pressure change.

- You may need to count calories. Your medicine may give you a bigger appetite and cause you to gain weight.
- You may have to eat less salt. Your medications may cause your body to retain sodium, leading to high blood pressure.

### Pros and Cons

Kidney transplantation has advantages and disadvantages.

Pros:

- A transplanted kidney works like a normal kidney.
- You may feel healthier or "more normal."
- You have fewer diet restrictions.
- You won't need dialysis.
- Patients who successfully go through the selection process have a higher chance of living a longer life.

Cons:

- It requires major surgery.
- You may need to wait for a donor.
- Your body may reject the new kidney, so one transplant may not last a lifetime.
- You'll need to take immunosuppressants, which may cause complications.

### Working with Your Health Care Team

Questions you may want to ask:

- Is transplantation the best treatment choice for me? Why?

- What are my chances of having a successful transplant?

- How do I find out whether a family member or friend can donate?

- What are the risks to a family member or friend who donates?

- If a family member or friend doesn't donate, how do I get placed on a waiting list for a kidney? How long will I have to wait?

- What symptoms does rejection cause?

- How long does a transplant work?

- What side effects do immunosuppressants cause?

- Who will be on my health care team? How can these people help me?

- Whom can I talk to about finances, sexuality, or family concerns?

- How or where can I talk to other people who have faced this decision?

## Treatment Choice: Refusing or Withdrawing from Treatment

For many people, dialysis and transplantation not only extend life but also improve quality of life. For others who have serious ailments in addition to kidney failure, dialysis may seem a burden that only prolongs suffering. You have the right to refuse or withdraw from dialysis if you feel you have no hope of leading a life with dignity and meaning. You may want to speak with your spouse, family, religious counselor, or social worker as you make this decision.

If you withdraw from dialysis treatments or refuse to begin them, you may live for a few days or for several weeks, depending on your health and your remaining kidney function. Your doctor can give you medicines to make you more comfortable during this period. Should you change your mind about refusing dialysis, you may start or resume your treatments at any time.

Even if you're satisfied with your quality of life on dialysis, you should think about circumstances that might make you want to stop dialysis treatments. At some point in a medical crisis, you might lose the ability to express your wishes to your doctor. An advance directive is a statement or document in which you give instructions either to withhold treatment or to provide it, depending on your wishes and the specific circumstances.

An advance directive may be a living will, a document that details the conditions under which you would want to refuse treatment. You may state that you want your health care team to use all available means to sustain your life. Or you may direct that you be withdrawn from dialysis if you become permanently unresponsive or fall into a coma from which you won't awake. In addition to dialysis, other life-sustaining treatments that you may choose or refuse include

- Cardiopulmonary resuscitation (CPR)
- Tube feedings
- Mechanical or artificial respiration
- Antibiotics
- Surgery
- Blood transfusions

Another form of advance directive is called a durable power of attorney for health care decisions or a health care proxy. In this type of advance directive, you assign a person to make health care decisions for you if you become unable to make them for yourself. Make sure the person you name understands your values and is willing to follow through on your instructions.

Each State has its own laws governing advance directives. You can obtain a form for an advance medical directive that's valid in your State from Partnership for Caring (see the "Resources" section).

## Paying for Treatment

Treatment for kidney failure is expensive, but Federal health insurance plans pay much of the cost, usually up to 80 percent. Often, private insurance or State programs pay the rest. For more information, see the NIDDK fact sheet Financial Help for Treatment of Kidney Failure.

## Conclusion

Deciding which type of treatment is best for you isn't easy. Your decision depends on your medical condition, lifestyle, and personal likes and dislikes. Discuss the pros and cons of each treatment with your health care team and family. You can switch between treatment methods during the course of your therapy. If you start one form of treatment and decide you'd like to try another, talk to your doctor. The key is to learn as much as you can about your choices first. With that knowledge, you and your doctor will choose the treatment that suits you best.

## Resources

**American Association of Kidney Patients**
3505 East Frontage Road
Suite 315
Tampa, FL 33607
Phone: 1-800-749-2257
Email: info@aakp.org
Internet: **www.aakp.org**

**American Kidney Fund**
6110 Executive Boulevard
Suite 1010
Rockville, MD 20852
Phone: 1-800-638-8299 or (301) 881-3052
Email: helpline@akfinc.org
Internet: **www.kidneyfund.org**

**Life Options/Rehabilitation Resource Center**
c/o Medical Education Institute, Inc.
414 D'Onofrio Drive
Suite 200
Madison, WI 53719
Phone: 1-800-468-7777
Email: lifeoptions@MEIresearch.org
Internet: **www.lifeoptions.org**
**www.kidneyschool.org**

**National Kidney Foundation Inc.**
30 East 33rd Street
Suite 1100
New York, NY 10016
Phone: 1-800-622-9010 or (212) 889-2210
Email: info@kidney.org
Internet: **www.kidney.org**

**Partnership for Caring: America's Voices for the Dying**
1620 Eye Street, NW
Suite 202
Washington, DC 20006
Phone: 1-800-989-9455
Email: pfc@partnershipforcaring.org
Internet: **www.partnershipforcaring.org**

**United Network for Organ Sharing**
P.O. Box 2484
Richmond, VA 23218
Phone: 1-888-894-6361 or (804) 782-4800
Internet: **www.unos.org**

## Additional Reading

If you would like to learn more about kidney failure and its treatment, you may be interested in reading the following:

**AAKP Patient Plan**
American Association of Kidney Patients
100 South Ashley Drive, Suite 280
Tampa, FL 33602
Phone: 1-800-749-2257 or (813) 223-7099
Email: AAKPnat@aol.com
Internet: **www.aakp.org**
This is a series of booklets and newsletters that cover the different phases of learning about kidney failure, choosing a treatment, and adjusting to changes.

**Financing Transplantation: What Every Patient Needs To Know, 2nd edition, 1996**
United Network for Organ Sharing
1100 Boulders Parkway
Suite 500
P.O. Box 13770
Richmond, VA 23225-8770
Phone: 1-888-894-6361 to order single copies
(804) 330-8541 to order bulk copies
Internet: **www.unos.org**

**Kidney Disease: A Guide for Patients and Their Families**
American Kidney Fund
6110 Executive Boulevard
Suite 1010
Rockville, MD 20852
Phone: 1-800-638-8299 or (301) 881-3052
Email: helpline@akfinc.org
Internet: **www.akfinc.org**

**Medicare Coverage of Kidney Dialysis and Kidney Transplant Services: A Supplement to Your Medicare Handbook**
Publication Number HCFA-10128
U.S. Department of Health and Human Services
Health Care Financing Administration
7500 Security Boulevard
Baltimore, MD 21244-1850
Phone: 1-800-MEDICARE (1-800-633-4227)
TDD: 1-877-486-2048
Internet:
**http://www.medicare.gov/publications/pubs/pdf/esrdcoverage.pdf**

**National Kidney Foundation (NKF) Patient Education Brochures**
(includes materials based on NKF's Dialysis Outcomes Quality Initiative)
National Kidney Foundation, Inc.
30 East 33rd Street
New York, NY 10016
Phone: 1-800-622-9010 or (212) 889-2210
Internet: **www.kidney.org**

**What Every Patient Needs To Know, 1997**
United Network for Organ Sharing
1100 Boulders Parkway
Suite 500
P.O. Box 13770
Richmond, VA 23225-8770
Phone: 1-888-894-6361 to order single copies
(804) 330-8541 to order bulk copies
Internet: **www.unos.org**

**Newsletters and Magazines**

**Family Focus Newsletter** (published quarterly)
National Kidney Foundation, Inc.
30 East 33rd Street
New York, NY 10016
Phone: 1-800-622-9010 or (212) 889-2210
Email: info@kidney.org
Internet: **www.kidney.org**

**For Patients Only** (published six times a year)
ATTN: Subscription Department
18 East 41st Street, 20th Floor
New York, NY 10017-6222

**Renalife** (published quarterly)
American Association of Kidney Patients
100 South Ashley Drive
Suite 280
Tampa, FL 33602
Phone: 1-800-749-2257 or (813) 223-7099
Email: AAKPnat@aol.com
Internet: **www.aakp.org**

## More Guideline Sources

The guideline above on kidney failure is only one example of the kind of material that you can find online and free of charge. The remainder of this chapter will direct you to other sources which either publish or can help you find additional guidelines on topics related to kidney failure. Many of the guidelines listed below address topics that may be of particular relevance to your specific situation or of special interest to only some patients with kidney failure. Due to space limitations these sources are listed in a concise manner. Do not hesitate to consult the following sources by either using the Internet hyperlink provided, or, in cases where the contact information is provided, contacting the publisher or author directly.

**Topic Pages: MEDLINEplus**

For patients wishing to go beyond guidelines published by specific Institutes of the NIH, the National Library of Medicine has created a vast and patient-oriented healthcare information portal called MEDLINEplus. Within this Internet-based system are "health topic pages." You can think of a health topic page as a guide to patient guides. To access this system, log on to **http://www.nlm.nih.gov/medlineplus/healthtopics.html**. From there you can either search using the alphabetical index or browse by broad topic areas. Recently, MEDLINEplus listed the following as being relevant to kidney failure:

**African-American Health**
http://www.nlm.nih.gov/medlineplus/africanamericanhealth.html

**Bile Duct Diseases**
http://www.nlm.nih.gov/medlineplus/bileductdiseases.html

**Cirrhosis**
http://www.nlm.nih.gov/medlineplus/cirrhosis.html

**Diabetic Kidney Problems**
http://www.nlm.nih.gov/medlineplus/diabetickidneyproblems.html

**Dietary Supplements**
http://www.nlm.nih.gov/medlineplus/dietarysupplements.html

**Heart Failure**
http://www.nlm.nih.gov/medlineplus/heartfailure.html

**Hepatitis**
http://www.nlm.nih.gov/medlineplus/hepatitis.html

**Hepatitis A**
http://www.nlm.nih.gov/medlineplus/hepatitisa.html

**Hepatitis B**
http://www.nlm.nih.gov/medlineplus/hepatitisb.html

**Hepatitis C**
http://www.nlm.nih.gov/medlineplus/hepatitisc.html

**Juvenile Rheumatoid Arthritis**
http://www.nlm.nih.gov/medlineplus/juvenilerheumatoidarthritis.html

**Kidney Cancer**
http://www.nlm.nih.gov/medlineplus/kidneycancer.html

**Kidney Diseases**
http://www.nlm.nih.gov/medlineplus/kidneydiseases.html

**Kidney Failure**
http://www.nlm.nih.gov/medlineplus/kidneyfailure.html

**Kidney Failure**
http://www.nlm.nih.gov/medlineplus/tutorials/kidneyfailureloade
r.html

**Kidney Transplantation**
http://www.nlm.nih.gov/medlineplus/kidneytransplantation.html

**Liver Diseases**
http://www.nlm.nih.gov/medlineplus/liverdiseases.html

**Liver Transplantation**
http://www.nlm.nih.gov/medlineplus/livertransplantation.html

**Lupus**
http://www.nlm.nih.gov/medlineplus/lupus.html

**Metabolic Disorders**
http://www.nlm.nih.gov/medlineplus/metabolicdisorders.html

**Neuromuscular Disorders**
http://www.nlm.nih.gov/medlineplus/neuromusculardisorders.htm
l

**Nutrition for Seniors**
http://www.nlm.nih.gov/medlineplus/nutritionforseniors.html

Within the health topic page dedicated to kidney failure, the following was recently recommended to patients:

- Nutrition

    **Eat Right to Feel Right on Hemodialysis**
    http://kidney.niddk.nih.gov/kudiseases/pubs/eatright/index.htm

    **Na-K-Phos Counter**
    Source: American Association of Kidney Patients
    http://www.aakp.org/AAKP/nakphos.htm

    **Nutrition and Peritoneal Dialysis**
    Source: National Kidney Foundation
    http://www.kidney.org/atoz/pdf/nutri_pd.pdf

    **Protein/Calorie Counter**
    Source: American Association of Kidney Patients
    http://www.aakp.org/AAKP/protcal.htm

- Children

    **Treatment Methods for Kidney Failure in Children**
    Source: National Kidney and Urologic Diseases Information Clearinghouse
    http://kidney.niddk.nih.gov/kudiseases/pubs/childkidneydiseases/treatment_methods/index.htm

    **What's the Deal with Dialysis?**
    Source: Nemours Foundation
    http://kidshealth.org/kid/feel_better/things/dialysis.html

- From the National Institutes of Health

    **Treatment Methods for Kidney Failure: Hemodialysis**
    Source: National Kidney and Urologic Diseases Information Clearinghouse
    http://kidney.niddk.nih.gov/kudiseases/pubs/hemodialysis/index.htm

    **Treatment Methods for Kidney Failure: Peritoneal Dialysis**
    Source: National Kidney and Urologic Diseases Information Clearinghouse
    http://kidney.niddk.nih.gov/kudiseases/pubs/peritoneal/index.htm

- Latest News

    **Possible West Nile Cases from Dialysis**
    Source: 08/19/2004, Reuters Health
    http://www.nlm.nih.gov//www.nlm.nih.gov/medlineplus/news/fullstory_19618.html

- Law and Policy

    **Medicare Coverage of Kidney Dialysis and Kidney Transplant Services**
    Source: Dept. of Health and Human Services
    http://www.medicare.gov/Publications/Pubs/pdf/esrdCoverage.pdf

- Organizations

    **Life Options Rehabilitation Program**
    http://www.lifeoptions.org/

**National Institute of Diabetes and Digestive and Kidney Diseases**
http://www.niddk.nih.gov/

**National Kidney and Urologic Diseases Information Clearinghouse**
Source: National Institute of Diabetes and Digestive and Kidney Diseases
http://kidney.niddk.nih.gov/

**National Kidney Foundation**
http://www.kidney.org/

- Research

  **Hemodialysis Study Results Published Confirms Current Recommended Practice**
  Source: National Institute of Diabetes and Digestive and Kidney Diseases
  http://www.nih.gov/news/pr/dec2002/niddk-18.htm

  **Preventing Worsening Kidney Function in Patients Receiving Peritoneal Dialysis**
  Source: American College of Physicians
  http://www.annals.org/cgi/content/full/139/2/I-32

You may also choose to use the search utility provided by MEDLINEplus at the following Web address: **http://www.nlm.nih.gov/medlineplus/**. Simply type a keyword into the search box and click "Search." This utility is similar to the NIH search utility, with the exception that it only includes materials that are linked within the MEDLINEplus system (mostly patient-oriented information). It also has the disadvantage of generating unstructured results. We recommend, therefore, that you use this method only if you have a very targeted search.

**The Combined Health Information Database (CHID)**

CHID Online is a reference tool that maintains a database directory of thousands of journal articles and patient education guidelines on kidney failure and related conditions. One of the advantages of CHID over other sources is that it offers summaries that describe the guidelines available, including contact information and pricing. CHID's general Web site is **http://chid.nih.gov/**. To search this database, go to **http://chid.nih.gov/detail/detail.html**. In particular, you can use the advanced search options to look up pamphlets, reports, brochures, and information kits. The following was recently posted in this archive:

- **1 Out of Every 3 People with Kidney Failure is African American: High Blood Pressure and Kidney Disease**

Source: Rockville, MD: American Kidney Fund. 199x. [6 p.].

Contact: Available from American Kidney Fund. 6110 Executive Blvd., Suite 1010, Rockville, MD 20852-9813. (800) 638-8299 or (301) 881-3052. Fax (301) 881-0898. PRICE: Single copy free.

Summary: High blood pressure is the leading cause of **kidney failure** in African Americans. This brochure encourages African Americans to learn about high blood pressure (hypertension) and kidney disease. The brochure emphasizes that **kidney failure** from hypertension is preventable; high blood pressure cannot be cured, but it can be controlled. Written in question and answer format, the brochure describes how blood pressure is monitored and measured, the risk factors for high blood pressure (including being African American, overweight, older, or in a family with high blood pressure, lack of exercise, eating too much salt, and smoking cigarettes), treatment options for hypertension, the complications that can arise from high blood pressure, how hypertension affects the kidneys, the role of the kidneys, what happens to the body in **kidney failure,** the warning signs of kidney disease, the role of diabetes in kidney disease, and the activities of the American Kidney Fund (AKF), an organization that helps people of all races cope with the effects of kidney disease. The warning signs of kidney disease include swelling of parts of the body (especially around the eyes or ankles), pain in the lower back, burning or unusual sensation during urination, bloody or coffee colored urine, urinating more often (especially at night), listless or tired feeling, and high blood pressure. The brochure includes a tear off card for readers to return to the AKF to obtain more information, to volunteer, or to contribute money. The brochure is written in nontechnical language.

- **1 Out of Every 3 People with Kidney Failure is African American: Diabetes and Kidney Disease**

Source: Rockville, MD: American Kidney Fund. 199x. [6 p.].

Contact: Available from American Kidney Fund. 6110 Executive Blvd., Suite 1010, Rockville, MD 20852-9813. (800) 638-8299 or (301) 881-3052. Fax (301) 881-0898. PRICE: Single copy free.

Summary: One out of every three people with **kidney failure** is African American, and diabetes is the second leading cause of **kidney failure** in African Americans. This brochure encourages African Americans to learn about diabetes and kidney disease. The brochure emphasizes that African Americans with diabetes develop **kidney failure** and other serious complications more often than other groups with diabetes. Written in question and answer format, the brochure describes the disease of diabetes, the different types of diabetes, the symptoms of diabetes, risk factors that may contribute to diabetes, treatment options, **kidney failure** as a result of uncontrolled diabetes, the role of the kidneys in good health, how to know if kidney disease is present, and the role of hypertension (high blood pressure) in causing kidney disease. The warning signs of kidney disease include swelling of parts of the body (especially around the eyes or ankles), pain in the lower back, burning or unusual sensation during urination, bloody or coffee colored urine, urinating more often (especially at night), listless or tired feeling, and high blood pressure. The brochure includes a tear off card for readers to return to the AKF to obtain more information, to volunteer, or to contribute money. The brochure is written in nontechnical language.

- **Fitness After Kidney Failure: Building Strength Through Exercise**

  Source: New York, NY: National Kidney Foundation. 1994. 4 p.

  Contact: Available from National Kidney Foundation, Inc. 30 East 33rd Street, New York, NY 10016. (800) 622-9010. PRICE: Single copy free.

  Summary: Recent studies with dialysis and transplant patients show that, for many kidney patients, exercise may be even more important than it is for the general population. This brochure provides general guidelines for the post-transplant patient who is interested in beginning a fitness program. After presenting a number of case stories, the brochure discusses the four areas to consider when planning an exercise program: mode or type of exercise; duration or length of time to be spent exercising; frequency, or how often to exercise; and intensity or how hard to work while exercising. Checklists detailing when not to exercise and when to stop exercising are included. The brochure concludes that working toward fitness is a way of gaining control over some of the many changes that sometimes affect a kidney patient's life.

- **Sexuality and Chronic Kidney Failure**

  Source: New York, NY: National Kidney Foundation. 1999. 15 p.

  Contact: National Kidney Foundation. 30 East 33rd Street, New York, NY 10016. (800) 622-9010. Fax (212) 689-9261. E-mail: info@kidney.org. Website: www.kidney.org. PRICE: Single copy free; contact organization for print copies.

  Summary: This booklet answers questions about the effects of chronic **kidney failure** on sexuality and encourages patients, families, and professionals to talk openly about these issues. Written in a question-and-answer format, the brochure covers many topics including a definition of sexuality; the physical and emotional changes that kidney disease can cause that may affect the patient's sex life; the safety of sexual intercourse for transplant recipients and for people with dialysis access sites; and suggestions for couples for whom intercourse is not possible. The booklet discusses several pregnancy-related issues including pregnancy for women who are on dialysis; fathering a child for men who are on dialysis; pregnancy in women who are kidney transplant recipients; how anti-rejection medicines may harm a fetus; and birth control. Other issues raised include the sexual development of children with **kidney failure;** the risks of contracting AIDS from transplants or blood transfusions; the sexual problems of transplant recipients versus those on dialysis; the long-term impact of dialysis on sexuality; how to tell whether sexual problems are due to a physical or emotional cause; treatment options for physical problems and for emotional problems; and the role of sex therapy. The authors offer suggestions for kidney patients who want to take an active approach in their care, and stress the importance of talking about sexual problems.

- **Treatment Methods for Kidney Failure: Peritoneal Dialysis**

  Source: Bethesda, MD: National Kidney and Urologic Diseases Information Clearinghouse (NKUDIC), National Institute of Diabetes and Digestive and Kidney Diseases (NIDDK), National Institutes of Health (NIH). 2001. 24 p.

  Contact: Available from National Kidney and Urologic Diseases Information Clearinghouse (NKUDIC). 3 Information Way, Bethesda, MD 20892-3580. (800) 891-5390 or (301) 654-4415. Fax (301)634-0716. E-mail: nkudic@info.niddk.nih.gov. Website: http://www.niddk.nih.gov/health/kidney/nkudic.htm. PRICE: Full-text available online at no charge; single copy free; bulk orders available. Order number: KU-153.

  Summary: This booklet describes the option of peritoneal dialysis (PD) as a treatment for people with advanced and permanent **kidney failure** (end stage renal disease or ESRD). Healthy kidneys clean the blood by removing excess fluid, minerals, and wastes. They also make hormones to keep the bones strong and the blood healthy. In **kidney failure,** medical treatments must be used to perform these functions of the kidneys. This booklet describes how PD works, getting ready for PD, the different types of PD, customizing PD to the individual patient, preventing problems, equipment and supplies for PD, testing the effectiveness of the dialysis, conditions related to **kidney failure** and their treatments, and the psychosocial adjustments that occur as one learns to cope with **kidney**

**failure.** In PD, a soft tube (catheter) is used to fill the abdomen with dialysis solution; the peritoneum (lining of the abdomen) serves as a membrane to allow waste products and extra fluid to pass from the blood into the dialysis solution. These wastes and fluid then leave the patient's body when the dialysis solution is drained. The most common form of PD, continuous ambulatory peritoneal dialysis (CAPD), does not require a machine; other forms use a cycler to perform the exchanges. Infection is the most common problem for people on PD, but equipment advances and strict adherence to infection control measures can reduce this complication. Monitoring tests are performed on the used solution, urine, and blood measurements to determine whether the dialysis is adequate. Conditions related to **kidney failure** and their treatments include anemia, renal osteodystrophy (bone disease associated with kidney failure), itching (pruritus), sleep disorders, and dialysis related amyloidosis. The booklet concludes with a description of current research efforts devoted to improving treatment for patients with progressive kidney disease and permanent **kidney failure.** The booklet also includes a list of resources (organizations and instructional materials) and a brief description of the National Kidney and Urologic Diseases Information Clearinghouse (NKUDIC) and its contact information. 4 figures.

- **Kidney Failure Glossary**

Source: Bethesda, MD: National Kidney and Urologic Diseases Information Clearinghouse (NKUDIC), National Institute of Diabetes and Digestive and Kidney Diseases (NIDDK), National Institutes of Health (NIH). 2001. 16 p.

Contact: Available from National Kidney and Urologic Diseases Information Clearinghouse (NKUDIC). 3 Information Way, Bethesda, MD 20892-3580. (800) 891-5390 or (301) 654-4415. Fax (301)634-0716. E-mail: nkudic@info.niddk.nih.gov. Website: http://www.niddk.nih.gov/health/kidney/nkudic.htm. PRICE: Full-text available online at no charge; single copy free; bulk orders available. Order number: KU-151.

Summary: This booklet offers a glossary of words that are often used when people talk or write about **kidney failure** and its treatments. It is designed for people whose kidneys have failed and for their families and friends. The words are listed in alphabetical order, and a guide to pronunciation is included for most words. Some words have many meanings; only those meanings that relate to kidney diseases are included. A term will refer the reader to another definition only when the second definition gives additional information about the topic that is directly related to the first term. Some terms include illustrations (arteriovenous fistula, catheters, hemodialysis, dialyzer, graft, glomerulus, urinary tract). The booklet concludes with a brief description of the National Kidney and Urologic Diseases Information Clearinghouse (NKUDIC) and its contact information. 7 figures.

- **Treating Kidney Failure**

Source: Montreal, Quebec: Kidney Foundation of Canada. 199x. [4 p.].

Contact: Available from Kidney Foundation of Canada. 300-5165, rue Sherbrooke Ouest, Montreal, QC H4A 1T6. (514) 369-4806. Fax (514) 369-2472. Website: www.kidney.ca. PRICE: Single copy free.

Summary: This brochure answers questions that readers may have as they face a diagnosis of **kidney failure.** The brochure first reviews the physiology of the kidneys, emphasizing that kidneys remove wastes from the blood via the urine. In the early stages of chronic **kidney failure,** the only treatment needed may be a special diet or medication. When kidney function is no longer adequate (end stage renal disease, or ESRD), dialysis treatment or a kidney transplant is required. Dialysis is a way to clean the blood by removing wastes and excess water. The brochure describes the two types: hemodialysis and peritoneal dialysis. A kidney transplant is a surgical procedure, in which a healthy kidney from either a living or deceased donor is placed in the recipient's lower abdomen. Choosing a treatment depends on what is available in the community, as well as what is most appropriate for each individual's particular needs. The health care team can provide information and support to help the patient make a decision about the best treatment. The brochure concludes with a brief description of the Kidney Foundation of Canada, including patient services and public education programs. 5 figures.

- **One Out of Every Three People with Kidney Failure is African American**

Source: Rockville, MD: American Kidney Fund. 1997. 4 p.

Contact: Available from American Kidney Fund. 6110 Executive Boulevard, Suite 1010, Rockville, MD 20852. (800) 638-8299 or (301) 881-3052. Fax (301) 881-0898. PRICE: Single copy free.

Summary: This brochure encourages black American readers to educate themselves about kidney disease and to take steps to prevent kidney problems. The brochure notes that although only one out of eight people in the general population is African American, one of every three people with **kidney failure** is African American. High blood pressure (hypertension) and diabetes are the leading causes of **kidney failure;** both of these problems are more prevalent among blacks than among whites. The brochure describes how both diabetes and hypertension should be monitored and treated. The remainder of the brochure describes **kidney failure** and the role of the American Kidney Fund (AKF) in helping people cope with the effects of kidney disease. A final section encourages readers to live healthy lives in order to improve their odds of avoiding kidney disease. The brochure features a tear-off self mailer, for readers who wish to request additional information about high blood pressure and kidney disease, diabetes and kidney disease, treatments for **kidney failure,** kidney donation, and the AKF. One sidebar lists the symptoms of kidney disease.

- **Living with Kidney Failure: A Guide for Patients and Their Families**

Source: New York, NY: National Kidney Foundation. 1999. 11 p.

Contact: Available from National Kidney Foundation. 30 East 33rd Street, Suite 1100, New York, NY 10016. (800) 622-9010 or (212) 889-2210. Fax (212) 689-9261. E-mail: info@kidney.org. Website: www.kidney.org. PRICE: Single copy free; bulk copies available.

Summary: This brochure from the National Kidney Foundation (NKF) offers patients and their families information for living with **kidney failure.** The brochure encourages patients to educate themselves and become an integral member of their own health care team. The brochure focuses on strategies for maintaining health and getting back to the activities of daily living, such as work, school, hobbies, and other activities. Topics covered include how to cope more effectively with kidney disease and its treatment; treatment methods that are available, including home hemodialysis, in-center hemodialysis, peritoneal dialysis, and kidney transplantation; how to gather adequate information to make treatment choices; how to choose a treatment center; how to build a good relationship with the health care team; the types of information that is available about kidney disease and rehabilitation and how to obtain it; where to get help for exercise and other independence strategies; strategies to keep working even while dealing with **kidney failure;** legal issues and laws that protect patients with **kidney failure;** how family members and other loved ones can work with the patient and health care team to encourage patient rehabilitation; aspects of care that impact rehabilitation, including the delivered dose of dialysis, treatments for anemia, diet therapy, and treatment for bone disease; the responsibilities of each member of the health care team in patient rehabilitation (nephrologist, administrator, nephrology nurse or patient care technician, dietitian, social worker); and patient rights and responsibilities. The brochure concludes with a list of instructional materials available from the NKF and a brief description of the activities of the organization (including their website at www.kidney.org).

- **Choosing a Treatment for Kidney Failure**

   Source: New York, NY: National Kidney Foundation (NKF). 2002. 15 p.

   Contact: Available from National Kidney Foundation (NKF). 30 East 33rd Street, New York, NY 10016. (800) 622-9010. Website: www.kidney.org. PRICE: Single copy free; $25.00 for 100 copies.

   Summary: This brochure outlines the treatment options for patients with a diagnosis of **kidney failure.** When the kidneys are not working well, as a result of disease or injury, wastes and excess fluid build up in the blood. Treatment is instigated at this point, taking into consideration the patient's general medical condition, how much kidney function he or she has left, and the patient's nutritional status. The treatments for chronic **kidney failure** are dialysis (hemodialysis or peritoneal) and kidney transplantation. Hemodialysis is a treatment during which the blood travels through soft tubes to a dialysis machine where it goes through a special filter (dialyzer) to be cleaned. As the blood is cleaned, it is returned to the bloodstream. Only a small amount of blood is out of the body at any time. Hemodialysis requires an access (entrance) to the bloodstream; this can be a fistula, a graft, or a catheter. The brochure describes each type. In peritoneal dialysis, the blood is cleansed inside the body. The lining of the abdomen (the peritoneum) acts as a natural filter. The dialysate (cleansing solution) is passed into the belly through a catheter, wastes and excess fluid pass from the blood into the cleansing solution, and the used solution is drained from the abdomen. There are different types of peritoneal dialysis. A kidney transplant is an operation that places a healthy kidney from another person into the patient with kidney disease. The kidney may come from someone who has died (a cadaver) or from a living donor (a close relative or spouse). The patient must take medications to prevent their body from rejecting the new kidney. The brochure describes each of these treatments in some detail and considers the impact of each on the patient's diet, the use of special medications, prognosis, the role of exercise, vocational rehabilitation (returning to work), coping and psychological issues, and cost issues. The brochure concludes with a list of publications available from the National Kidney Foundation. 3 figures.

- **Planning for the Treatment of Kidney Failure**

   Source: New York, NY: National Kidney Foundation. 1994. 5 p.

Contact: Available from National Kidney Foundation. 30 East 33rd Street, New York, NY 10016. (800) 622-9010. PRICE: Single copy free.

Summary: This brochure provides information for kidney patients and their families about kidney disease and the different treatments for chronic **kidney failure.** Written in a question and answer format, the brochure covers topics including the role of the kidneys and the determination to start kidney replacement therapy; hemodialysis; peritoneal dialysis; kidney transplantation; receiving a transplant before going on dialysis; diet therapy and the dietary recommendations associated with each of the treatment options; drug therapy for each of the treatment options; how treatment impacts the patient's quality of life; the prognosis for regular lifespan; the role of exercise; rehabilitation to work; paying for kidney replacement treatment; and coping with kidney disease and its treatment. The brochure stresses the importance of working in close collaboration with one's physician and other members of the health care team in order to ensure the best outcome.

- **Help Your Family Prevent Kidney Failure**

Source: Bethesda, MD: National Kidney Disease Education Program. 2004. 2 p.

Contact: Available from NKDEP ( National Kidney Disease Education Program). Office of Communications and Public Liaison, NIDDK, NIH, Building31, Room 9A06, Center Drive, MSC2560, Bethesda, MD 20892-2560. (800) 891-5390 or (301) 654-4415. Fax: (301) 897-9587. Email: nkdep@info.niddk.nih.gov. Website: www.nkdep.nih.gov. PRICE: Full-text available online at no charge.

Summary: This brochure reminds readers with kidney disease of the importance of getting their family members tested for kidney function. Kidney disease runs in families and even if only one person in a family has **kidney failure,** all blood relatives should be tested for kidney disease. With early treatment, kidney disease can be slowed and dialysis or a transplant may be avoided. The brochure outlines what the patient should tell his or her family, and explains what the family members should tell their physicians. The brochure is part of the National Kidney Disease Education Program, characterized by the acronym TEST: Teach that kidney disease runs in families; Encourage testing; Support efforts to control diabetes and high blood pressure (hypertension); and Tell family members where to get more information. The brochure includes a tear-off mailer card to give to family members. Both the brochure and the card have the contact information for the NKDEP (www.nkdep.nih.gov or 866-454-3639).

- **Social Work Services: For the Patient with Chronic Renal Failure**

  Source: New York, NY: National Kidney Foundation. 1991. 2 p.

  Contact: Available from National Kidney Foundation. 30 East 33rd Street, New York, NY 10016. (212) 889-2210 or (800) 622-9010. PRICE: Single copy free. Order Number 08-01-PP.

  Summary: This brochure reviews the role of the nephrology social worker as a member of the treatment team at all transplant and dialysis facilities. Among the many services provided by the social worker are helping the patient adjust to chronic kidney disease by providing counseling to the patient and family, identifying community services, providing resources, and making referrals.

- **Bone Disease in Chronic Kidney Failure**

  Source: New York, NY: The National Kidney Foundation. 1996. [4 p.].

  Contact: National Kidney Foundation. 30 East 33rd Street, New York, NY 10016. (800) 622-9010. Website: www.kidney.org. PRICE: Single copy free; bulk copies available.

  Summary: This brochure, written in question and answer format, presents patient information about bone disease in chronic **kidney failure.** Topics include the causes of bone disease in people with **kidney failure,** the different types of bone disease, how phosphorus levels affect the bones, the role of the parathyroid glands, how aluminum levels in the bones are related to bone disease, the role of vitamin D, how diet and exercise can contribute to healthy bones, guidelines for calcium supplementation, how a kidney transplant will affect bone disease problems, and risk factors for bone disease. The brochure concludes with a list of patient education publications available from the National Kidney Foundation.

- **Acute Renal Failure**

  Source: in Kerestes-Smith, J.; Chua, G.; Sullivan, K. Guidelines for Nutritional Care. Ann Arbor, MI: Food and Nutrition Services, University of Michigan Medical Center. 1995. Chapter 53, p. 53.1-53.4.

  Contact: Available from Guidelines for Nutritional Care. Food and Nutrition Services, 2C227-0056, University of Michigan Hospitals, 1500 East Medical Center Drive, Ann Arbor, MI 48109-0056. (313) 936-5199. Fax (313) 936-5195. PRICE: $79.00 including shipping and handling (as of 1996). ISBN: 0964799405.

  Summary: This chapter on dietary recommendations for individuals with acute **renal failure** (ARF) is from a manual of the impact nutrition has on promoting health and in preventing and treating disease. Included are sections detailing indications for use, contraindications, a description of the diet including a brief physiological and/or biochemical rationale, guidelines for nutritional management, nutrient adequacy, ordering procedures, and references for both the health care providers and the layperson. 1 table. 19 references.

- **Financial Help for Treatment of Kidney Failure**

    Source: Bethesda, MD: National Kidney and Urologic Diseases Information Clearinghouse (NKUDIC), National Institute of Diabetes and Digestive and Kidney Diseases (NIDDK), National Institutes of Health (NIH). 2001. 4 p.

    Contact: Available from National Kidney and Urologic Diseases Information Clearinghouse (NKUDIC). 3 Information Way, Bethesda, MD 20892-3580. (800) 891-5390 or (301) 654-4415. Fax (301)634-0716. E-mail: nkudic@info.niddk.nih.gov. Website: http://www.niddk.nih.gov/health/kidney/nkudic.htm. PRICE: Full-text available online at no charge; single copy free; bulk orders available. Order number: KU-147.

    Summary: This fact sheet describes the types of financial assistance available for the treatment of chronic **kidney failure** (end stage renal disease, or ESRD). In 1972, Congress passed legislation making people of any age with permanent **kidney failure** eligible for Medicare, a program that helps people over 65 and people with disabilities pay for medical care, usually up to 80 percent. Other public and private resources can help with the remaining 20 percent of the costs. The fact sheet encourages readers to consult with dialysis or transplant center social workers who can help patients locate and apply for financial assistance. The fact sheet details how Medicare works, the role of private insurance, Medicaid, benefits available through the Department of Veterans Affairs (VA), Social Security Disability Income (SSDI) and Supplemental Security Income (SSI) programs, and patient assistance programs from prescription drug companies. The fact sheet includes a list of resource organizations for more information, a few resources for additional reading (with availability details), and a brief description of the National Kidney and Urologic Diseases Information Clearinghouse (NKUDIC) and its contact information. 2 references.

- **Renal Failure, Acute (Kidney Failure, Acute)**

    Source: in Griffith, H.W. Instructions for Patients. 5th ed. Philadelphia, PA: W.B. Saunders Company. 1994. p. 395.

Contact: Available from W.B. Saunders Company. Book Order Fulfillment, 6277 Sea Harbor Drive, Orlando, FL 32887-4430. (800) 545-2522. Fax (800) 874-6418. PRICE: $49.95. ISBN: 0721649300 (English); 0721669972 (Spanish).

Summary: This fact sheet on acute **renal failure** is from a compilation of instructions for patients, published in book format. The fact sheet covers a description of the condition, frequent signs and symptoms, causes, risk factors, preventive measures, expected outcome, and possible complications; treatment, including general measures, medication, activity guidelines, and diet; and when to contact one's health care provider. The fact sheet can be photocopied and distributed to patients as a reinforcement of oral instructions and as a teaching tool. The book in which the fact sheet appears is available in English or Spanish.

- **Renal Failure, Chronic (Kidney Failure, Chronic)**

  Source: in Griffith, H.W. Instructions for Patients. 5th ed. Philadelphia, PA: W.B. Saunders Company. 1994. p. 396.

  Contact: Available from W.B. Saunders Company. Book Order Fulfillment, 6277 Sea Harbor Drive, Orlando, FL 32887-4430. (800) 545-2522. Fax (800) 874-6418. PRICE: $49.95. ISBN: 0721649300 (English); 0721669972 (Spanish).

  Summary: This fact sheet on chronic **kidney failure** is from a compilation of instructions for patients, published in book format. The fact sheet covers a description of the condition, frequent signs and symptoms, causes, risk factors, preventive measures, expected outcome, and possible complications; treatment, including general measures, medication, activity guidelines, and diet; and when to contact one's health care provider. The fact sheet can be photocopied and distributed to patients as a reinforcement of oral instructions and as a teaching tool. The book in which the fact sheet appears is available in English or Spanish.

- **Nutrition for Children with Chronic Kidney Failure**

  Source: New York, NY: National Kidney Foundation, Inc. 1991. 3 p.

  Contact: Available from National Kidney Foundation, Inc. 30 East 33rd Street, New York, NY 10016. (800) 622-9010. PRICE: Single copy free.

  Summary: This fact sheet presents a brief overview of nutrition for children with chronic **kidney failure.** The goals in feeding a child with **kidney failure** are to promote normal growth and to protect his or her health as much as possible. Written in a question-and-answer format, the fact sheet includes information about special diets and diet therapy, diet changes before dialysis, a diet recommended for children on peritoneal dialysis, restrictions needed on hemodialysis, what to expect after a transplant, and the activities of the National Kidney Foundation.

- **It's Just a Part of My Life: A Guide for Young Adults with Chronic Kidney Failure**

Source: New York, NY: National Kidney Foundation. 1998. 14 p.

Contact: Available from National Kidney Foundation. 30 East 33rd Street, Suite 1100, New York, NY 10016. (800) 622-9010 or (212) 889-2210. Fax (212) 689-9261. E-mail: info@kidney.org. Website: www.kidney.org. PRICE: $2.25.

Summary: This patient education handbook offers information for young adults with chronic **kidney failure.** The handbook focuses on the feelings that an adolescent may have as he or she adjusts to chronic **kidney failure,** including the need to be on dialysis. Sections address learning to accept the illness, the role of support groups, special concerns that young people with chronic disease must face, physical development, changing emotions, nutrition, sexual development, dealing with the side effects of steroids (for young people who have had a transplant), diabetes, fitting in, the patient care team, the physiology of the kidneys, the development of kidney disease, hemodialysis, peritoneal dialysis, and kidney transplantation. An additional section offers strategies for learning more about treatment and patient care management, including medications for blood pressure, phosphorus binding, and anemia (erythropoietin); diet therapy, handling any restrictions that are necessary (sodium, potassium, protein), and eating at restaurants; the role of exercise; and finding the energy for outside interests. The handbook concludes with a section of recipes that might be particularly appealing to young people, including marshnut squares, peanut butterscotch treats, mallow bars, quick mix nibbles, dressing, baked tortillas, and Italian pasta salad. The handbook includes a list of other resources available from the National Kidney Foundation (NKF) and a glossary of terms. The handbook is illustrated with bold graphics of young people involved in a variety of lifestyle and health related activities.

- **Accelerating Recovery From Acute Renal Failure: News Briefings for Science Writers on Transplantation, Dialysis and Kidney Research (memorandum)**

Source: New York, NY: National Kidney Foundation, Inc. March 26-27, 1990. 5 p.

Contact: Available from National Kidney Foundation, Inc. 30 East 33rd Street, New York, NY 10016. (800) 622-9010 or (212) 889-2210.

Summary: This technical paper prepared for the National Kidney Foundation's 1990 science writers news briefing on transplantation, dialysis, and kidney/urology research discusses ways to accelerate recovery from acute **renal failure.** The paper reports on recent work demonstrating that a single dose of two growth factors to animals whose kidneys have been severely damaged, either from ischemia or administered toxins, substantially accelerates the repair of damaged kidney tissue and leads to accelerated recovery of kidney function. The two growth factors are epidermal growth factor and transforming growth factor-alpha. This finding is the initial demonstration that certain growth factors can accelerate the repair of injured tissue in a visceral organ, similar to recent clinical and experimental demonstrations that various growth factors can speed the repair of cutaneous wounds. Clinical use of growth factors to speed the regenerative repair of damaged kidney tissue will have the potential to limit hospital length of stay, minimize expensive dialytic therapy, or diminish mortality rates. The use of growth factors during the harvesting process for kidneys for transplantation may also lessen the rate of acute **kidney failure** following transplantation to a recipient.

- **Facts About Kidney Failure: A Guide for Employers**

Source: New York, NY: National Kidney Foundation. 1999. 3 p.

Contact: Available from National Kidney Foundation. 30 East 33rd Street, Suite 1100, New York, NY 10016. (800) 622-9010 or (212) 889-2210. Fax (212) 689-9261. E-mail: info@kidney.org. Website: www.kidney.org. PRICE: Single copy free; bulk copies available.

Summary: Treatments such as dialysis and kidney transplantation enable people with **kidney failure** to live normal lives, including working. Working is very important because it makes people feel valuable to their families, to society, and to themselves. This publication, one in a series developed to help the members of the renal (kidney) treatment team better understand all aspects of ESRD patient rehabilitation and increase their involvement in rehabilitation, focuses on the role of the employer. The brochure answers questions about **kidney failure** and demonstrates that an employee with **kidney failure** can be a valuable worker who contributes to the organization. The brochure reminds readers that Medicare helps pay for the cost of treating **kidney failure** regardless of the employee's age; Medicare becomes the primary payer 30 months after the employee becomes eligible for Medicare. Employers are reassured that studies have shown that employees with **kidney failure** are no different from other employees with regard to attendance, conscientiousness, and productivity. Employees who choose hemodialysis or peritoneal dialysis may need a temporary reduction of hours while they are getting used to their new home. The brochure outlines strategies for accommodating employees with **kidney failure,** the benefits (tax credits) that may be available, and laws that cover employment of people with **kidney failure.** A list of publications from the National Kidney Foundation (NKF) is offered, with a brief description of the organization and its activities.

- **Facts About End Stage Renal Disease: A Guide for Employers**

Source: New York, NY: National Kidney Foundation, Inc. 1996. 6 p.

Contact: Available from National Kidney Foundation. U.S. Materials Orders, 30 East 33rd Street, New York, NY 10016. (212) 889-2210. Fax (212) 689-9261. PRICE: $7.00 for 25 copies. Item number: 05-14.

Summary: Working is very important to many people who have **kidney failure,** also known as **end-stage renal disease** (ESRD). This fact sheet answers common questions that employers may have about ESRD, allays their fears about employing people with this problem , and helps employers understand the important contribution that employment can make to the patient's quality of life, self-esteem, and livelihood. Topics covered include a definition of ESRD, treatment options for the disease (hemodialysis, peritoneal dialysis, and transplantation), how ESRD and its treatments affect a person's ability to work, how businesses accommodate people with ESRD, who pays for ESRD treatments, benefits for employing a person with ESRD, laws that pertain to the employment of people with ESRD (including the Americans With Disabilities Act), understanding why someone who can qualify for disability payments would prefer to work, and where to get more information. The fact sheet concludes with a brief list of related brochures available from the National Kidney Foundation (NKF). (AA-M).

- **EPO: Treating Anemia in Chronic Renal Failure**

Source: New York, NY: National Kidney Foundation. 1990. 4 p.

Contact: Available from National Kidney Foundation. 30 East 33rd Street, New York, NY 10016. (800) 622-9010. PRICE: Single copy free ($12 per 100 copies). Order Number 08-75.

Summary: Written in a question-and-answer format, this brochure provides basic information about the use of erythropoietin (EPO) in treating the anemia frequently resulting from chronic **renal failure.** Topics covered include the development of kidney disease, obtaining and using EPO, dosage information, complications and side effects of EPO, and the impact of EPO on the daily lifestyle of the patient. The brochure notes that rehabilitation and adjustment to **kidney failure** require hard work, determination, and close cooperation between patient and doctor. EPO can be an important adjunct to successfully living with chronic **renal failure.**

### Healthfinder™

Healthfinder™ is an additional source sponsored by the U.S. Department of Health and Human Services which offers links to hundreds of other sites that contain healthcare information. This Web site is located at **http://www.healthfinder.gov**. Again, keyword searches can be used to find guidelines. The following was recently found in this database:

- **Kidney Failure Glossary**

  Summary: This glossary defines words that are often used when people talk or write about kidney failure and its treatments.

  Source: National Institute of Diabetes and Digestive and Kidney Diseases, National Institutes of Health

  http://www.healthfinder.gov/scripts/recordpass.asp?RecordType=0&RecordID=6517

### The NIH Search Utility

After browsing the references listed at the beginning of this chapter, you may want to explore the NIH search utility. This allows you to search for documents on over 100 selected Web sites that comprise the NIH-WEB-SPACE. Each of these servers is "crawled" and indexed on an ongoing basis. Your search will produce a list of various documents, all of which will relate in some way to kidney failure. The drawbacks of this approach are that the information is not organized by theme and that the references are often a mix of information for professionals and patients. Nevertheless, a large number of the listed Web sites provide useful background information. We can only recommend this route, therefore, for relatively rare or specific disorders, or when using highly targeted searches. To use the NIH search utility, visit the following Web page: **http://search.nih.gov/index.html**.

**Additional Web Sources**

A number of Web sites that often link to government sites are available to the public. These can also point you in the direction of essential information. The following is a representative sample:

- AOL: **http://search.aol.com/cat.adp?id=168&layer=&from=subcats**

- Family Village: **http://www.familyvillage.wisc.edu/specific.htm**

- Google: **http://directory.google.com/Top/Health/Conditions_and_Diseases/**

- Med Help International: **http://www.medhelp.org/HealthTopics/A.html**

- Open Directory Project: **http://dmoz.org/Health/Conditions_and_Diseases/**

- Yahoo.com: **http://dir.yahoo.com/Health/Diseases_and_Conditions/**

- WebMD®Health: **http://my.webmd.com/health_topics**

# Vocabulary Builder

The material in this chapter may have contained a number of unfamiliar words. The following Vocabulary Builder introduces you to terms used in this chapter that have not been covered in the previous chapter:

**Adjustment:**  The dynamic process wherein the thoughts, feelings, behavior, and biophysiological mechanisms of the individual continually change to adjust to the environment. [NIH]

**Antibiotic:**  A substance usually produced by vegetal micro-organisms capable of inhibiting the growth of or killing bacteria. [NIH]

**Cataracts:**  In medicine, an opacity of the crystalline lens of the eye obstructing partially or totally its transmission of light. [NIH]

**Catheters:**  A small, flexible tube that may be inserted into various parts of the body to inject or remove liquids. [NIH]

**Contraindications:**  Any factor or sign that it is unwise to pursue a certain kind of action or treatment, e. g. giving a general anesthetic to a person with pneumonia. [NIH]

**Forearm:**  The part between the elbow and the wrist. [NIH]

**Hepatitis:**  Infectious disease of the liver. [NIH]

**HLA:**  A glycoprotein found on the surface of all human leucocytes. The HLA region of chromosome 6 produces four such glycoproteins-A, B, C and

D. [NIH]

**Infections:**  The illnesses caused by an organism that usually does not cause disease in a person with a normal immune system. [NIH]

**Monitor:**  An apparatus which automatically records such physiological signs as respiration, pulse, and blood pressure in an anesthetized patient or one undergoing surgical or other procedures. [NIH]

**Nerve:**  A cordlike structure of nervous tissue that connects parts of the nervous system with other tissues of the body and conveys nervous impulses to, or away from, these tissues. [NIH]

**Outpatient:**  A patient who is not an inmate of a hospital but receives diagnosis or treatment in a clinic or dispensary connected with the hospital. [NIH]

**Physiology:**  The science that deals with the life processes and functions of organismus, their cells, tissues, and organs. [NIH]

**Potassium:**  It is essential to the ability of muscle cells to contract. [NIH]

**Race:**  A population within a species which exhibits general similarities within itself, but is both discontinuous and distinct from other populations of that species, though not sufficiently so as to achieve the status of a taxon. [NIH]

# CHAPTER 2. SEEKING GUIDANCE

## Overview

Some patients are comforted by the knowledge that a number of organizations dedicate their resources to helping people with kidney failure. These associations can become invaluable sources of information and advice. Many associations offer aftercare support, financial assistance, and other important services. Furthermore, healthcare research has shown that support groups often help people to better cope with their conditions.[8] In addition to support groups, your physician can be a valuable source of guidance and support. Therefore, finding a physician that can work with your unique situation is a very important aspect of your care.

In this chapter, we direct you to resources that can help you find patient organizations and medical specialists. We begin by describing how to find associations and peer groups that can help you better understand and cope with kidney failure. The chapter ends with a discussion on how to find a doctor that is right for you.

## Finding Associations

There are a several Internet directories that provide lists of medical associations with information on or resources relating to kidney failure. By consulting all of associations listed in this chapter, you will have nearly exhausted all sources for patient associations concerned with kidney failure.

---

[8] Churches, synagogues, and other houses of worship might also have groups that can offer you the social support you need.

### The National Health Information Center (NHIC)

The National Health Information Center (NHIC) offers a free referral service to help people find organizations that provide information about kidney failure. For more information, see the NHIC's Web site at **http://www.health.gov/NHIC/** or contact an information specialist by calling 1-800-336-4797.

### DIRLINE

A comprehensive source of information on associations is the DIRLINE database maintained by the National Library of Medicine. The database comprises some 10,000 records of organizations, research centers, and government institutes and associations which primarily focus on health and biomedicine. DIRLINE is available via the Internet at the following Web site: **http://dirline.nlm.nih.gov/**. Simply type in "kidney failure" (or a synonym) or the name of a topic, and the site will list information contained in the database on all relevant organizations.

### The Combined Health Information Database

Another comprehensive source of information on healthcare associations is the Combined Health Information Database. Using the "Detailed Search" option, you will need to limit your search to "Organizations" and "kidney failure". Type the following hyperlink into your Web browser: **http://chid.nih.gov/detail/detail.html**. To find associations, use the drop boxes at the bottom of the search page where "You may refine your search by." For publication date, select "All Years." Then, select your preferred language and the format option "Organization Resource Sheet." By making these selections and typing in "kidney failure" (or synonyms) into the "For these words:" box, you will only receive results on organizations dealing with kidney failure. You should check back periodically with this database since it is updated every 3 months.

### The National Organization for Rare Disorders, Inc.

The National Organization for Rare Disorders, Inc. has prepared a Web site that provides, at no charge, lists of associations organized by specific diseases. You can access this database at the following Web site:

**http://www.rarediseases.org/search/orgsearch.html**. Type "kidney failure" (or a synonym) in the search box, and click "Submit Query."

### Online Support Groups

In addition to support groups, commercial Internet service providers offer forums and chat rooms for people with different illnesses and conditions. WebMD®, for example, offers such a service at its Web site: **http://boards.webmd.com/roundtable**. These online self-help communities can help you connect with a network of people whose concerns are similar to yours. Online support groups are places where people can talk informally. If you read about a novel approach, consult with your doctor or other healthcare providers, as the treatments or discoveries you hear about may not be scientifically proven to be safe and effective.

## Finding Doctors

One of the most important aspects of your treatment will be the relationship between you and your doctor or specialist. All patients with kidney failure must go through the process of selecting a physician. While this process will vary from person to person, the Agency for Healthcare Research and Quality makes a number of suggestions, including the following:[9]

- If you are in a managed care plan, check the plan's list of doctors first.

- Ask doctors or other health professionals who work with doctors, such as hospital nurses, for referrals.

- Call a hospital's doctor referral service, but keep in mind that these services usually refer you to doctors on staff at that particular hospital. The services do not have information on the quality of care that these doctors provide.

- Some local medical societies offer lists of member doctors. Again, these lists do not have information on the quality of care that these doctors provide.

---

[9] This section has been adapted from the AHRQ: **www.ahrq.gov/consumer/qntascii/qntdr.htm**.

Additional steps you can take to locate doctors include the following:

- Information on doctors in some states is available on the Internet at **http://www.docboard.org**. This Web site is run by "Administrators in Medicine," a group of state medical board directors.

- The American Board of Medical Specialties can tell you if your doctor is board certified. "Certified" means that the doctor has completed a training program in a specialty and has passed an exam, or "board," to assess his or her knowledge, skills, and experience to provide quality patient care in that specialty. Primary care doctors may also be certified as specialists. The AMBS Web site is located at **http://www.abms.org/newsearch.asp**.[10] You can also contact the ABMS by phone at 1-866-ASK-ABMS.

- You can call the American Medical Association (AMA) at 800-665-2882 for information on training, specialties, and board certification for many licensed doctors in the United States. This information also can be found in "Physician Select" at the AMA's Web site: **http://www.ama-assn.org/aps/amahg.htm**.

## Finding a Urologist

The American Urological Association (AUA) provides the public with a free-to-use "Find A Urologist" service to help patients find member urologists in their area. The database can be searched by physician name, city, U.S. State, or country and is available via the AUA's Web site located at **http://www.auanet.org/patient_info/find_urologist/index.cfm**. According to the AUA: "The American Urological Association is the professional association for urologists. As the premier professional association for the advancement of urologic patient care, the AUA is pleased to provide Find A Urologist, an on-line referral service for patients to use when looking for a urologist. All of our active members are certified by the American Board of Urology, which is an important distinction of the urologist's commitment to continuing education and superior patient care."[11]

If the previous sources did not meet your needs, you may want to log on to the Web site of the National Organization for Rare Disorders (NORD) at **http://www.rarediseases.org/**. NORD maintains a database of doctors with expertise in various rare diseases. The Metabolic Information Network

---

[10] While board certification is a good measure of a doctor's knowledge, it is possible to receive quality care from doctors who are not board certified.

[11] Quotation taken from the AACE's Web site: **http://www.aace.com/memsearch.php**.

(MIN), 800-945-2188, also maintains a database of physicians with expertise in various metabolic diseases.

## Selecting Your Doctor[12]

When you have compiled a list of prospective doctors, call each of their offices. First, ask if the doctor accepts your health insurance plan and if he or she is taking new patients. If the doctor is not covered by your plan, ask yourself if you are prepared to pay the extra costs. The next step is to schedule a visit with your chosen physician. During the first visit you will have the opportunity to evaluate your doctor and to find out if you feel comfortable with him or her. Ask yourself, did the doctor:

- Give me a chance to ask questions about kidney failure?

- Really listen to my questions?

- Answer in terms I understood?

- Show respect for me?

- Ask me questions?

- Make me feel comfortable?

- Address the health problem(s) I came with?

- Ask me my preferences about different kinds of treatments for kidney failure?

- Spend enough time with me?

Trust your instincts when deciding if the doctor is right for you. But remember, it might take time for the relationship to develop. It takes more than one visit for you and your doctor to get to know each other.

---

[12] This section has been adapted from the AHRQ:
www.ahrq.gov/consumer/qntascii/qntdr.htm.

## Working with Your Doctor[13]

Research has shown that patients who have good relationships with their doctors tend to be more satisfied with their care and have better results. Here are some tips to help you and your doctor become partners:

- You know important things about your symptoms and your health history. Tell your doctor what you think he or she needs to know.

- It is important to tell your doctor personal information, even if it makes you feel embarrassed or uncomfortable.

- Bring a "health history" list with you (and keep it up to date).

- Always bring any medications you are currently taking with you to the appointment, or you can bring a list of your medications including dosage and frequency information. Talk about any allergies or reactions you have had to your medications.

- Tell your doctor about any natural or alternative medicines you are taking.

- Bring other medical information, such as x-ray films, test results, and medical records.

- Ask questions. If you don't, your doctor will assume that you understood everything that was said.

- Write down your questions before your visit. List the most important ones first to make sure that they are addressed.

- Consider bringing a friend with you to the appointment to help you ask questions. This person can also help you understand and/or remember the answers.

- Ask your doctor to draw pictures if you think that this would help you understand.

- Take notes. Some doctors do not mind if you bring a tape recorder to help you remember things, but always ask first.

- Let your doctor know if you need more time. If there is not time that day, perhaps you can speak to a nurse or physician assistant on staff or schedule a telephone appointment.

- Take information home. Ask for written instructions. Your doctor may also have brochures and audio and videotapes that can help you.

---

[13] This section has been adapted from the AHRQ: **www.ahrq.gov/consumer/qntascii/qntdr.htm.**

- After leaving the doctor's office, take responsibility for your care. If you have questions, call. If your symptoms get worse or if you have problems with your medication, call. If you had tests and do not hear from your doctor, call for your test results. If your doctor recommended that you have certain tests, schedule an appointment to get them done. If your doctor said you should see an additional specialist, make an appointment.

By following these steps, you will enhance the relationship you will have with your physician.

## Broader Health-Related Resources

In addition to the references above, the NIH has set up guidance Web sites that can help patients find healthcare professionals. These include:[14]

- Caregivers:
  **http://www.nlm.nih.gov/medlineplus/caregivers.html**

- Choosing a Doctor or Healthcare Service:
  **http://www.nlm.nih.gov/medlineplus/choosingadoctororhealthcareserv ice.html**

- Hospitals and Health Facilities:
  **http://www.nlm.nih.gov/medlineplus/healthfacilities.html**

---

[14] You can access this information at
**http://www.nlm.nih.gov/medlineplus/healthsystem.html**.

# PART II: ADDITIONAL RESOURCES AND ADVANCED MATERIAL

## ABOUT PART II

In Part II, we introduce you to additional resources and advanced research on kidney failure. All too often, patients who conduct their own research are overwhelmed by the difficulty in finding and organizing information. The purpose of the following chapters is to provide you an organized and structured format to help you find additional information resources on kidney failure. In Part II, as in Part I, our objective is not to interpret the latest advances on kidney failure or render an opinion. Rather, our goal is to give you access to original research and to increase your awareness of sources you may not have already considered. In this way, you will come across the advanced materials often referred to in pamphlets, books, or other general works. Once again, some of this material is technical in nature, so consultation with a professional familiar with kidney failure is suggested.

# CHAPTER 3. STUDIES ON KIDNEY FAILURE

## Overview

Every year, academic studies are published on kidney failure or related conditions. Broadly speaking, there are two types of studies. The first are peer reviewed. Generally, the content of these studies has been reviewed by scientists or physicians. Peer-reviewed studies are typically published in scientific journals and are usually available at medical libraries. The second type of studies is non-peer reviewed. These works include summary articles that do not use or report scientific results. These often appear in the popular press, newsletters, or similar periodicals.

In this chapter, we will show you how to locate peer-reviewed references and studies on kidney failure. We will begin by discussing research that has been summarized and is free to view by the public via the Internet. We then show you how to generate a bibliography on kidney failure and teach you how to keep current on new studies as they are published or undertaken by the scientific community.

## The Combined Health Information Database

The Combined Health Information Database summarizes studies across numerous federal agencies. To limit your investigation to research studies and kidney failure, you will need to use the advanced search options. First, go to **http://chid.nih.gov/index.html**. From there, select the "Detailed Search" option (or go directly to that page with the following hyperlink: **http://chid.nih.gov/detail/detail.html**). The trick in extracting studies is found in the drop boxes at the bottom of the search page where "You may refine your search by." Select the dates and language you prefer, and the format option "Journal Article." At the top of the search form, select the number of records you would like to see (we recommend 100) and check the box to display "whole records." We recommend that you type in "kidney failure" (or synonyms) into the "For these words:" box. Consider using the option "anywhere in record" to make your search as broad as possible. If you want to limit the search to only a particular field, such as the title of the journal, then select this option in the "Search in these fields" drop box. The following is a sample of what you can expect from this type of search:

- **Prevention and Treatment of Acute Renal Failure in Sepsis**

  Source: JASN. Journal of the American Society of Nephrology. 14(3): 792-805 March 2003.

  Contact: Available from Lippincott Williams and Wilkins. 12107 Insurance Way, Hagerstown, MD 21740. (800) 638-6423. Website: www.jasn.org/.

  Summary: Acute **renal failure** (ARF) is a common complication of sepsis and has a poor prognosis. Mortality (death) was reported higher in patients with septic ARF (74.5 percent) than in those whose renal (kidney) failure did not result from sepsis (45.2 percent). This article discusses the use of drug therapy to interfere with each of the dysfunctional pathways to improve the course of septic ARF. These include inhibition of inflammatory mediators, improvement of renal hemodynamics (blood flow) by amplifying vasodilator mechanisms and blocking vasoconstrictor mechanisms, interruption of leukocyte infiltration, inhibition of the coagulation cascade, and administration of growth factors to accelerate renal recovery. The author also highlights the available supportive measures, including dialysis, that can be used for septic patients with ARF. The author notes that, unfortunately, treatment of ARF in sepsis is still only supportive; there have been no conclusive drug therapies available to treat the condition. 1 figure. 1 table. 136 references.

- **Impact of Burn Size and Initial Serum Albumin Level on Acute Renal Failure Occurring in Major Burn**

  Source: American Journal of Nephrology. 23: 55-60. January-February 2003.

  Contact: Available from S. Karger Publishers, Inc. 26 West Avon Road, P.O. Box 529, Farmington, CT 06085. (800) 828-5479. Website: www.karger.com.

  Summary: Acute renal (kidney) failure (ARF) is not a rare occurrence in severe burns and is an important complication leading to an increase in mortality (death). The severity of the burn is largely determined by the burn size, and severe burns are likely to cause enough loss of extracellular fluid and albumin from plasma volume to produce shock and hypoalbuminemia (low levels of the protein albumin in the blood). This article reports on a study in which the authors hypothesized that initial serum albumin level may be useful as an indicator of prognosis and severity of injury in burned patients. The authors retrospectively analyzed the clinical characteristics of 147 adult patients with second-and third-degree burns covering 30 percent or more of their body surface area. Of the 147 patients, 27 (19 percent) experienced ARF, defined as a serum creatinine greater than 2 milligrams per deciliter, during the admission. The patients with ARF had larger burn size and lower serum albumin concentration at admission, compared with those without ARF. All patients with ARF expired, whereas 29.4 percent (35 of 119 patients) of the patients without ARF died. The burn size greater than 65 percent was associated with a risk of ARF that was 9.9 times and with a risk of death that was 14.2 times as high as that for burn size less than 65 percent. The authors conclude that when major burns are complicated by ARF, the mortality rate increases significantly. Burn size is an independent predictor of ARF occurring in major burns. Initially depressed serum albumin level is associated with an increase in mortality in the major burn patients. 3 figures. 4 tables. 21 references.

- **Quality of Prereferral Care in Patients with Chronic Renal Insufficiency**

Source: American Journal of Kidney Diseases. 40(1): 30-36. July 2002.

Contact: Available from W.B. Saunders Company. Periodicals Department, 6277 Sea Harbor Drive, Orlando, FL 32887-4800. (800) 654-2452 or (407) 345-4000.

Summary: Appropriate care in **chronic renal insufficiency** (CRI) includes blood pressure and diabetes control, as well as the investigation and management of anemia, acidosis, and bone disease. There is a lack of data on the control of these parameters at the time of referral to a nephrologist. Similarly, early referral has been emphasized in the literature, yet very little published has examined current referral patterns. This article reports on a review of all new outpatient referrals to nephrologists in Halifax, Canada in 1998 and 1999; the review was conducted to identify patients with CRI. Quality of pre-referral care was based on data from the initial clinic visit. Of 1,050 charts reviewed, 411 patients met the study criteria. Twenty-six percent of patients had diabetes mellitus, 18 percent were referred with a calculated glomerular filtration rate (GFR) less than 15 milliliters per minute, and blood pressure was optimally controlled in only 24 percent. Only 44 percent of patients were administered an ACE inhibitor. Patients were administered an average of 1.9 antihypertensive agents. Significant anemia was present in 21 percent and appropriate investigations (diagnostic tests) were performed in only 35 percent of these patients. Calcium levels less than 8.6 milligrams per deciliter were found in 19 percent of patients, and only 14 percent of these patients were started on calcium supplement therapy. Phosphate levels greater than 5.0 milligrams per deciliter were seen in 20 percent of patients, and 14 percent of these patients were on phosphate-binder therapy. Parathyroid hormone levels were more than five times normal values in 18 percent of patients. The authors conclude that a significant proportion of patients referred with CRI receive inadequate pre-referral care. Continuing education programs and referral guidelines must not only emphasize the importance of early referral, but also address the related consequences of CRI to delay the progression of renal (kidney) disease and avoid complications. 3 tables. 34 references.

- **Slowing the Progression of Chronic Renal Failure: Economic Benefits and Patients' Perspectives**

Source: American Journal of Kidney Diseases. 39(4): 721-729. April 2002.

Contact: Available from W.B. Saunders Company. Periodicals Department, 6277 Sea Harbor Drive, Orlando, FL 32887-4800. (800) 654-2452 or (407) 345-4000.

Summary: Because of the predicted increase in **end stage renal disease** (ESRD) incidence, prevalence, and cost, a cohesive national effort is needed to develop strategies to slow the progression of chronic renal (kidney) failure (CRF). The question arises of how much reduction in the progression of CRF would lead to a meaningful decrease in the prevalence and cost of ESRD. This article reports on the development of a mathematical model to assess the economic impact of decreasing the progression of CRF by 10 percent, 20 percent, and 30 percent. United States Renal Data System (USRDS) projections were used to model the rate of increase in ESRD incidence and prevalence. Glomerular filtration rate (GFR, a measure of kidney function) at the initiation of ESRD therapy and cost per patient year were based on USRDS data. The authors also determined how much slowing of the progression of CRF is important from patients' perspectives by means of a written questionnaire (which inquired about willingness to go on a restricted diet, take six extra medications per day, and make six extra office visits per year). The authors note that their data suggest that the cumulative economic impact of slowing the progression of CRF, even by as little as 10 percent, would be staggering. The authors call for the development and implementation of intensive renoprotective (protecting the kidney) efforts beginning at the early stages of chronic renal disease and continued throughout its course. 2 figures. 5 tables. 48 references.

- **Assessing Glycemic Control in Patients with Diabetes and End-Stage Renal Failure**

  Source: American Journal of Kidney Diseases. 41(3): 523-531. March 2003.

  Summary: Blood glucose monitoring is important in optimizing long-term outcomes in patients with diabetes. Reliance on near-patient testing and the use of longer term measures of glycation (glycosylated hemoglobin) are the current cornerstones. This review article considers the assessment of glycemic control in patients with diabetes and **end-stage renal disease** (ESRD). The authors caution that there are significant problems using blood tests as measures of metabolic control in diabetes patients who are uremic. The authors advocate the use of patient glucose diaries, catering for individualized dialysis regimens, to supplement the information that can be derived from metabolic parameters. They do not advocate the abandonment of measurements of glycosylated hemoglobin (HbA1c) and fructosamine in **uremia,** but encourage a recognition of their limitations. 4 figures. 1 table. 60 references.

- **Renal Failure and Deafness: Branchio-Oto-Renal Syndrome**

  Source: American Journal of Kidney Diseases. 32(2): 334-337. August 1998.

  Contact: Available from W.B. Saunders Company. P.O. Box 628239, Orlando, FL 32862-8239. (800) 654-2452. Fax (800) 225-6030. E-mail: wbspcs@harcourtbrace.com. Website: www.ajkd.org.

  Summary: Branchio oto renal (BOR) syndrome is a rare autosomal dominant condition that may present with hearing loss, branchial cysts, and **renal failure.** The characteristic phenotypic expression of the full syndrome may be partial or complete, and a whole range of renal (kidney) abnormalities may be present. The similarity of BOR to Alport's syndrome may lead to misdiagnosis. This article presents a case report of adult onset **renal failure** in a 44 year old white man with deafness, previously believed to have Alport's syndrome. The patient's hearing loss was believed to be congenital, and he was prescribed hearing aids. By the age of 19 years, deafness had worsened significantly, and a diagnosis of bilateral moderately severe mixed hearing loss was made. The authors review the relevant literature. The authors note that it is not clear why there is an association between renal malformation and abnormalities of the ear. 2 figures. 18 references.

- **Growth in Children with Chronic Renal Failure on Intermittent Versus Daily Calcitriol**

Source: Pediatric Nephrology. 18(5): 440-444. May 2003.

Summary: Calcitriol treatment strategies for secondary hyperparathyroidism remain controversial regarding efficacy and safety. In children, intermittent calcitriol administration has been suspected of impairing body growth. This article reports on a prospective, randomized study in which the authors compared the effect of daily versus twice weekly calcitriol on plasma intact parathyroid hormone (iPTH) levels and growth in 24 prepubertal children with **chronic renal insufficiency** (CRI). After a 3-week washout period, the patients were randomly assigned to two different doses of daily or twice a week oral calcitriol. The calcitriol dose was kept constant for 2 months and was then be adapted to maintain iPTH target ranges. The change in height standard deviation score during the study period was not affected by either treatment modality. The authors conclude that daily and intermittent calcitriol do not differentially affect growth rate and are equally effective in controlling secondary hyperparathyroidism in children with chronic **renal failure.** 4 figures. 2 tables. 29 references.

- **Varicella Vaccination in Children with Chronic Renal Failure: A Report of the Southwest Pediatric Nephrology Study Group**

Source: Pediatric Nephrology 18(1): 33-38. January 2003.

Contact: Available from Springer-Verlag. Service Center Secaucus, 44 Hartz Way, Secaucus, NJ 07094. (201) 348-4033.

Summary: Children with kidney disease are at risk for serious varicella related complications. This article reports on a study undertaken to evaluate the safety and immunogenicity of a two-dose regimen of varicella (the virus that causes chickenpox) vaccine in children (aged 1 to 19 years, n = 96) with chronic renal (kidney) insufficiency and on dialysis. Of the 96 patients, 50 (mean age 4.2 years) had no detectable varicella zoster virus (VZV) antibody; 98 percent sero-converted after the two-dose vaccine regimen. At 1, 2, and 3 years' follow up, all patients studied maintained VZV antibody, including 16 who received a transplant. No significant vaccine-associated adverse events were seen. One subject developed mild varicella 16 months post transplant. In multivariate regression analysis, patients vaccinated after 6 years of age had VZV antibody levels 73 percent lower than patients vaccinated before 6 years of age. The authors conclude that a two-dose varicella vaccination regimen was generally well tolerated and highly immunogenic in children with chronic kidney disease. 1 figure. 2 tables. 25 references.

- **Hepatitis C and Renal Failure**

  Source: American Journal of Medicine. 107(6B): 90S-94S. December 27, 1999.

  Contact: Available from Exerpta Medica, Inc. American Journal of Medicine, P.O. Box 7247-7197, Philadelphia, PA 19170-7197. (800) 606-0023 or (609) 786-0841. Fax (609) 786-7032.

  Summary: Chronic hepatitis C virus (HCV) infection is common among patients with chronic renal (kidney) failure (CRF). This article reviews the interplay between HCV and **kidney failure.** The chronic viral infection can result in significant morbidity (illness) and mortality (death). Liver failure from chronic hepatitis C is one of the leading causes of death among long term survivors of kidney transplantation. Between 10 and 20 percent of patients on hemodialysis are chronically infected with HCV. HCV infection also can be a cause of glomerulonephritis (and infection of the kidneys) and nephrotic syndrome (edema, or fluid accumulation, protein in the urine or proteinuria, and susceptibility to infections). The author stresses that primary care physicians need to recognize these conditions in order to optimize the management of patients with CRF. 45 references.

- **Resistance Training to Counteract the Catabolism of a Low-Protein Diet in Patients with Chronic Renal Insufficiency**

  Source: Annals of Internal Medicine. 135(11): 965-976. December 4, 2001.

  Contact: Available from American College of Physicians. American Society of Internal Medicine. 190 North Independence Mall West, Philadelphia, PA 19106-1572. Website: www.acponline.org.

  Summary: Chronic renal insufficiency (CRI) leads to muscle wasting, which may be exacerbated by low-protein diets prescribed to delay or slow disease progression. Resistance training increases protein utilization and muscle mass. This article reports on a study undertaken to determine the efficacy of resistance training in improving protein utilization and muscle mass in patients with CRI treated with a low protein diet. Results that show that resistance exercise training can preserve lean body mass, nutritional status, and muscle function in patients with moderate chronic kidney disease. The study's results suggest that resistance training is a safe and effective countermeasure to the negative effects of protein restriction on muscle mass accretion, protein utilization, nutritional status, and muscle function in patients with chronic kidney disease. 3 figures. 4 tables. 43 references.

- **Some Medical Aspects of Nutritional Therapy in Elderly Chronic Renal Failure Patients**

Source: Dialysis and Transplantation. 31(9): 607-608, 610-614. September 2002.

Contact: Available from Dialysis and Transplantation, Attn.: Subscriptions. P.O. Box 10535, Riverton, NJ 08076. (800) 624-4196 or (609) 786-0871.

Summary: Elderly chronic renal (kidney) failure (CRF) patients present special problems to the renal team. This article focuses on some medical aspects of nutritional therapy in elderly CRF patients. The authors note that signs due to aging often superimpose on symptoms related to CRF. There are some specific age-associated problems in geriatric patients, such as diminished taste and smell perception, loss of teeth, constipation, poor physical condition, and psychosocial problems including economic limitations, social isolation, and depression. All of these conditions can have a negative impact on the nutritional status in elderly CRF patients. The authors advise a moderate protein restriction and an increased calorie intake in elderly renal patients who are in the Predialysis stage. Metabolic acidosis should be treated to prevent further catabolism, and more intensive nutritional monitoring is advocated to avoid occult (hidden) malnutrition. The authors also discuss the nutritional recommendations for elderly patients on hemodialysis and comment on a new therapeutic trend for the treatment of malnutrition in CRF patients, i.e., the use of recombinant forms of human growth hormone and insulin-like growth factor 1. 3 figures. 1 table. 25 references.

- **Twenty-Eight-Year-Old Female with Primary Amenorrhea and Chronic Renal Failure: A Case of Frasier Syndrome?**

Source: Journal of the American Medical Association. 96(2): 256-261. February 2004.

Summary: Frasier syndrome is a very rare developmental disorder of autosomal recessive inheritance. Frasier syndrome is characterized by male hermaphroditism, primary amenorrhea, chronic **renal failure** (CRF), and a number of other abnormalities. In this article, a 28 year old Nigerian female who was considered as a possible case of Frasier syndrome was described; she first presented to the authors in July 2002 with primary amenorrhea, congenital bilateral absence of middle toes, elevated blood pressure, and the uremic syndrome. The management of the case was mainly conservative, including blood pressure control with appropriate antihypertensives. The problems inherent in this index case are discussed while proffering appropriate management approach in a near-ideal situation, which unfortunately is nonexistent in the author's local environment (Nigeria). 10 references.

- **Growth Failure, Risk of Hospitalization and Death of Children with End-stage Renal Disease**

Source: Pediatric Nephrology. 17(6): 450-455. June 2002.

Contact: Available from Springer-Verlag. Service Center Secaucus, 44 Hartz Way, Secaucus, NJ 07094. (201) 348-4033.

Summary: Growth failure remains a significant problem for children with **chronic renal insufficiency** and **end stage renal disease** (ESRD). This article reports on a study that examined whether growth failure is associated with more-frequent hospitalizations or higher mortality in children with kidney disease. The authors studied data on prevalent United States pediatric patients with ESRD in 1990 who were followed through 1995. Patients were categorized according to the standard deviation score (SDS) of their incremental growth during 1990. Among 1,112 prevalent pediatric dialysis and transplant patients, those with severe and moderate growth failure had higher hospitalization rates respectively than those with normal growth after adjustment for age, gender, race, cause and duration of ESRD, and treatment modality in 1990. Survival analysis showed 5 year survival rates of 85 percent and 90 percent for patients with severe and moderate growth failure, respectively, compared with 96 percent for patients with normal growth. A higher proportion of deaths in the severe and moderate growth failure groups were attributed to infectious causes (22 percent and 18.7 percent, respectively) than in the normal growth group (15.6 percent). The authors conclude that growth failure is associated with a more complicated clinical course and increased risk of death for children with **kidney failure.** 1 figure. 3 tables. 15 references.

- **Randomized Trial of Folic Acid for Prevention of Cardiovascular Events in End-Stage Renal Disease**

Source: Journal of the American Society of Nephrology. 15(2): 420-426. February 2004.

Summary: High serum total homocysteine (tHcy) is gaining scrutiny as a risk factor for cardiovascular disease in the general population. The relationship between tHcy and mortality and cardiovascular events in patients with **end stage renal disease** (ESRD) is unsettled. This article reports on a randomized trial that evaluated the effectiveness of high dose folic acid in preventing events in ESRD. A total of 510 patients on chronic dialysis were randomized to 1, 5, or 15 milligrams of folic acid contained in a renal multivitamin, with a median follow-up of 24 months. Mortality, cardiovascular events, and homocysteine levels were assessed. There were 189 deaths, and 121 patients experienced at least one cardiovascular event. Composite rates of mortality and cardiovascular events among the folic acid groups did not differ. Unexpectedly, high baseline tHcy was associated with lower event rates. The authors conclude that, in contrast to some studies describing tHcy as a risk factor for mortality and cardiovascular events, this study found a reverse relationship between tHcy and events in ESRD patients. Administration of high-dose folic acid did not affect event rates. 4 figures. 2 tables. 27 references.

- **Atherosclerosis in Patients with End-Stage Renal Failure Prior to Initiation of Hemodialysis**

Source: Renal Failure. 25(2): 247-254. 2003.

Summary: In patients on dialysis, cardiovascular mortality (death) is 10 to 20 times higher than in the general population. It remains uncertain whether atherosclerosis of dialysis patients is effectively accelerated because many dialysis patients have more or less marked vascular lesions present at the start of dialysis treatment. This article reports on a study in which the authors compared intima-media thickness (IMT) and plaque occurrence (indicators of atherosclerosis) in the common carotid arteries (CC) in the area of bifurcation (CB) and in the proximal part of internal carotid arteries (CI) in 28 hemodialysis patients (14 men and 14 women, mean age 49.4 years, mean duration of HD treatment 66.6 months) with that in 28 age-matched patients prior to initiation of hemodialysis. The authors found that the IMT values of CC, CB, and CI were not significantly different in dialysis patients and patients starting dialysis treatment. The results also showed no difference in plaque occurrence and in atherosclerotic risk factors (hypertension, smoking, lipids) between groups. The authors recommend earlier and more aggressive intervention before dialysis treatment in order to reduce the atherosclerotic risk factors. 31 references.

- **Survival of Patients with AIDS and End-Stage Renal Disease Receiving Hemodialysis**

Source: Dialysis and Transplantation. 33(4): 176, 178, 180-181, 184-186. April 2004.

Summary: In the 1980s, most patients with AIDS who progressed to **end stage renal disease** (ESRD) survived for less than 6 months on maintenance hemodialysis. This article reports on a 68 month (1995 to 2001) prospective, multicenter, case-control cohort study undertaken to determine the present course and survival of patients with AIDS and ESRD receiving hemodialysis in four outpatient dialysis facilities in Brooklyn, NY. The course of all 34 patients with both ESRD and HIV infection in the four outpatient dialysis facilities was compared to that of 131 ESRD patients without known HIV infection who were randomly selected from the same dialysis facilities. At initiation, the mean age of the 34 patients with ESRD and HIV infection was 42 years, compared to 56 years for the control cohort (ESRD alone). During the 68-month observation period, 17 (50 percent) of the 34 patients with HIV and ESRD died, compared with 65 (50 percent) of the 131 patients with ESRD alone. Mean survival was equivalent between groups. Analyses showed that with adjustment for age, patients with both ESRD and HIV infection had a 97 percent higher risk of death than did their counterparts with ESRD alone. The authors conclude that the survival of patients with HIV infection and ESRD receiving hemodialysis has improved significantly compared with the uniformly dismal outcomes in the 1980s. The combination of HIV infection and ESRD no longer signals near-term death; thus, clinicians should not hesitate to refer HIV-infected patients with **renal failure** for **uremia** therapy.

- **Impact of Simultaneous Pancreas and Kidney Transplantation on Progression of Coronary Atherosclerosis in Patients with End-Stage Renal Failure due to Type 1 Diabetes**

Source: Diabetes Care. 25(5): 906-911. May 2002.

Contact: Available from American Diabetes Association. 1701 North Beauregard Street, Alexandria, VA 22311. (800) 232-3472. Website: www.diabetes.org.

Summary: Mortality (death) in type 1 diabetes patients with end stage **renal failure** is high and is dominated by coronary (heart) atherosclerotic events. With regard to prognosis, simultaneous transplantation of pancreas and kidney (SPK) may be superior to kidney transplantation alone (KTA) in these patients, because normalization of blood glucose levels may reduce progression of coronary atherosclerosis and because it is well known that progression of coronary atherosclerosis is one of the major factors that determines clinical prognosis. This article reports on a study that compared progression of coronary atherosclerosis in patients with (n = 26) and those without (n = 6) a functioning pancreas graft after SPK. Mean follow up was 3.9 years. Average glucose control was significantly worse for the patients without a pancreas graft than for patients with a functioning pancreas graft. Regression of atherosclerosis occurred in 38 percent of patients with a functioning pancreas graft compared with 0 percent of patients in whom the pancreas graft was lost.

The authors conclude that this observation is an important part of the explanation for the observed improved mortality rates reported in type 1 diabetes patients with end stage **renal failure** after SPK compared with KTA. In light of these findings, the authors recommend that SPK be carefully considered for all diabetes transplant candidates. 3 figures. 1 table. 40 references.

- **Nutrition in Children with Preterminal Chronic Renal Failure: Myth or Important Therapeutic Aid?**

Source: Pediatric Nephrology. 17(2): 111-120. February 2002.

Contact: Available from Springer-Verlag. Service Center Secaucus, 44 Hartz Way, Secaucus, NJ 07094. (201) 348-4033.

Summary: Nutrition has been believed to be an important therapeutic instrument in children with chronic renal (kidney) failure for improving growth and for slowing down the deterioration of renal function. The therapeutic strategies for both targets may be conflicting, at least in part, since a high caloric intake is needed for optimal growth, whereas a low protein diet, which was believed to protect renal function, places patients at risk of low calorie intake. This review article considers the role of nutrition in children with preterminal chronic **renal failure** (CRF). Dietary manipulations for optimal growth are mainly effective in infants with CRF. However, growth remains suboptimal even with an energy intake above 80 percent of RDA. Although a low protein diet is able to slow down the rate of deterioration in renal function in rodent studies, the results of prospective clinical studies were disappointing, at least for an observation period up to three years. The conclusions from dracon meta-analyses of these clinical studies in adults are contradictory. The progression rate was not significantly influenced by protein restriction, whereas renal replacement therapy could be postponed. However, the latter seems to be the effect of weakening uremic symptoms during the phase of end stage **renal failure.** The authors conclude that, according to present knowledge, it is not justified to prescribe special diets to children early in the course of CRF, but the composition of their nutrition should follow the general concept of an optimal mixed diet. 2 figures. 2 tables. 143 references.

- **Dialysis, Kidney Transplantation, or Pancreas Transplantation for Patients with Diabetes Mellitus and Renal Failure: A Decision Analysis of Treatment Options**

Source: Journal of the American Society of Nephrology. 14(2): 500-515. February 2003.

Contact: Available from Lippincott Williams and Wilkins. 12107 Insurance Way, Hagerstown, MD 21740. (800) 638-6423. Website: www.jasn.org/.

Summary: Patients with type 1 diabetes mellitus and end stage renal (kidney) disease (ESRD) may remain on dialysis or undergo cadaveric kidney transplantation, living kidney transplantation, sequential pancreas-after-living kidney transplantation, or simultaneous pancreas-kidney transplantation. This article reports on a study undertaken to determine the optimal treatment strategy for type 1 diabetes patients with **kidney failure.** The outcome measures were life expectancy in life-years (LY) and quality-adjusted life expectancy in quality-adjusted life-years (QALY). Living kidney transplantation was associated with 18.30 LY and 10.29 QALY; pancreas after kidney transplantation, 17.21 LY and 10.00 QALY; simultaneous pancreas-kidney transplantation, 15.74 LY and 9.09 QALY; cadaveric kidney transplantation, 11.44 LY and 6.53 QALY; dialysis, 7.82 LY and 4.52 QALY. The results were sensitive to the value of several key variables. Simultaneous pancreas-kidney transplantation had the greatest life expectancy and quality-adjusted life expectancy when living kidney transplantation was excluded from the analysis. The data indicate that living kidney transplantation is associated with the greatest life expectancy and quality-adjusted life expectancy for type 1 diabetes patients with **renal failure.** Treatment strategies involving pancreas transplantation should be considered for patients with frequent metabolic complications of diabetes. For patients without a living donor, simultaneous pancreas-kidney transplantation is associated with the greatest life expectancy. 5 figures. 4 tables. 162 references.

- **Erythropoietin Therapy in Pre-Dialysis Patients with Chronic Renal Failure: Lack of Need for Parenteral Iron**

Source: American Journal of Nephrology. 23(3): 78-85. 2003.

Summary: Scant information exists regarding the optimal target percent saturation of transferrin (TSAT), ferritin, and the mode and amount of iron supplementation during erythropoietin therapy in pre-dialysis patients with anemia due to chronic kidney disease (CKD). Pre-dialysis CKD patients may have different needs for iron supplementation than **end-stage renal disease** (ESRD) subjects during erythropoietin therapy. This article reports on a retrospective analysis of pre-dialysis CKD subjects (n = 31) treated with erythropoietin at the authors' institution. In this population, target hematocrit (33 to 36 percent) was achievable with erythropoietin without parenteral iron therapy. This response extends even to subgroups with TSAT or ferritin levels deemed to indicate iron deficiency in CKD subjects, and may mean that no functional iron deficiency exists in this group of patients. 3 figures. 2 tables. 34 references.

- **Effects of Secondary Hyperparathyroidism Treatments on Blood Pressure and Lipid Levels in Chronic Renal Failure Patients**

Source: Transplantation Proceedings. 34(6): 2041-2043. September 2002.

Contact: Available from Elsevier Science Inc. 655 Avenue of the Americas, New York, NY 10010. (212) 633-3730. Website: www.elsevier.com.

Summary: Secondary hyperparathyroidism, a frequent complication in chronic renal (kidney) failure (CRF) patients, is generally managed by controlling hyperphosphatemia, normalizing serum calcium levels, and administering oral or intravenous active vitamin D metabolites. Parathyroidectomy (PTX) is another treatment option when medical therapy fails to control the disease. This article reports on a study undertaken to investigate the effects of medical and surgical therapy on blood pressure and lipid levels in CRF patients. In this study, both medical and surgical therapies resulted in a significant decline in systolic and diastolic blood pressure. The authors conclude that treatment of secondary hyperparathyroidism has beneficial effects not only on renal osteodystrophy (bone disease associated with kidney disease), but also on blood pressure and triglyceride levels. They emphasize the need for surgical treatment of patients who are unresponsive to medical therapy. 4 figures. 13 references.

- **Gastrointestinal Complications of Renal Failure**

Source: Gastroenterology Clinics of North America. 27(4): 875-892. December 1998.

Contact: Available from W.B. Saunders. 6277 Sea Harbor Drive, Orlando, FL 32887-4800. (800) 654-2452 or (407) 345-4000.

Summary: Seventy-five percent of patients with **end-stage renal disease** (ESRD) have gastrointestinal complaints. Although some of these complaints may be specifically related to the techniques and procedures of the dialysis method itself, the physiologic state of chronic **uremia** is likely to contribute to the development of the majority of symptoms. **Uremia** is the presence of excessive amounts of urea and other nitrogen waste products in the blood. This article begins with a brief review of the systemic effects of uremic toxins followed by a review of the effects of the uremic state on the esophagus, stomach, duodenum, and pancreas. The effects of ESRD on the gastrointestinal (GI) tract can be divided into complications directly attributable to dialysis and complications that are more systemically related. The majority of complications are likely to be related to the latter. Dialysis related GI complications include peritonitis and sclerosing peritonitis. Esophageal abnormalities associated with the uremic state include esophagitis, motility disorders, and hiatal hernia. Stomach involvement in ESRD can include gastritis and duodenitis (infections), abnormal gastric emptying, peptic ulcer disease, and vascular ectasias (blood vessel distension). Other problems can include amyloidosis, abnormal pancreatic morphology, and pancreatitis. The author concludes that unless the supply of donor kidneys increases dramatically, these complications of ESRD will continue to be an important clinical issue for gastroenterologists, given the large percentage of patients with symptoms. 4 tables. 99 references.

- **Acute Renal Failure Mortality in Hospitalized African Americans: Age and Gender Considerations**

Source: Journal of the National Medical Association. 94(3): 127-134. March 2002.

Summary: The aging kidney is at risk for both toxic and hemodynamic induced acute damage, resulting in a high incidence of acute renal (kidney) failure (ARF) in elderly patients. This article reports on a 3 year computer assisted retrospective review in which the effect of age and or gender in ARF mortality in African Americans (AA) was studied. In an inner city medical center, 100 patients classified as ARF at discharge or death were included in the study. Patients were classified into 3 age categories: younger than 40 years, 40 to 64 years, and older than 64 years. The incidence of ARF was 35 percent, 28 percent, and 37 percent, respectively. Patients greater than 64 years of age were less likely to be put on dialysis. Both pre and post renal causes of ARF were more common in patients greater than 64 years of age than in younger patients. Hospital length of stay increased progressively with age. Mortality (rate of death) was lower in patients older than 64 years of age than in younger patients. The incidence of ARF was higher in male than female patients and the incidence of sepsis (generalized infection) was higher in female than male patients. Dialysis need was greater in male patients, but mortality was higher in female than male patients. Analyses showed that in the presence of sepsis, oliguria (decreased ability to form urine) and mechanical ventilatory support, the relative risk of mortality associated with advanced age was 16.5, the relative risk of mortality associated with female gender was 0.2. In summary, hospitalized elderly AA patients have a high incidence of ARF, and patients less than 40 years of age are equally at risk. Although mortality was higher in female patients, gender and advanced age did not independently contribute to high mortality. Neither age nor gender considerations should replace sound clinical judgement in the management of and decision making in elderly African American patients with ARF. 5 figures. 3 tables. 25 references.

- **Preventing Hepatitis B and Hepatitis C Virus Infections in End-Stage Renal Disease Patients: Back to Basics (editorial)**

Source: Hepatology. 29(1): 291-293. January 1999.

Contact: Available from W.B. Saunders Company. 6277 Sea Harbor Drive, Orlando, FL 19106-3399. (800) 654-2452 or (407) 345-4000.

Summary: The impact of hepatitis B (HBV) and C (HCV) on patient survival after kidney transplantation is controversial. This article comments on a study published in the journal that assessed the independent prognostic values of HBsAg and anti-HCV in a large renal transplant population. At 10 years, among all patients with HCV screening (n = 834), 4 variables had independent prognostic values in patient survival: age at transplantation, year of transplantation, biopsy proven cirrhosis, and presence of HCV antibodies. The authors of the commentary note that the findings of the study underscore the importance of preventing hepatitis B and C virus infections in **end stage renal disease** (ESRD). Patients with ESRD on chronic hemodialysis are at risk for both HBV and HCV infection, despite the success of longstanding infection control practices in the dialysis setting. The authors consider the reasons why infection control strategies are no longer universally implemented and discuss routine hemodialysis unit precautions that could prevent transmission of HBV if the precautions are routinely and rigorously followed. The transmission of HCV infection among chronic hemodialysis patients also might be related to failure to follow routine hemodialysis unit precautions. The authors conclude by reiterating that those responsible for the care of chronic hemodialysis patients should reacquaint themselves with the recommendations for preventing bloodborne pathogen transmission in this setting and ensure that they are performed. 17 references.

- **Cell Therapy of Renal Failure**

Source: Transplantation Proceedings. 35(8): 2837-2842. December 2003.

Summary: The kidney is unique in that it is the first organ for which long term ex vivo (outside the body) substitutive therapy has been available. Hemodialysis and transplantation methods in use today were pioneered in the 1940s and 1950s. There is ample evidence that the small solute clearance function provided by hemodialysis does not confer the same survival advantage as a functional kidney, both in acute and in chronic renal (kidney) failure. In this article, the authors describe the use of a bioartificial device that can improve the results of dialysis. To mimic the metabolic, endocrine, and immunologic functions of the kidney, the authors' group has successfully engineered a bioartificial device that includes a conventional dialysis filter and a bioreactor containing renal proximal tubule cells. Their group has demonstrated differentiated activity of these cells both in vitro and ex vivo in a large animal model. The bioreactor has been shown to confer a survival advantage in two large animal models of gram-negative sepsis, seemingly due to modulation of inflammatory mediators. This bioartificial kidney has now completed a Phase I clinical trial in acute **renal failure.** 6 figures. 17 references.

- **Renal Replacement Therapy in Patients with Diabetes and End-Stage Renal Disease**

Source: Journal of the American Society of Nephrology. 15(1): S25-S29. January 2004.

Summary: The number of patients who have diabetes and **end stage renal disease** (ESRD) and who are being admitted to renal replacement therapy (RRT) is increasing dramatically worldwide; in many countries, diabetes has become the single most frequent cause of ESRD. This article explores RRT (dialysis or transplantation) in patients with diabetes and ESRD. Although the prognosis of patients who have diabetes and are receiving RRT has greatly improved, survival and medical rehabilitation rates continue to be significantly worse than those of nondiabetic patients, mainly because of preexisting severely compromised cardiovascular conditions. The most common RRT modality in patients with diabetes is still hemodialysis, but it gives rise to a number of clinical problems, in particular, difficulties in the management of the vascular access and high frequency of intradialytic hypotension. However, patients who have diabetes and who are on peritoneal dialysis have to face a progressive increase in peritoneal permeability, loss of ultrafiltration, and peritoneal fibrosis, all phenomena being accelerated in patients with diabetes and ultimately leading to an increased technique failure. Accumulating evidence shows that both survival and medical rehabilitation of patients with diabetes are significantly better after renal transplantation, which should be the first-choice option for patients who have diabetes and reach ESRD. 2 figures. 28 references.

- **Early Initiation of Dialysis Fails to Prolong Survival in Patients With End-Stage Renal Failure**

Source: JASN. Journal of the American Society of Nephrology. 13 (8): 2125-2132. August 2002.

Contact: Available from Lippincott Williams and Wilkins. 12107 Insurance Way, Hagerstown, MD 21740. (800) 638-6423.

Summary: There is a trend to start dialysis earlier in patients with chronic renal (kidney) failure (CRF). Studies that suggest improved survival from earlier initiation are flawed in that they have measured survival from start of dialysis rather than from a time point before dialysis, when patients have the same renal function. This flaw is termed lead-time bias. This article reports on a study that used the electronic patient record at the renal unit of Glasgow Royal Infirmary to identify all patients who had received dialysis for CRF and who had sufficient data to calculate the time point that they reached a certain level of creatinine clearance (a measure of kidney function). This date was used to time survival. Results showed no significant benefit in patient survival from earlier initiation of dialysis. Patients who started dialysis with a lower estimated creatinine clearance tended to survive longer. This relationship retained significance when gender, age, weight, presence of diabetes, mode of first dialysis, initial dialysis access, hemoglobin, serum albumin, blood leukocyte count, Wright Khan index, and estimated creatinine clearance at the start of dialysis were taken into account. The authors conclude that their study fails to support a policy of earlier initiation of dialysis for patients with **end stage renal disease** (ESRD). 3 figures. 4 tables. 30 references.

- **Eight-Year-Old Boy with Recurrent Macroscopic Hematuria, Weight Loss, and Kidney Failure**

  Source: The Journal of Pediatrics. 142(3): 342-345. March 2003.

  Contact: Mosby, Inc. Periodicals Department, 6277 Sea Harbor Drive, Orlando, FL 32887-4800. (800) 654-2452.

  Summary: This article describes a case of an 8 year old boy who was examined by the authors in the emergency department; the boy had a third episode of macroscopic hematuria (visible blood in the urine), which had lasted for 6 days. This symptom was accompanied by a dull, bilateral back and paraumbilical abdominal pain of moderate intensity. The color of the urine was dark brown (tea-colored). The authors describe the case in detail and then consider the differential diagnosis. When the boy's clinical course deteriorated and a rapidly progressive renal insufficiency ensued, a definite histologic diagnosis was sought with kidney biopsy. The histopathologic diagnosis was a primary malignant non-Hodgkin lymphoma with a precursor T-cell phenotype. 3 figures. 19 references.

- **Hypokalemic Salt-Losing Tubulopathy with Chronic Renal Failure and Sensorineural Deafness**

  Source: Pediatrics. 108(1): [9 p.]. July 2001.

  Contact: Available from American Academy of Pediatrics. 141 Northwest Point Boulevard, Elk Grove Village, IL 60007-1098. (888) 227-1773. Fax (847) 434-8000. E-mail: journals@aap.org. Website: www.pediatrics.org. Full text of this article is available at www.pediatrics.org/cgi/content/full/108/1/e5.

  Summary: This article describes a rare inherited hypokalemic (low levels of potassium) salt losing tubulopathy (kidney disease) with linkage to chromosome 1p31. The authors conducted a retrospective analysis of the clinical data for 7 patients in whom cosegregation of the disease with chromosome 1p31 had been demonstrated. In addition, in 1 kindred, prenatal diagnosis in the second child was established, allowing a prospective clinical evaluation. Clinical presentation (symptoms) of the patients was similar and included premature birth attributable to polyhydramnios, severe renal (kidney) salt loss, normotensive hyperreninemia, hypokalemic alkalosis, and excessive hyperprostaglandin E urea, which suggested the diagnosis of hyperprostaglandin E syndrome and antenatal Bartter syndrome. However, the response to indomethacin was only poor, accounting for a more severe variant of the disease. The patients invariably developed chronic **renal failure.** The majority had extreme growth retardation, and motor development was markedly delayed. In addition, all patients turned out to be deaf. The authors conclude that this hypokalemic salt losing tubulopathy with chronic **kidney failure** and sensorineural deafness represents not only genetically but also clinically a disease entity distinct from hyperprostaglandin E syndrome and antenatal Bartter syndrome. A pleiotropic (causing multiple, seemingly unrelated symptoms) effect of a single gene defect is most likely causative for syndromic hearing loss. 6 figures. 1 table. 41 references.

- **Chronic Renal Failure: Slowing the Onset, Changing the Course**

  Source: Patient Care. 33(19): 76, 78, 83-88. November 30, 1999.

  Contact: Available from Medical Economics. 5 Paragon Drive, Montvale, NJ 07645. (800) 432-4570. Fax (201) 573-4956.

  Summary: This article provides health professionals with guidelines for detecting and managing chronic renal disease. Patients who have diabetes mellitus or hypertension are at greatest risk for developing **end stage renal disease** (ESRD). Patients who have diabetes and microalbuminuria are at substantially increased risk for developing overt renal disease and for death from cardiovascular disease. The early markers of kidney disease, urine protein and serum creatinine levels, can provide valuable information about kidney function. Although proteinuria/albuminuria indicates the onset of diabetic nephropathy, it is also an important early independent marker for kidney disease in patients who have essential hypertension and perhaps other nondiabetic renal diseases. The magnitude of protein in the urine appears to predict rate of progression to ESRD. Patients who have persistent protein excretion of 3 grams per day or more seem to progress to ESRD the fastest. The American Diabetes Association suggests that screening for microalbuminuria begin at diagnosis in patients who have type 2 diabetes, at puberty for children who have type 1 diabetes, and 5 years after onset of type 1 diabetes in older patients. Although serum creatinine is one of the best measures of kidney function, minor elevations are often considered insignificant, and a significantly elevated level is frequently overlooked as an important disease marker. Women with creatinine levels greater than 1.2 milligrams (mg) per deciliter (dL) and men with levels greater than 1.4 mg/dL should undergo further evaluation for kidney dysfunction. Other tests for kidney disease include kidney biopsy. Although whether to order a kidney biopsy for diabetic patients is controversial, a reasonable approach is to obtain a biopsy if there is any doubt or clinical findings are not typical for diabetic nephropathy. Strategies for slowing the progression of renal disease in people who have diabetic nephropathy include controlling blood pressure using angiotensin converting enzyme inhibitors. Sodium restriction may be beneficial for all patients who have renal insufficiency and proteinuria. Complications of ESRD include anemia, metabolic acidosis, and osteodystrophy. Early assessment by a nephrology specialist is important. 3 figures. 2 tables. 9 references.

- **End-Stage Renal Disease Attributable to Diabetes Mellitus**

  Source: Annals of Internal Medicine. 121(12): 912-918. December 15, 1994.

  Summary: This article reports on a case-control study to determine the proportion of **end-stage renal disease** (ESRD) associated with diabetes mellitus in a biracial population, using population-attributable risk estimates. The participants were 716 patients newly-diagnosed with **kidney failure,** aged 20 to 64 years, and 361 age-matched controls. The measurement was a self-reported history of diabetes mellitus, including type, duration, treatment, and complications. Persons with insulin-dependent diabetes mellitus (IDDM) and noninsulin-dependent diabetes mellitus (NIDDM) were at greater risk for ESRD than were persons without diabetes. The odds ratio was only slightly increased for diabetes lasting less than 15 years, but the ratio increased more than 20-fold for diabetes lasting 15 years or more. The population-attributable risk for **kidney failure** was 21 percent for IDDM and 21 percent for NIDDM. A similar proportion of ESRD was attributed to diabetes in whites (44 percent) and in blacks (41 percent). IDDM had a relatively greater effect on the incidence of **kidney failure** in whites; in contrast, NIDDM had a relatively greater effect on **kidney failure** in blacks. 2 figures. 3 tables. 27 references. (AA-M).

- **Selection of Triple Therapy for Helicobacter Pylori Eradication in Chronic Renal Insufficiency**

Source: Alimentary Pharmacology and Therapeutics. 17(10): 1283-1290. May 2003.

Summary: This article reports on a study undertaken to establish a triple therapy regimen for Helicobacter pylori eradication in patients with **chronic renal insufficiency** (CRI). The study included 88 patients with CRI and H. pylori infection who were evenly randomized into two groups receiving 1 week lansoprazole, 30 milligrams, clarithromycin, 500 milligrams, and either amoxicillin, 750 milligrams or metronidazole, 500 milligrams, twice daily. The adverse events and compliance with triple therapy were reviewed at the week 1 visit. The success of H. pylori eradication was higher in the lansoprazole-clarithromycin-metronidazole group than in the lansoprazole-clarithromycin-amoxicillin group. Complete drug compliance was also better in the lansoprazole-clarithromycin-metronidazole group than in the lansoprazole-clarithromycin-amoxicillin group (77 percent versus 52 percent, respectively). The lansoprazole-clarithromycin-metronidazole group had a lower risk of acute **renal failure** than those in the lansoprazole-clarithromycin-amoxicillin group (2 percent versus 18 percent, respectively). The authors conclude that triple therapy with metronidazole and clarithromycin, but not amoxicillin, can be used for H. pylori eradication in patients with CRI, because it is more effective, well tolerated, and less likely to cause deterioration of renal (kidney) function. 3 figures. 4 tables. 29 references.

- **Role of Parenteral Nutrition in Inflammatory Bowel Disease, Acute Renal Failure, and Hepatic Encephalopathy**

Source: International Journal of Technology Assessment in Health Care. 6(4): 655-662. 1990.

Summary: This article reviews the evidence concerning efficacy and safety of the use of parenteral nutritional support (also called total parenteral nutrition or TPN) in three clinical situations: as a primary therapy for patients with inflammatory bowel disease, for patients with acute **renal failure,** and for patients with hepatic cirrhosis resulting in encephalopathy. For each of the three situations, the rationale, efficacy, safety, and recommendations for using TPN are given. The authors conclude that the true value of parenteral nutritional support in these three clinical indications remains unknown. It is possible that future clinical trials will demonstrate the value of parenteral nutrition for these patients or for subgroups of these patients. 32 references.

- **Early Detection, Treatment May Prevent, Slow Kidney Failure**

Source: Diabetes in the News. 10(6): 42-43. December 1991.

Summary: This article reviews the importance of early detection and treatment of diabetes-related kidney disease in preventing and slowing **kidney failure.** Topics include diabetic retinopathy, risk factors for **kidney failure,** the role of hypertension, diagnostic tests, limited protein intake diets, and treatment options including hemodialysis, peritoneal dialysis, and transplantation. 2 figures.

- **Current Issues and Future Perspectives of Chronic Renal Failure**

Source: JASN. Journal of the American Society of Nephrology. 13 (Supplement 1): S3-S6. January 2002.

Contact: Available from Lippincott Williams and Wilkins. 12107 Insurance Way, Hagerstown, MD 21740. (800) 638-6423.

Summary: This brief review article discusses some key issues of **end stage renal disease** (ESRD) and the prevention strategy for chronic progressive renal disease. The authors focus primarily on the issues in Japan and the United States because they represent and illustrate common problems pertaining to ESRD. Although some dialysis patients live longer than 5 to 10 years and are able to work and contribute to the society in which they live, others fare poorly and die within 2 to 3 years of going on dialysis. In addition to mortality (death), another issue surrounding ESRD is a rapidly aging dialysis population, in part related to the fact that the major proportion of new patients entering dialysis programs comprise people with type 2 diabetes. These problems require the worldwide nephrology community to rededicate itself to the retardation and prevention of the progression of all forms of renal disease. The authors discuss kidney transplantation, peritoneal dialysis, the complications of chronic dialysis, control of hypertension (high blood pressure), the role of dietary protein intake, and the potential impact of advances in molecular biology and genetic engineering. 2 tables. 8 references.

- **Nutritional Status of Chronic Renal Failure Patients Following the Initiation of Hemodialysis Treatment. (editorial)**

Source: American Journal of Kidney Diseases. 40(1): 205-207. July 2002.

Contact: Available from W.B. Saunders Company. Periodicals Department, 6277 Sea Harbor Drive, Orlando, FL 32887-4800. (800) 654-2452 or (407) 345-4000.

Summary: This editorial serves as an introduction to two related articles in this journal on the nutritional status of chronic **renal failure** (CRF) patients following the initiation of hemodialysis treatment. The author notes that the two papers have virtually identical titles and nearly the same conclusion; namely, that the initiation of chronic hemodialysis therapy in incident CRF patients is associated with improvement in nutritional status. The author discusses how these observations are important in a number of areas, including the predialysis management of chronic renal (kidney) insufficiency, when to initiate hemodialysis, subsequent nutritional status of patients on hemodialysis, and the influence of all of these on the long term outcome of patients with **chronic renal insufficiency.**. The author concludes that until further information regarding nutrition, early start, dose and flux is obtained, these current studies certainly give credence to the National Kidney Foundation KDOQI recommendations on the initiation of dialysis therapy on malnourished patients with advanced chronic **renal failure** in whom other interventions have failed to result in nutritional improvement. 10 references.

- **Oral Health in Children with Chronic Renal Failure**

Source: Pediatric Nephrology 18(1): 39-45. January 2003.

Contact: Available from Springer-Verlag. Service Center Secaucus, 44 Hartz Way, Secaucus, NJ 07094. (201) 348-4033.

Summary: This study investigated oral health in 70 children (aged 4 to 13.6 years) with chronic renal (kidney) failure (CRF). Indices were recorded for dental caries (cavities), dental plaque, gingival (gum) inflammation, gingival enlargement, and enamel defects. Salivary urea, buffering capacity, and the oral streptococcal flora were determined for 25 of the children. A significantly greater proportion of the CRF children was caries free, 40 percent compared with 8.5 percent of the controls. The mean plaque score was significantly greater in the CF group for both the primary (12.7) and permanent dentition (22.0) compared with the controls: 5.3 and 15.5, respectively. Eight CRF children had gingival enlargement. Enamel defects affecting the permanent teeth were observed in 57 percent of the CRF children compared with 33 percent of the controls. The buffering capacity was significantly greater in the CRF group, pH 6.4 compared with the controls' pH 5.6. The mean salivary urea level was significantly greater in the CRF children. The isolation frequency of Streptococcus mutans was significantly greater from controls compared with the CRF children. The authors conclude that an integrated dental service needs to be developed with emphasis on toothbrushing to prevent gingival hyperplasia and periodontal disease after puberty in this population. 7 tables. 34 references.

## Federally Funded Research on Kidney Failure

The U.S. Government supports a variety of research studies relating to kidney failure and associated conditions. These studies are tracked by the Office of Extramural Research at the National Institutes of Health.[15] CRISP (Computerized Retrieval of Information on Scientific Projects) is a searchable database of federally funded biomedical research projects conducted at universities, hospitals, and other institutions. Visit CRISP at **http://crisp.cit.nih.gov/crisp/crisp_query.generate_screen**. You can perform targeted searches by various criteria including geography, date, as well as topics related to kidney failure and related conditions.

For most of the studies, the agencies reporting into CRISP provide summaries or abstracts. As opposed to clinical trial research using patients, many federally funded studies use animals or simulated models to explore kidney failure and related conditions. In some cases, therefore, it may be difficult to understand how some basic or fundamental research could eventually translate into medical practice. The following sample is typical of the type of information found when searching the CRISP database for kidney failure:

- **Project Title: A PHARMACOGENETICS APPROACH TO DRUG INDUCED WEIGHT GAIN**

  Principal Investigator & Institution: Coe, Natalie R.; Jackson Laboratory 600 Main St Bar Harbor, Me 04609

  Timing: Fiscal Year 2002; Project Start 26-MAY-2002

---

[15] Healthcare projects are funded by the National Institutes of Health (NIH), Substance Abuse and Mental Health Services (SAMHSA), Health Resources and Services Administration (HRSA), Food and Drug Administration (FDA), Centers for Disease Control and Prevention (CDCP), Agency for Healthcare Research and Quality (AHRQ), and Office of Assistant Secretary of Health (OASH).

Summary: (Scanned from the applicant?s description) Obesity, often the result of a person?s genetic predisposition, can lead to serious medical conditions, including non-insulin dependent diabetes, heart disease, stroke, high blood pressure, **kidney failure,** and depression. Clozapine is a highly prescribed anti-psychotic drug, but unfortunately, many patients become obese within several months after initiation of this drug therapy. Identification of the clozapine weight responsive genetic locus and subsequent gene identification will 1) further enhance our understanding of obesity, including genetic suscepibility and onset as well as the its underlying molecular basis, 2) allow psychiatric patients to be screened prior to clozapine treatment to avoid potential health risks brought on by obesity, 3) identify potential cross talk of neuronal and obesity-related metabolic pathways, and 4) help aid in the design of new anti-psychotic drugs that do not interfere with metabolic weight homeostasis. The potential correlation (positive or negative) between formation of the principal active metabolite of clozapine(N-desmethyl-clozapine) and the onset of obesity will be explored as a viable tool to screen psychiatric patients genetically predisposed to clozapine induced weight gain. The involvement of histamine (H1) receptors and the neuroleptic induced obesity phenotype has abeen eluded to but not formally addressed in the literature. The potential role of the H1 receptor will be examined directly by the proposed work.

Website: http://crisp.cit.nih.gov/crisp/Crisp_Query.Generate_Screen

- **Project Title: ACUTE ISCHEMIC RENAL FAILURE AND KIDNEY-LIVER CROSSTALK**

Principal Investigator & Institution: Kielar, Mariusz; Internal Medicine; University of Texas Sw Med Ctr/Dallas Dallas, Tx 753909105

Timing: Fiscal Year 2002; Project Start 01-SEP-2000; Project End 31-AUG-2005

Summary: (adapted from the application): Recovery from ischemic renal injury is affected by several cytokines and growth factors including interleukin 10 (IL-10), tumor necrosis factor (TNFa), and hepatocyte growth factor (HGF). Previous studies have focused on production of these molecules by the kidney. However, after severe ischemia, the renal cells may be too damaged to make the molecules necessary to regulate repair. We suggest that such molecules may be produced outside the kidney in the liver. The proposed studies will test the existence of a kidney-liver axis that regulates the response to renal ischemia. We propose that the ischemic kidney produces IL-6, which stimulates hepatic production of IL-10 and induces renal expression of the IL-10 receptor (IL-10R) enabling the kidney to respond to IL-10. This hypothesis is supported by our Preliminary Data, demonstrating that renal ischemia results in renal production of IL-6, followed by expression of IL-10R, and hepatic production of IL-10. Others have shown that hepatic IL-10 is produced by hepatic macrophages; we found that IL-6 stimulates macrophages to produce IL-10. IL-10 has been shown to ameliorate ischemic injury to kidney and other organs. Specific Aim 1 will: 1) determine if IL-6 is the signal from the ischemic kidney that stimulates the liver to produce IL-10; 2) test whether IL-6 is produced in response to hypoxia, or to other cytokines, such as TNFa and IL-1b; 3) test IL-6 production in hypoxic renal tubular cells in vitro; 4) determine the role of the putative hypoxia response element (NF-IL-6); 5) localize sites of IL-6 production in the kidney; and 6) evaluate whether the NF-IL-6 response element activates IL-6 gene in the ischemic kidney and use a gene therapy vector to drive IL-10 expression in the kidney. Specific Aim 2 will: 1) determine IL-10 protein presence in the liver and blood and then 2) determine whether IL-10 inhibits four genes (TNFU, ICAM-1, IL-8 and iNOS) known to exacerbate ischemic renal injury; 3a) investigate IL-10 effects on SOCS-3 (suppressor of cytokine signaling-3) upregulation in the ischemic kidney by comparing SOCS-3 expression in the ischemic kidney of wild-type, IL-10 knockout and anti-IL-10 antibody-treated mice; and 3b) determine if over expression of SOCS-3 in renal cells in vitro inhibits production of TNFa, ICAM-1,IL-8 and iNOS during hypoxia-reoxygenation. This novel proposal is an excellent vehicle for Dr. Kielar to learn new techniques, including organ specific gene therapy and in vivo reporter gene assay. The sponsor for the training grant, Dr. Chris Lu, is an authority on renal immunology and inflammation. The co-sponsor, Dr. Robert Munford, is an expert in physiologically responsive gene therapy. The training program will include formal course work in immunology and immunogenetics to prepare the applicant for an investigative career.

Website: http://crisp.cit.nih.gov/crisp/Crisp_Query.Generate_Screen

- **Project Title: ADHERENCE AND ADJUSTMENT IN END-STAGE RENAL DISEASE**

Principal Investigator & Institution: Christensen, Alan J.; Professor; Psychology; University of Iowa Iowa City, Ia 52242

Timing: Fiscal Year 2002; Project Start 01-JAN-1995; Project End 31-DEC-2003

Summary: (adapted from investigator's abstract): Increased quality assurance concerns associated with the Medicare **End-Stage Renal Disease** (ESRD) program underscore the need for research addressing the adaptation and quality of life of ESRD patients. Patients' levels of psychological adjustment and their degree of adherence with ESRD treatment regimen reflect two important criteria that are examined in the present continuation proposal. One central objective of the research involves identifying psychological characteristics that influence medical regimen adherence and emotional adjustment among patients treated with renal dialysis. This will be accomplished using a longitudinal study design that considers the effects of patient individual differences (i.e., coping style) and contextual differences among the available dialysis treatment modalities. A key aspect of the study involves the assessment of patients at an early stage of progressive renal insufficiency, before renal dialysis is clinically necessary. We hypothesize that adherence and adjustment will vary as a joint function of the type of dialysis prescribed and patient individual differences assessed at baseline. For example, we predict that patients' possessing a more active or vigilant style of coping will exhibit more favorable adherence when undergoing a self-administered dialysis treatment modality (e.g., continuous ambulatory peritoneal dialysis) but poorer adherence when receiving staff administered dialysis (e.g., center hemodialysis). A second objective involves identifying patient characteristics that are related to adherence to adjustment among renal transplantation patients. Initial psychosocial assessment will be conducted during the pre-transplant evaluation process. A set of hypotheses regarding psychological predictors of patient adherence and changes in emotional well being after transplantation will be tested in a prospective manner. For Example, we hypothesize that patients with a more active style of coping with health-related stress will exhibit better regimen adherence and better emotional adjustment than other transplant patients. We believe the proposed research will extend the role of psychological theory and practice in contributing to the care of ESRD patients. The knowledge generated will add to a growing body of literature that suggests psychosocial assessment information can be useful in the selection f the most beneficial renal treatment modality for a particular patient.

Website: http://crisp.cit.nih.gov/crisp/Crisp_Query.Generate_Screen

- **Project Title: ASSESSING FUNCTIONAL OUTCOMES IN ADOLESCENT WITH ESRD**

Principal Investigator & Institution: Furth, Susan L.; Associate Professor; Pediatrics; Johns Hopkins University 3400 N Charles St Baltimore, Md 21218

Timing: Fiscal Year 2002; Project Start 01-JUL-2001; Project End 31-MAR-2004

Summary: provided by applicant): Dr. Furth is seeking the Small Grant Award to expand the study of clinical outcomes for children with **end stage renal disease** (ESRD) initiated under her KO8 Award DK 02586-01A1. With the support of the KO8 funding, Dr. Furth has completed her PhD in Clinical Investigation and has begun the transition to an independent research career. She has published a number of manuscripts using her training in epidemiology and clinical investigation: examining how clinical and socio-economic factors affect access to different treatment regimens for children with **kidney failure,** and how clinical experience with ESRD care for children affects treatment decisions. She has examined how poor growth, a crucial pediatric issue, affects mortality, hospitalization rates and educational achievement. She has also initiated a multi-center, cross-sectional study comparing functional outcomes/ health related quality of life (HRQL) for pediatric patients with chronic **renal failure** or ESRD treated with hemodialysis, peritoneal dialysis or transplant. Resources provided by the RO3 award will allow Dr. Furth to expand the multi-center study of health related quality of life in adolescents with ESRD to a prospective study. A prospective study will allow Dr. Furth to determine whether specific measures of health related quality of life are sensitive to clinical changes, as patients proceed from dialysis to transplantation. The supplementary funding of the R03, additionally will allow Dr. Furth to examine the link between clinical measures such as hematocrit, serum albumin, and dialysis adequacy (Kt/V) and functional outcome/HRQL. Furthermore, the prospective study will assess whether high risk behavior characterized by patterns of response on an adolescent health status questionnaire can predict non-compliance with therapy, increased hospitalization rates, acute rejection or transplant failure. The measures of functional outcome studied will include the Child Health and Illness Profile-Adolescent Edition, and the Child Health Questionnaire (Parent report). This research will provide an in-depth analysis of a measure of functional outcome in children with ESRD, and will provide valuable information regarding optimal treatment choices for children with kidney disease. If assessments of high risk behavior predict increased rates of hospitalization, rejection or transplant failure, results of this study will allow identification of a high risk population of adolescents with ESRD, who can be targeted for early intervention and close follow-up to improve long term outcomes of care. The proposal addresses several priority areas for Clinical Research highlighted in the NIH Task Force publication, Research Needs in Pediatric Kidney Disease: 2000 and beyond. During this project, Dr. Furth will gain new skills in organizing and coordinating a prospective multi-center clinical research study. This experience will give Dr. Furth the tools she needs to develop into an independent clinical investigator in a nurturing academic environment.

Website: http://crisp.cit.nih.gov/crisp/Crisp_Query.Generate_Screen

- **Project Title: BRIDGES TO THE BACCALAUREATE DEGREEE PROGRAM**

Principal Investigator & Institution: Cameron, Joseph A.; Professor and Director; Biology; Jackson State University Jackson, Ms 39217

Timing: Fiscal Year 2002; Project Start 01-APR-1994; Project End 31-AUG-2005

Summary: (provided by the applicant): Cancer, diabetes, **kidney failure** and cardiovascular, lung and blood diseases are annually responsible for several million deaths, high morbidity and tremendous economic costs in the United States alone. Minorities and blacks in particular, suffer unporportionally higher devastating effects from the aforementioned diseases than whites. The exceptionally high impact of these disorders on minority populations, results from a multitude of factors including a high percentage of economically disadvantaged minority families and an inadequate number of minority health care professionals and basic science researchers trained in biomedical science areas. The purpose of the proposed Bridges to the Baccalaureate Degree Program (BBDP) is to motivate and prepare 2-year baccalaureate degree in Biomedical areas. The program will expand established cooperative, inter-institutional and interdisciplinary training program between Jackson State University, (a historically black institution) and Hinds Community College (a 2-year college). The Program will utilize Faculty and Administrators at each institution in the planning, implementation and programmatic aspects including 1. Provision of functional steering and Advisory committees 2. Development and implementation of student selection and advisement procedures, and 3. Conceptualization, implementation and publicity of research finding. All HCC students will enroll in an Introduction to Research course that wilt provide training in research and laboratory methodologies, literature survey mechanisms, and scientific writing techniques. Students will engage in specific individualized research projects and present their research finding at local seminar and professional meetings. They will also be encouraged to submit research manuscripts to travel to local scientific conferences with student trainees where appropriate. Students will be exposed to biomedical, professional, and career experiences. They will also receive assistance in application procedures for baccalaureate degree programs in biomedical schools.

Website: http://crisp.cit.nih.gov/crisp/Crisp_Query.Generate_Screen

- **Project Title: CALCINEURIN IN CONGENITAL NEPHROPATHY**

Principal Investigator & Institution: Chen, Feng; Medicine; Washington University Lindell and Skinker Blvd St. Louis, Mo 63130

Timing: Fiscal Year 2003; Project Start 01-JUL-2003; Project End 31-MAY-2005

Summary: (provided by applicant): Congenital obstructive nephropathy is the most frequent cause of **renal failure** in infants and children. The molecular and cellular lesions leading to the congenital obstruction, however, are still largely undetermined. We hypothesize that calcineurin, a serine/threonine phosphatase, is indispensable for the normal development of the excretory system. We have generated a mouse strain with deletion of the CnB gene in a subset of Pax3 positive cells and their derivatives by Cre-mediated LoxP recombination. These mice have deletion of CnB in the excretory system, including the smooth muscle cells in the ureter. The affected mice have hydronephrosis and hydroureter and die from postnatal **renal failure.** We plan to further determine the nature, the spectrum, as well as the prenatal and postnatal progression of the congenital nephropathy in the mutants. Of particular interests, our previous experiments have demonstrated an indispensable role of calcineurin in the formation of the vascular smooth muscle layer around the major blood vessels. Based on this finding and our preliminary results, we further hypothesize that the disruption of calcineurin function in the ureteral smooth muscle or in the innervating nerves causes a defective peristalsis, leading to the obstructive nephropathy. To test this hypothesis, we will determine whether the mutants have anatomical or functional defects preventing effective peristalsis and will identify the causative cellular lesions. Finally, we will study the ontogeny of the urinary tract smooth muscle cells and the potential neuronal contribution to the congenital nephropathy. The Pax3Cre-CnB mutants we generated have defined genetic modifications and a consistent early onset congenital obstructive nephropathy leading to **kidney failure.** These mice will serve as a good animal model to study the causes of congenital obstructive nephropathy. Results from the proposed study will also enhance our understanding of the pyeloureteral peristalsis, the ontogeny of ureteral smooth muscle cells, and the role of calcineurin signaling in these processes.

Website: http://crisp.cit.nih.gov/crisp/Crisp_Query.Generate_Screen

- **Project Title: CELLULAR PATHOPHYSIOLOGY OF ACUTE RENAL FAILURE**

Principal Investigator & Institution: Weinberg, Joel M.; Professor; Internal Medicine; University of Michigan at Ann Arbor 3003 South State, Room 1040 Ann Arbor, Mi 481091274

Timing: Fiscal Year 2002; Project Start 01-JUL-1984; Project End 31-AUG-2005

Summary: Recently there has been a renewal of interest in mitochondrial dysfunction as a mediator of diverse forms of cell injury as a result of new insights into the mechanism for the mitochondrial permeability transition and recognition of the role of mitochondrial cytochrome c release in apoptosis. ATP production in the proximal tubule, a major site of injury during ischemic and toxic forms of acute **renal failure,** is especially sensitive to mitochondrial dysfunction because, depending on the segment, glcolysis is absent or minimal in proximal tubule cells in vivo. In studies during the present funding period, we have identified a mitochondrial lesion characterized by inhibition of electron transport in complex I associated with matrix condensation and partial deenergization as a functionally important form of mitochondrial injury during hypoxia/reoxygenation of freshly isolated rabbit proximal tubules that play a pivtal role in overall cellular recovery. The lesion: a) precedes the mitochondrial permeability transition and cytochrome c release; b) depresses energetic function of otherwise viable tubules for sustained periods; and c) is highly amenable to prevention and reversal by specific citric acid cycle metabolites that promote anaerobic pathways of intramitochondrial ATP production and electron transport or, under aerobic conditions, bypass the complex I block. The mitochondrial lesion is expressed both in freshly isolated tubules subjected to hypoxia/reoxygeation, and based on ultrastructural changes and modification by citric acid cycle metabolites, during ischemia/reperfusion in vivo. Our general hypothesis is that this form of mitochondrial dysfunction plays a critical role in the outcome of ischemic insults to the kidney and that its amelioration will beneficially impact on cell and tissue recovery from these insults. To test this hypothesis and further investigate its implications for understanding and treating ischemic acute **renal failure** we propose studies to: 1) Characterize the energetic deficit as it evolves during extended durations of hypoxia/reoxygenation and the effects of protective substrates to ameliorate it under those conditions. 2) Better define the mechanisms for the mitochondrial inner membrane abnormalities during the insult and their relative contributions to the energetic deficit. 3) Assess expression of the lesion and test efficacy of protective metabolites during ischemia/reperfusion of the kidney in vivo.

Website: http://crisp.cit.nih.gov/crisp/Crisp_Query.Generate_Screen

- **Project Title: CHANGES IN KIDNEY MRNA PROFILES AFTER ACUTE RENAL FAILURE**

Principal Investigator & Institution: Price, Peter M.; Professor; University of Arkansas Med Scis Ltl Rock Little Rock, Ar 72205

Timing: Fiscal Year 2002

Summary: (Provided by the applicant) Mortality rates from acute **renal failure** have changed little since 1960, with little progress made in the underlying mechanism(s) for injury or repair. We and others have proposed that there are molecular pathways activated by a variety of renal stresses that result in the syndrome's phenotype. For example, we have found that the gene for p21, a cyclin-dependent kinase inhibitor, is activated to high levels in all types of **renal failure** and that expression of this gene is protective, both after cisplatin treatment and ischemia-reperfusion. We hypothesized that p21 acts as a cell cycle inhibitor after its induction and that this is the mechanism of its participation and protective effect after acute **renal failure.** Understanding other pathways and the interrelationships between these pathways is essential before a rational treatment of this syndrome can be approached. Many of these pathways will be dependent on activation and repression of gene transcription, which will be reflected in the change of abundance of mRNAs in the kidney after injury. For this project, we will quantify mRNA profiles in kidneys from untreated mice and compare these profiles with those obtained in kidneys after injury. Inasmuch as we have found that severity of the **renal failure** phenotype is affected by the presence of p21, we will also compare mRNA profiles from kidneys of injured mice of wild-type genotype and of an isogenic population lacking the p21 gene. Comparison of these two genotypes will establish which genes could contribute either to the increased severity of **renal failure** seen in p21 (-/-) mice or the lesser damage seen in p21 (+/+) mice. The mRNA profiles obtained from these mice could also reveal genes important for acute **renal failure** development in general. These profiles will first be approximately by the Serial Analysis of Gene Expression (SAGE) protocol in which the detailed analysis of thousands of transcripts can be assayed and quantified. The SAGE analyses will also provide information about the mRNA coding potential of the untreated and injured kidney. Data from the SAGE analysis will be used to design arrays of genes to be assayed by DNA microarray. The microarray will be used to establish mRNA profiles as well as to reveal pathways affected by acute **renal failure.**

Website: http://crisp.cit.nih.gov/crisp/Crisp_Query.Generate_Screen

- **Project Title: CHRONIC RENAL INSUFFICIENCY COHORT (CRIC) STUDY**

Principal Investigator & Institution: Appel, Lawrence J.; Associate Professor; Medicine; Johns Hopkins University 3400 N Charles St Baltimore, Md 21218

Timing: Fiscal Year 2002; Project Start 28-SEP-2001; Project End 30-JUN-2008

Summary: (provided by applicant): This proposal describes the Johns Hopkins-University of Maryland field center for the Prospective Cohort Study of **Chronic Renal Insufficiency,** also termed CRIC. The incidence and prevalence of end stage kidney disease are relentlessly increasing, along with attendant co-morbidities, particularly cardiovascular disease. CRIC is a longitudinal, observational study that will determine the risk factors for progression of **chronic renal insufficiency** and the risk factors for cardiovascular disease in a cohort of individuals with impaired kidney function. Participants will be 3,000 individuals (250 at Hopkins, 250 at Maryland), 50% diabetic and 50% non-diabetic, with an estimated glomerular filtration rate (GFR) of 30-70 ml/min/1.73 m2. The primary recruitment strategy will be to identify individuals with an elevated creatinine that corresponds to this GFR range. Both Hopkins and U.Maryland have the proven capacity to generate lists of such individuals. These 2 medical centers are the largest health care delivery systems in the Baltimore metropolitan area, which is populated by 1.6 million persons. The locations of the two institutions should facilitate enrollment of a diverse cohort, many of whom will be indigent. Baseline data will be collected over3 visits (a brief eligibility visit and 2 subsequent visits). Outcomes will be ascertained at an annual in-person follow-up visit and by telephone surveillance. Core measurements will include questionnaires, GFRs, echocardiograms, and biological specimens. Study investigators have a proven track record of successfully designing and conducting large-scale, collaborative research studies. Specifically, they have successfully recruited large cohorts of participants, have achieved high follow-up rates, have collected virtually all of the major measurements proposed in this study, and have made substantive scientific contributions through publication and presentation of their findings. The impressive infrastructure of the two institutions and the large population of the Baltimore metropolitan area will further enhance the potential for success. In short, the Hopkins-U.Maryland field center is extremely well positioned to accomplish each of the major task required of the CRIC field centers and to contribute to the overall success of this vitally important study.

Website: http://crisp.cit.nih.gov/crisp/Crisp_Query.Generate_Screen

- **Project Title: CONSEQUENCES OF CHRONIC RENAL INSUFFICIENCY**

Principal Investigator & Institution: Hsu, Chi-Yuan; Medicine; University of California San Francisco 3333 California Street, Suite 315 San Francisco, Ca 941430962

Timing: Fiscal Year 2002; Project Start 01-JUL-2002; Project End 30-JUN-2007

Summary: (provided by applicant) Currently 300,000 Americans suffer from **end-stage renal disease** (ESRD), which is associated with substantial morbidity and mortality. Recent data suggest there is a much larger number of individuals who have impaired kidney function not requiring dialysis or transplantation (i.e., chronic renal insufficiency). However, the health consequences and public health burden of **chronic renal insufficiency** (CRI) are incompletely defined. We hypothesize that the relationship between CRI prevalence and subsequent ESRD incidence varies across demographic and disease subgroups because of differences in rates of decline of renal function and competing mortality risks. We hypothesize that the metabolic and homeostatic disturbances of CRI lead to osteopenia, periodontal disease and blood pressure elevation. Expression of these consequences of CRI may be influenced by dietary factors such as intake of sodium, calcium and other dietary components. We hypothesize that CRI is associated with reduced physical functioning. We will analyze the nationally representative Second (1976-80) and Third (1988-94) National Health and Nutrition Examination Survey (NHANES II and III) databases which contain information on renal function as well as detailed assessment of health and nutrition status. We will use the nationwide and comprehensive US Renal Data System ESRD registry (1988-present) to examine the relationship between CRI prevalence and subsequent ESRD incidence in specific birth cohorts. We will collect longitudinal data on physical functioning, body composition and nutritional status in a separate cohort of CRI subjects. Linear, logistic and Poisson regression and longitudinal data analysis techniques will be used to assess the independent association of CRI with outcomes. The overall objective of this application is to support my development in a career focused on patient-oriented research in nephrology. To accomplish this objective, the proposed program has both scientific and career development components. The scientific component is outlined above.

The first career development objective is to strengthen my analytic skills and increase my sophistication as a clinical researcher through formal course work, directed reading and one-on-one tutorials. The second career development objective is to obtain training in creating and following a cohort of subjects with CRI and conducting primary data collection. These will contribute greatly to my development into an independent investigator.

Website: http://crisp.cit.nih.gov/crisp/Crisp_Query.Generate_Screen

- **Project Title: EARLY GLOMERULAR CHANGES IN DIABETIC AFRICAN-AMERICANS**

Principal Investigator & Institution: Guasch, Antonio; Medicine; Emory University 1784 North Decatur Road Atlanta, Ga 30322

Timing: Fiscal Year 2003; Project Start 01-SEP-2003; Project End 30-JUN-2005

Summary: (provided by applicant): Diabetic nephropathy is the leading cause of **kidney failure** in the U.S. **Kidney failure** occurs more often in diabetic African-Americans than in Caucasians with diabetes. The cause for this higher propensity to **kidney failure** in African-Americans is not known. Recently, certain types of antihypertensive medications have been shown to slow down the rate of development of **kidney failure** once damage has occurred, however, to date, no treatment can prevent the development of **kidney failure** once a certain degree of kidney is present. Very little is known about the early stages of the disease, when kidney damage could be reversible or about possible differences in kidney function between African-Americans and Caucasians with early diabetes that could explain the propensity to kidney disease in African-Americans. We postulate that there are differences in intraglomerular hemodynamics and the hormonal regulation of the glomerular circulation, at the renin-angiotensin and nitric oxide systems level, between African-Americans and Caucasians that underlie the susceptibility to kidney disease in the African-American population. We plan to compare glomerular function and glomerular permselectivity between African-Americans and Caucasians with early diabetes and to study the role the renin angiotensin and nitric oxide systems in the regulation of the glomerular circulation. This may lead to therapies that could be started very early on in diabetic patients targeted at preventing the development of kidney complications.

Website: http://crisp.cit.nih.gov/crisp/Crisp_Query.Generate_Screen

- **Project Title: ENDOTHELIAL CELL INJURY: QUANTIFYING ITS ROLE IN ISCHEMIC ACUTE RENAL FAILURE**

Principal Investigator & Institution: Molitoris, Bruce A.; Professor of Medicine and Chief,; Indiana Univ-Purdue Univ at Indianapolis 620 Union Drive, Room 618 Indianapolis, in 462025167

Timing: Fiscal Year 2002; Project Start 01-APR-2002; Project End 31-MAR-2007

Summary: (Taken directly from the application) Ischemia/reperfusion injury (IRI) is a major contributor to the organ damage that results in acute **renal failure,** one of the major causes of morbidity and mortality in hospitalized patients in the United States. We propose endothelial cell injury during the initiation phase of ARF (anoxia resulting from decreased vascular perfusion of the organ) occurs and is compounded thereafter by continued hypoxia in the cortical medullary region of the kidney. This results in further endothelial cell injury mediating epithelial cell injury and worsening organ dysfunction. Many factors are known to be involved in ischemia/reperfusion injury, but considerable data point to an important role for endothelial cells, as agents of injury in the kidney as well as other organs. Furthermore there is evidence that actin cytoskeletal alterations, occurring during cellular ATP depletion, mediate many of the structural and functional changes known to occur in ischemic cells. However, documentation of endothelial damage in the kidney is lacking. Therefore, we propose to test our hypothesis using an experimental model of ischemia/reperfusion injury in the mouse, and to determine the extent of initial and subsequent ischemia-induced endothelial injury and endothelial actin alterations. We will exploit recent advances in gene therapy and imaging technologies to image endothelial cell dynamics in live animals whose endothelial cells have been labeled with green fluorescent protein (GFP). We will also use this system to investigate the effect of ischemia/reperfusion on the dynamics of renal microvascular blood flow. Finally we will isolate GFP labeled microvascular endothelial cells and study the effects of ATP depletion on the actin cytoskeleton, actin depolymerizing factor (ADF) and expression of ADF using an adenoviral system to express a GFP-ADF chimera in cultured endothelial cells and in in vivo studies. These studies will provide a better understanding of the clinically important phenomenon of ischemia/reperfusion injury, and provide new methods for testing potential therapeutic approaches.

Website: http://crisp.cit.nih.gov/crisp/Crisp_Query.Generate_Screen

- **Project Title: HYPERTENSION PHARMACOGENETICS**

Principal Investigator & Institution: Johnson, Julie A.; Professor and Chair, Pharmacy Practice; Pharmacy Practice; University of Florida Gainesville, Fl 32611

Timing: Fiscal Year 2003; Project Start 26-SEP-2003; Project End 31-AUG-2007

Summary: (provided by applicant): Hypertension (HTN) is the most common chronic disease in the United States, and is a leading cause of stroke, acute myocardial infarction (MI), heart failure and **kidney failure.** There are numerous effective antihypertensive drug classes, but only about half of patients have a good response to any given drug. Pharmacogenetics might significantly improve BP control and outcomes, as genetically-guided drug therapy selection could dramatically increase the number of patients who receive the best drug for their HTN. We propose to test pharmacogenetic hypotheses that center on BP response and outcomes (death, MI, stroke) in HTN, using 5,871 genomic DNA samples we have collected from participants in INVEST, a large, international trial in patients with HTN and ischemic heart disease. We propose to test the following hypotheses: Hypothesis 1: Genetic variability in the proteins important to verapamil's pharmacologic action contribute to interpatient variability in verapamil's antihypertensive effect. Specific Aim 1A. Identify sequence variability in the genes for the major L-type Ca channel (LTCC) subunits alpha1C and beta, the sarcoplasmlc retlculum Ca2+-ATPase 2, the Ca2+-activated K channel, and critical portions of the ryanodine receptor by resequencing the genes in Corriel DNA from 60 individuals. Predict those polymorphisms most likely to be functionally significant using various bioinformatics techniques. Specific Aim lB. Perform in vitro functional studies, including ion channel patch-clamp studies, to test for functional significance of polymorphisms in the LTCC a1C subunit. Specific Aim 1C. Determine the association between verapamil's antihypertensive effect and genetic polymorphisms of interest, as identified in Aim 1A. Hypothesis 2: Antihypertensives that target the underlying molecular/genetic basis of a patient's HTN will result in better outcomes than antihypertensives that do not target the underlying pathophysiology. Specific Aim 2. Determine whether drug therapy that is targeted at a "drug response" polymorphism or haplotype results in better patient outcomes (specifically fewer deaths, strokes, MIs) than therapy that does not target the "drug response" polymorphism(s). This hypothesis will be tested for all four study drugs: atenolol, verapamil, hydrochlorothiazide and trandolapril. Because of the diversity of the INVEST genetics sample (47% Hispanic (mostly Puerto Ricans), 38% Caucasian and 11% African American), we will test

Hypothesis 3: Use of molecular markers to define genetic heterogeneity in the study population is superior to race/ethnicity information in genetic associations with drug response. Specific Aim 3A. Determine whether models of genetic association with drug response perform better with use of genetic marker-defined population cluster and individual ancestral proportion information than with clinician-defined information on race/ethnicity. Specific Aim 3B. Document that any positive associations between drug response and genotype are not the result of population stratification or admixture. These aims will be accomplished by genotyping patients for at least 50 Ancestral Informative Markers. The proposed studies will provide considerable new evidence regarding the pharmacogenetics of verapamil, and will significantly further our understanding of the pharmacogenetics of p-blockers, thiazide diuretics, and ACE inhibitors. They will substantially enhance our understanding of the genetic variability in proteins important to Ca ++ regulation and response to CCBs and other drugs, and the functional significance of this genetic variability. Finally, the proposed studies will increase our understanding of the role of molecular markers for defining population stratification and admixture in pharmacogenetic studies. The proposed studies should add substantial new information about antihypertensive pharmacogenetics, and could influence how antihypertensive medications are prescribed in the future.

Website: http://crisp.cit.nih.gov/crisp/Crisp_Query.Generate_Screen

- **Project Title: IGF-I AND PROGRESSION OF CHRONIC RENAL FAILURE IN RATS**

Principal Investigator & Institution: Moore, Leon C.; Physiology and Biophysics; State University New York Stony Brook Stony Brook, Ny 11794

Timing: Fiscal Year 2002; Project Start 01-MAY-1999; Project End 30-SEP-2003

Summary: In chronic **renal failure** (CRF), glomerular sclerosis (GS), tubulointerstitial fibrosis, and microvascular injury are thought to be consequences of elevated intravascular pressures that injure the kidney. The progression of CRF is accelerated by hypertension and loss of renal autoregulation. Insulin-like growth factor-1 (IGF-I) increases glomerular filtration rate, and is under investigation for therapeutic use in children with CRF with growth hormone (GH) insensitivity. IGF-I activity is low in CRF owing to high serum levels of inhibitory IGF-I binding proteins. We have developed a hypertensive, rapidly-progressing model of CRF in growing rats that may be relevant to **renal failure** in those children most at risk for hypertension and renal insufficiency, including African-

American children, and those with low birth weight and congenital low nephron number. We found that treatment with IGF-I lowers blood pressure, preserves renal function, reduces the severity of GS, and completely prevents vascular injury, suggesting that IGF-I could slow the progression of CRF in children. The specific aims are: 1. To further characterize our model of CRF in young rats and the impact of IGF-I therapy by a) conducting longer-term (8 week) studies of the effect of IGF-I therapy on the progression of CRF, b) examining the effects of IGF-I therapy in young rats with established progressive CRF, c) to define residual renal function in untreated and IGF-I treated growing rats with CRF and how this is influenced by food intake, and d) defining the effects of IGF-I therapy in adult rats with CRF. 2. To test the hypothesis that the beneficial effects of IGF-I in CRF can not be fully attributed to its antihypertensive action. To determine if endothelin-1 receptor blockade reduces hypertension and progression CRF. 3. To test the hypothesis that the loss of renal autoregulation is an early event that precedes the development of both vascular injury and glomerular injury in CRF. 4. To determine if the beneficial effects of IGF-I on the progression of CRF are compromised by co-treatment with GH. 5. To identify the mechanisms through which acute treatment with IGF-I is able to restore autoregulatory ability in growing rats with CRF, and the extent to which abnormalities in vascular reactivity in CRF are mediated by elevated NO production. Rats will be 5/6 nephrectomized shortly after weaning, and studied 4-8 weeks later. A variety of techniques will be used, including vessel perfusion in vitro, renal clearance analysis in vivo, and histological, immunocytochemical, and Western analyses. The proposed studies will be the first comprehensive, direct investigations of the pathophysiology of the renal microvasculature in CRF, and of the effects of chronic IGF- I therapy on progressive CRF in growing rats. The results may have therapeutic implications for children with progressive renal insufficiency.

Website: http://crisp.cit.nih.gov/crisp/Crisp_Query.Generate_Screen

- **Project Title: IMMUNOGENETICS OF TYPE 1 DIABETES IN A BEDOUIN FAMILY**

Principal Investigator & Institution: Fain, Pamela R.; Associate Professor; Medicine; University of Colorado Hlth Sciences Ctr P.O. Box 6508, Grants and Contracts Aurora, Co 800450508

Timing: Fiscal Year 2002; Project Start 15-AUG-2000; Project End 31-MAY-2004

Summary: (Adapted from the Investigator's abstract): Over 2 million Americans suffer from type 1 diabetes, most of the them children and young adults. In addition to the burden of daily insulin injection to sustain life, patients with diabetes face a high risk for blindness, **kidney failure,** heart disease, stroke, and amputations. A better understanding of the genetic causes of type 1 diabetes should lead to novel gene therapies for halting beta-cell destruction during the pediatric period or for preventing the destruction of residual beta -cells in patients who are already affected with the disease. Further, the ability to predict who will develop the disease depends on the ability to test for each of the multiple genes that are thought to be involved. These high-risk individuals represent the best target populations for testing experimental treatment and prevention strategies in the most efficient manner. Individuals carrying HLA-DR3 and/or DR4 are at high risk for disease, but there is general agreement that other, unknown genes are also involved. However, it has been difficult to identify non-MHC genes, most likely due to genetic heterogeneity of type 1 diabetes in the population under study. Based on genetic linkage studies in a remarkable Bedouin Arab family with 20 relatives affected with type 1 diabetes, a diabetes susceptibility locus (IDDM17) has been mapped to the long arm of chromosome 10 (10q25.1). Significant (p=0.00004) nonparametric linkage scores (NPLs) and parametric LOD scores were observed for marker D10S554, which was also in linkage disequilibrium with IDDM17. D10S554 and flanking markers map to a 1,240 kb YAC. The family previously studied consists of about 200 members, who are members of a large Bedouin Arab tribe with about 15,000 members. Remarkably, 8 of the 20 affected relatives were diagnosed between 1990 and 1999. Another, closely related branch of the tribe have a similarly high incidence of type 1 diabetes. The specific aims of this study are: (1) to determine the ability to predict the development of type 1 diabetes in the extended family based on HLA genotype, chromosome 10 haplotype (IDDM17), and the expression of islet-cell autoantibodies; and (2) identify the gene corresponding to IDDM17 by the position cloning.

Website: http://crisp.cit.nih.gov/crisp/Crisp_Query.Generate_Screen

- **Project Title: INNER-CITY NEPHROLOGY**

Principal Investigator & Institution: Ifudu, Onyekachi; Medicine; Suny Downstate Medical Center 450 Clarkson Ave New York, Ny 11203

Timing: Fiscal Year 2002; Project Start 15-MAY-2002; Project End 30-APR-2003

Summary: The Renal Disease Division of SUNY Downstate Medical Center at Brooklyn proposes to sponsor a series of one-day conferences entitled "Inner-City Nephrology". The tentative date for the first in a series of five annual conferences is May 3rd, 2002. The conference is necessitated by the unique issues associated with kidney diseases in the inner0city, ranging from the very high rates of **kidney failure** among US blacks, suboptimal pre-end state renal disease (ESRD) care, and epidemic of HIV-associated **renal failure** to lack of awareness about and access to kidney transplantation. Furthermore, issues specific to inner-city nephrology are rarely addressed in-depth at the key national and international nephrology meetings. The conference will tackle these issues and provide strategies for improving outcomes in renal care among inner-city residents. The target audience is non-nephrologist primary care providers, nephrologists and nurses-practicing in the inner-cities in the US. About 400 people are expected to attend. The overall goals of the conference are: 1) to raise the awareness of providers treating patients in the inner-city of the specific issues related to renal diseases in inner-city residents; and 2) to increase and enhance the level of nephrologic services they provide in order to improve outcomes. Speakers with requisite expertise in inner-city healthcare will address topics such as i): the burden of diabetes and hypertension and current status of pre-ESRD care in the inner-city; ii) Prevention, identification, and early detection of **renal failure** in inner-city residents; iii) Interventions to slow progression of **renal failure** in inner-city residents; iv) increasing awareness about kidney **renal failure** in inner-city residents; iv) increasing awareness about kidney transplantation/facilitating access to kidney transplants; v) Role of HIV infection in **renal failure** in the inner-city and vi) The intertwined role of nephrologist and non-nephrologist in care of inner city residents with **renal failure.**

Website: http://crisp.cit.nih.gov/crisp/Crisp_Query.Generate_Screen

- **Project Title: MANAGING DIABETES: USE OF A DIGITAL INTERCOM SYSTEM**

Principal Investigator & Institution: Flax, Stephen W.; Flextech Systems, Inc. 333 Bishops Way, Ste 109 Brookfield, Wi 53005

Timing: Fiscal Year 2003; Project Start 30-SEP-2001; Project End 31-JUL-2005

Summary: (provided by applicant): The long-term objective of this project is to develop a new and novel medical monitoring device aimed at benefiting a large class of diabetic individuals. The new device is being called an "Assisted Self- Management Monitor." There are many diseases, such as diabetes, which are considered "self-managed" diseases. With diabetes, it is expected that patients measure and monitor their own blood glucose levels, their own medication administration, and their own diet and exercise programs. When patients properly and actively manage their own disease, they will minimize the disease progression. Otherwise, the effects can be tragic in terms of disease progression and health care costs. Mismanaged diabetes will eventually put the patient at risk for coronary artery disease, stroke, **kidney failure**, blindness, and peripheral vascular disease. Furthermore, there is often a significant time lag between when a patient collects self-care information and when a medical staff is made aware of that information. The new device underdevelopment is designed to actually monitor and evaluate how well patients are self-managing their disease, and then provide feedback to the care staff and the patient when irregularities are detected. Initially, the system is intended to help diabetic patients living in an assisted living setting. The new device will automatically transfer a patient's glucose reading and medication usage information from his or her quarters to a central station. There, the information will be compared to a personal profile that has been developed for each individual patient. When something of concern is detected, the monitor will notify the care staff with an appropriate message on a computer screen. However, the resident will also be notified with a prerecorded voice message that pertains to the given condition.

Website: http://crisp.cit.nih.gov/crisp/Crisp_Query.Generate_Screen

- **Project Title: MOLECULAR CHANGES IN SLIT DIAPHRAGM RELATED PROTEINURIA**

Principal Investigator & Institution: Chugh, Sumant S.; Medicine; Northwestern University Office of Sponsored Research Chicago, Il 60611

Timing: Fiscal Year 2004; Project Start 01-AUG-2004; Project End 31-JUL-2006

Summary: (provided by applicant): Proteinuria is a major manifestation of glomerular disease, and reducing proteinuria has been conclusively shown to retard the progression of **kidney failure.** Our research effort is directed towards investigating the pathogenesis of proteinuria, with the long term goal of developing specific anti-proteinuric therapies based disease mechanisms. The slit diaphragm plays a major role in maintaining glomerular permeability characteristics. We have recently shown that injecting a combination of anti-neph1 and anti-nephrin antibodies in individual sub-nephritogenic doses into rats results in proteinuria / albuminuria. In this proposal, we plan to use this new model to study changes in the expression of podocyte genes and proteins during selective slit diaphragm injury and proteinuria. Specific aim1: To characterize the full range of complement- and leukocyte-independent heterologous phase proteinuria induced in rats as a result of slit diaphragm injury using a combination of affinity purified anti-neph1 and anti-nephrin antibodies, and study its effect on the expression and phosphorylation of slit diaphragm proteins. Specific aim 2: To identify and characterize genes that are differentially expressed in the podocyte in this model using a combination of supression subtractive hybridization, real time PCR, in situ hybridization, Western blot and cultured cell transfection studies. This study will bring us one step closer to understanding the pathogenesis of proteinuria, and will also help to correlate our existing knowledge of the in vitro characteristics of slit diaphragm proteins with in vivo function.

Website: http://crisp.cit.nih.gov/crisp/Crisp_Query.Generate_Screen

- **Project Title: MULTICENTER TRIAL OF FOCAL GLOMERULOSCLEROSIS**

Principal Investigator & Institution: Gipson, Debbie S.; Medicine; University of North Carolina Chapel Hill Aob 104 Airport Drive Cb#1350 Chapel Hill, Nc 27599

Timing: Fiscal Year 2002; Project Start 30-SEP-2002; Project End 31-AUG-2007

Summary: (provided by applicant): Idiopathic focal segmental glomerulosclerosis (FSGS) is a progressive scarring disorder that causes proteinuria and **kidney failure** in the majority of affected individuals. There is considerable controversy regarding the best therapeutic intervention and the definition of pathological variants of FSGS that may impact therapeutic response rates. This proposal focuses on the design and conduct of a collaborative multicenter trial that will evaluate response rates of children and young adults with the nephrotic syndrome due to FSGS treated with cyclosporin A as compared to corticosteroids plus angiotensin receptor blocker therapy. It will utilize a newly determined FSGS classification scheme as defined by the NY Pathology Consensus Group that includes one of our collaborators. In addition, since incidence of idiopathic FSGS has been increasing over the past 2 decades, a case-control study that will evaluate risk factors for FSGS is proposed to run concurrently with the trial. Our proposed southeastern clinical coordinating center will provide strength to the planned nation-wide trial through our large patient population with FSGS, the strength of the UNC nephropathology service, and the investigators' long track record of clinical trial and epidemiologic research in glomerular diseases through the UNC-Chapel Hill based Glomerular Disease Collaborative Network. In conjunction with committed collaborating sites, our group has over 400 FSGS patients who would be eligible for the proposed trial, as well as established mechanisms for including prospectively identified patients. The proposed case-control study will evaluate risk factors for the development of FSGS such as body mass, birth weight, viral illnesses and smoking in all patients screened for entry into the trial.

Website: http://crisp.cit.nih.gov/crisp/Crisp_Query.Generate_Screen

- **Project Title: NITRIC OXIDE AND ENDOTHELIN IN ENDOTOXEMIC RENAL FAILURE**

Principal Investigator & Institution: Poole, Brian D.; Medicine; University of Colorado Hlth Sciences Ctr P.O. Box 6508, Grants and Contracts Aurora, Co 800450508

Timing: Fiscal Year 2002; Project Start 30-MAY-2003

Summary: (provided by applicant): Sepsis and septic shock are associated with a high incidence of acute **renal failure** (ARF). Moreover, the combination of sepsis and ARF leads to a very high mortality ranging from 50-80%. Endotoxemia during sepsis is associated with systemic arterial vasodilation secondary to 1) a large increase in vasodilating nitric oxide (NO) generated by the inducible isoform of nitric oxide synthase (iNOS) and 2) reduced plasma volume due to increased endothelin (ET-1)-induced capillary leak. The resultant relative underfilling of the arterial circulation initiates compensatory vasoconstrictors of the sympathetic nervous system and renin angiotensin system which maintain mean arterial pressure at the expense of renal vasoconstriction, an important predisposing factor to ARF. ET-1 may also exert a vasoconstrictor effect systemically and on the kidney. In Specific Aim 1, the effect on renal function of specific iNOS versus non-specific NOS inhibition during endotoxemia will be studied; the role of eNOS will be examined in eNOS knockout mice. In Specific Aim 2, the role of ET-1 will be examined by assessment of renal function and capillary leak during early endotoxemia in ET-1 knockout mice and mice treated with an ET receptor antagonist. Specific Aim 3 will study the role of the interaction of the NO and ET-1 systems by examining the result of non-specific versus specific iNOS inhibition on ET-1 gene and protein expression. Understanding the early vasoactive events which cause ARF during endotoxemia would be a major medical advance, thereby allowing the development of pathogenetic-based interventions.

Website: http://crisp.cit.nih.gov/crisp/Crisp_Query.Generate_Screen

- **Project Title: PATHOGENESIS OF ENDOTOXIN-INDUCED ACUTE RENAL FAILURE**

Principal Investigator & Institution: Cunningham, Patrick N.; Associate Professor; Medicine; University of Chicago 5801 S Ellis Ave Chicago, Il 60637

Timing: Fiscal Year 2002; Project Start 01-MAY-2002; Project End 30-APR-2007

Summary: My ultimate goal is to head an idependent research laboratory in an academic setting directed towards a better understanding of acute **renal failure** (ARF). I have spent the last three years of my nephrology fellowship investigating a mouse model of endotoxin-induced ARF is mediated by tumor necrosis factor (TNF) acting on its principal receptor, TNFRI, in kidney. This topic is highly relevant from a clinical perspective, as ARF is a common and serious syndrome with no effective therapy, and is frequently a consequence of sepsis. With the support of this Career Development Award, and the guidance and support of the University of Chicago's Section of Nephrology under the sponsorship of Dr. Richard Quigg, I hope to expand my skills into new areas such as cell biology, to advance towards this long-term goal. This proposal will test the hypothesis that endotoxin- induced ARF is a consequence of renal neutrophil infiltration, renal cell apoptosis, and other forms of neurotic or sublytic injury by the direct action of TNF on renal tubular cells. The first specific aim seeks to characterize the time course of leukocyte accumulation in the kidney after endotoxin administration, to identify key adhesion molecules and chemokines mediating this process, and to evaluate their pathogenic role with the use of inhibitory antibodies and genetic "knockout" mice. The second specific aim seeks to better characterize the time course of renal cell apoptosis after endotoxin administration and to evaluate its pathogenic role through the use of specific pharmacologic agents. The third specific aim seeks to describe the effects of TNF on renal proximal tubular cells in culture, and specifically to access their effects on cell viability, apoptosis, morphology, cell-cell adhesion, and metabolism. The fourth specific aim of this study seeks to characterize the renal hemodynamic effects which occur after the administration of endotoxin, specifically the effects on systematic blood pressure, renal blood flow, and renal vascular resistance. It is hoped that the answers to these scientific questions can be assembled into a overall paradigm of how endotoxin injures the kidney, and that this work can be translated into the design of effective therapies for ARF.

Website: http://crisp.cit.nih.gov/crisp/Crisp_Query.Generate_Screen

- **Project Title: PATHOGENESIS OF FAMILIAL JUVENILE NEPHRONOPHTHISIS**

Principal Investigator & Institution: Hanks, Steven K.; Professor; Cell and Developmental Biology; Vanderbilt University 3319 West End Ave. Nashville, Tn 372036917

Timing: Fiscal Year 2002; Project Start 01-MAY-2000; Project End 30-APR-2004

Summary: The long-term objective of this proposal is to understand the nature of the cellular defects underlying the pathogenesis of familial juvenile nephronophthisis (NPH) -- a common genetic cause of **kidney failure** in children. Although clinical and histological observations indicate NPH results from a loss of normal excretory tubule function, the pathogenesis of the disease remains obscure. Recently a human gene mutated in the majority of NPH cases was isolated and the sequence of its encoded protein ("nephrocystin") was determined. A clue to the biochemical function of nephrocystin is the presence of a "Src homology 3" (SH3) domain known for mediating specific protein-protein interactions. New insight into the pathogenesis of NPH will now come from further study of nephrocystin. In preliminary studies, cDNAs encoding mouse nephrocystin have been isolated and the transcripts have been detected during post-implantation mouse embryogenesis and in a variety of adult tissues including the kidney. New information concerning the biochemical function of nephrocystin was obtained by identifying a tyrosine kinase substrate, p130Cas, as a protein bound by the nephrocystin SH3 domain and by showing that nephrocystin localizes to lateral membranes of polarized epithelial cells. These observations led to our general hypothesis that nephrocystin functions in the morphogenesis and/or maintenance of the kidney tubular epithelium, requiring specific interactions with p130Cas and other proteins involved in cell adhesive interactions. To test and expand the hypothesis, specific aims are proposed to: 1) determine the spatial pattern of expression of nephrocystin in developing mouse embryos and in the adult kidney, 2) further identify and characterize relevant nephrocystin-interacting proteins, and 3) determine the effects of nephrocystin on adhesion regulated p130Cas tyrosine phosphorylation and epithelial cell tight junction formation and tubulogenesis.

Website: http://crisp.cit.nih.gov/crisp/Crisp_Query.Generate_Screen

- **Project Title: PHASE II TRIAL OF DHEA IN CHRONIC RENAL FAILURE**

Principal Investigator & Institution: Walser, Mackenzie; Johns Hopkins University 3400 N Charles St Baltimore, Md 21218

Timing: Fiscal Year 2002

Summary: We have observed, in previous GCRC-supported studies of patients with chronic **renal failure,** that progression in negatively correlated with serum level of DHEA-S; i.e., patients with relatively low levels of this hormone (for their age and gender) progress rapidly while patients with relatively high levels progress slowly. Based on this finding, we have instituted a double-blind, randomized, crossover, dose-adjustment trial of DHEA supplementation in patients with chronic **renal failure.** After establishing (by sequential determinations of glomerular filtration rate) (GFR) that progression is occurring, we randomize patients to receive either placebo or DHEA first, followed by the opposite, in two equal periods of observation, varying in length from 2 to 6 months (depending on the prior rate of progression). Serum levels of DHEA-S are measured weekly for the first four weeks of both periods, and reported to an unblinded individual, who adjusts the dosage of DHEA capsules vs. placebo capsules so as to achieve a serum DHEA-S level approximating 12 ug/ml (in those receiving DHEA). So far 8 patients have entered this protocol. Two patients, one with non- insulin-dependent diabetes mellitus and one with IgA nephropathy, have shown accelerated progression during DHEA supplementation. One patient with insulin-dependent diabetes mellitus and one with polycystic kidney disease have shown slowed progression during DHEA supplementation. Our future studies will be limited to these latter two disorders. DHEA toxicity has not been noted otherwise.

Website: http://crisp.cit.nih.gov/crisp/Crisp_Query.Generate_Screen

- **Project Title: PILOT STUDY--CYCLOSPORINE & ISLET CELL TRANSPLANTATION**

Principal Investigator & Institution: Colgan, John; Columbia University Health Sciences Po Box 49 New York, Ny 10032

Timing: Fiscal Year 2003; Project Start 01-MAY-2003; Project End 31-JAN-2008

Summary: Recent advances have shown that beta islet cell transplantation can provide long term, insulin independent control of type-1 diabetes. However, transplant recipients must undergo immunosuppressive therapy that causes islet cell dysfunction among other serious complications. Thus understanding how conventional immunosuppressive drugs affect islet cells as well as identifying alternative immunosuppressive therapies could greatly facilitate the routine use of islet cell transplantation as a curative. Cyclosporine is a clinically used immunosuppressant that causes diabetes and **kidney failure.** As an approach toward defining the mechanisms underlying the toxic and immunosuppressive effects of the drug, targeted disruption was used to create mice lacking cyclophilin A (CypA), an abundant cyctosolic protein that functions as the receptor for cyclosporine. CypA-deficient mice display normal immune function, but are resistant to immunosuppression by cyclosporine and suffer less toxicity. Thus,

CypA-deficient mice provide a tool for dissecting the various effects of the drug. Regarding islet cell dysfunction, glucose regulation by wildtype and CypA-deficient islet cells in cyclosporine-treated mice can be compared. Maintenance of glucose regulation by CypA-deficient islet cells subjected to cyclosporine would indicate that the drug affects islet cells via interactions with CypA, and would point towards the involvement of specific regulatory pathways. How these pathways and their target genes are affected by cyclosporine could be further examined through molecular analysis of cultured wild-type and CypA-deficient islet cells. CypA-deficient mice also provide a way to identify the immune cells that must be targeted by cyclosporine in order to suppress transplant rejection. Genetically modified mice that are unable to generate specific immune cell types can be reconstituted with CypA-deficient cells via adoptive transfer. Reconstituted mice can then be treated with cyclosporine and challenged with allogeneic tissue in parallel with identically reconstituted animals not subjected to immunosuppression. The inability or ablility of mice reconstituted in different immune cell compartments to reject allogeneic tissue would provide an assay for determining the specific cell types that must be inhibited to prevent allograft rejection. Such knowledge could be applied toward the design of alternative immunosuppressive therapies.

Website: http://crisp.cit.nih.gov/crisp/Crisp_Query.Generate_Screen

- **Project Title: PREVENTION OF TYPE I DIABETES MELLITUS USING A CELL VAC\***

Principal Investigator & Institution: Giannoukakis, Nick; Children's Hosp Pittsburgh/Upmc Hlth Sys of Upmc Health Systems Pittsburgh, Pa 152132583

Timing: Fiscal Year 2002; Project Start 01-SEP-2001; Project End 31-JUL-2004

Summary: (provided by applicant): Type I diabetes mellitus is an autoimmune disease whose etiopathogenesis lies in the selective destruction of the insulin-producing beta cells of the islets of Langerhans in the pancreas. The current insulin replacement therapy strategies are not fully effective at recapitulating tight glucose control and consequently, many patients eventually succumb to debilitating and life-threatening complications such as **kidney failure** and heart disease. While transplantation of intact islets of Langerhans offers the potential to restore physiologic glycemic control, the requirement for life-long immunosuppressive interventions carries with it significant risks of rendering the islet transplants dysfunctional. Moreover, these strategies can lead to an array of other problems including **kidney failure** and a risk of malignancy. In contrast, preventing autoimmunity altogether will prevent beta cell destruction, thereby obviating the need for life-long insulin therapy or transplantation concomitant with chronic immunosuppressive therapy. Most of the preventive strategies in experimental animals to date have focused on the induction of tolerance to either soluble islet antigens or putative autoantigens like insulin and glutamic acid decarboxylase. Intrathymic injection of islet lysates or putative autoantigens has resulted in either the prevention of diabetes or prolongation of time to onset in diabetic rodent models. Intrathymic injection, however, is not practical in humans, and the candidate autoantigen approach is risky in that the identity of the causative diabetogenic autoantigens remains unknown. This application focuses on developing proof-of-principle studies of an alternative means of achieving tolerance to autoantigens by manipulating a subtype of the diabetic host's immune cells in order to educate the host immune system to ignore beta cell antigens before the onset of disease. The subtype of immune cells that this application aims to manipulate into a cell vaccine are dendritic cells, considered to be the body's natural adjuvant. These cells normally initiate potent immune responses against foreign tissue. Dendritic cells however, have also been manipulated to tolerise the host immune system to foreign antigens, including allogeneic, and it is possible that similar manipulation may promote tolerance to autoantigens in diabetes. By blocking co-stimulatory pathways in which dendritic cells figure prominently, it has been possible to achieve long-term acceptance of both allogeneic and xenogeneic transplants. The central hypothesis that this application will test is whether administration of a prediabetic animal host's dendritic cells, rendered unable to provide adequate costimulatory signals by ex vivo gene transfer technology and presenting islet antigens, can prevent or prolong the time to onset of diabetes when reintroduced into the host. Oligonucleotide decoys for NF-kappaB, a transcriptional regulator of dendritic cell activation, as well as antisense oligonucleotides against the transcripts encoding the costimulation molecules CD80 and CD86 will be used to engineer the host's dendritic cells into a cell vaccine for autoimmune diabetes.

Website: http://crisp.cit.nih.gov/crisp/Crisp_Query.Generate_Screen

- **Project Title: PTEN REGULATION DURING ISCHEMIC ACUTE RENAL FAILURE**

Principal Investigator & Institution: Venkatachalam, Manjeri A.; Professor; Pathology; University of Texas Hlth Sci Ctr San Ant 7703 Floyd Curl Dr San Antonio, Tx 78229

Timing: Fiscal Year 2004; Project Start 01-JUL-1987; Project End 30-JUN-2009

Summary: (provided by applicant): Following ischemic injury, surviving kidney proximal tubule cells dedifferentiate and proliferate to regenerate the tubules. After reaching critical cell densities, growth arrest and differentiation follow. The signaling mechanisms that govern this process are important and critically determine structural and functional recovery from ischemic injury. Our research suggests that the phosphatidylinositol 3-kinase (PI3K) signaling pathway may play an important role in proximal tubule cell proliferation and regeneration. We observed that the suppression of PI3K signaling associated with growth arrest of cultured proximal tubule cells is accompanied by an increase in the cellular content of the tumor suppressor protein PTEN. This suggests that PTEN might regulate proximal tubule proliferation through the lipid phosphatase actions of PTEN that would decrease the levels of D-3 phosphorylated inositol phospholipids made by PI3K. Our preliminary studies suggest that the increase of PTEN associated with growth inhibition is caused by at least two feedback mechanisms of autoregulatory signaling: one is driven by Akt, a downstream member of the PI3K pathway and the other by intercellular contact as cell numbers increase. We plan to use cell culture and in vivo models to unravel molecular mechanisms of proximal tubule cell growth regulation. Our research will use 5 approaches to study how PTEN regulates growth, and how PTEN is regulated. (1) We will employ PTEN vectors and siRNA methods to increase or decrease PTEN protein and activity. (2) We will use a constitutively expressed Akt construct that permits rapid and selective induction of Akt kinase activity to study how Akt activation leads to PTEN upregulation. (3) We will disrupt and restore cell junctions in cultured proximal tubule cells to study how cell contact leads to regulation of PTEN. Regulation of PTEN will be studied at the levels of transcription, mRNA stability and protein turnover. (4) We will use genomics and proteomics approaches to identify novel proteins involved in PTEN regulation. (5) We will study regulation of PI3K signaling by PTEN in vivo in rats and mice with ischemic acute **renal failure** using biochemical methods, immuno histochemistry and in situ hybridization. We will employ PTEN antisense oligonucleotides to suppress kidney PTEN in vivo to study how this intervention affects the course of proximal tubule regeneration and recovery.

Website: http://crisp.cit.nih.gov/crisp/Crisp_Query.Generate_Screen

- **Project Title: REGULATION OF EXTRACELLULAR MATRIX IN KIDNEY DISEASE**

Principal Investigator & Institution: Border, Wayne A.; Professor; Internal Medicine; University of Utah Salt Lake City, Ut 84102

Timing: Fiscal Year 2002; Project Start 30-SEP-1990; Project End 30-AUG-2004

Summary: The cytokine transforming growth factor-beta (TGF-beta) is a key biological mediator of extracellular matrix deposition in health and in fibrotic diseases, especially of the kidney. We have demonstrated a central role for TGF-beta in the pathogenesis of experimental and/or human forms of acute and chronic glomerulonephritis, diabetic nephropathy, hypertensive nephropathy, acute and chronic allograft rejection, cyclosporine nephropathy and HIV-associated nephropathy. TGF-beta is also implicated in numerous fibrotic disorders involving other tissues and organs and is considered to be a principal target for designing novel therapeutic agents to block fibrotic disease. An important question is what is the cause of the persistent TGF-beta overexpression that leads to progressive fibrosis and kidney failure? In the course of our work we have discovered a complex interconnection between TGF-beta and the renin-angiotensin system (RAS) in the kidney. The RAS acts to stimulate the production and activation of TGF-beta and to increase the expression of TGF-beta receptors which greatly enhances TGF-beta's fibrotic effects. We hypothesize that continued stimulation of TGF-beta by the RAS may be a molecular mechanism for the continued overexpression of TGF-beta in kidney diseases. In this application we propose to investigate the molecular interconnections by which the RAS may perpetuate the actions of TGF-beta and to explore in vivo therapeutic strategies to block these effects by doing the following: 1) Investigate a molecular mechanism by which angiotensin II may up-regulate TGF-beta receptors by analyzing the functional elements of the TGF-beta type I receptor promoter in the kidney, 2) Investigate the possibility that renin or prorenin may be up-stream effectors that, especially in the presence of angiotensin II blockade, induce TGF-beta overexpression and thus contribute to progressive fibrotic disease and 3) Continue investigation of the role of interactions between the renin-angiotensin system, TGF-beta overexpression and TGF-beta receptor expression in the pathogenesis of fibrosis using a model of acute glomerulonephritis and to compare the findings with parallel studies in a model of chronic glomerulonephritis. The significance of this application is that it will apply new knowledge and technology to an area of investigation that is directly relevant to improved understanding of the pathogenesis of kidney fibrosis and will likely provide insights that suggest new therapeutic strategies to prevent progressive **kidney failure** in humans suffering from kidney disease.

Website: http://crisp.cit.nih.gov/crisp/Crisp_Query.Generate_Screen

- **Project Title: REGULATION OF POLYCYSTIN-2**

Principal Investigator & Institution: Anyatonwu, Georgia I.; Pharmacology; Yale University 47 College Street, Suite 203 New Haven, Ct 065208047

Timing: Fiscal Year 2003; Project Start 01-SEP-2003; Project End 31-AUG-2006

Summary: (provided by applicant): Autosomal dominant polycystic kidney disease (ADPKD) affects millions of people and it is the fourth leading cause of **kidney failure** in the United States. The two genes encoded in this disease are PKD1 and PKD2, and mutations in either gene are associated with the phoenotype seen in ADPKD. The long-term objective entails PKD2 gene product, polycystin-2, functions as a calcium permeable nonselective cation channel. Dysregulation of this channel provides mechanism for the onset and progression of ADPKD. The specific aims of this research include to (1) Determine the interaction between polycystin-2 and the ryanodine receptor (RYR); (2) What effects mutated variants of polycystin-2 would impact on the function of polycystin-2; (3) Develop a screening assay for putative agonists and antagonists of PKD2. Since these channels are intracellular calcium channels, planar lipid bilayer and calcium imaging techniques will be used to perform this study.

Website: http://crisp.cit.nih.gov/crisp/Crisp_Query.Generate_Screen

- **Project Title: REGULATION OF THIAZIDE-SENSITIVE NACL TRANSPORT**

Principal Investigator & Institution: Ellison, David H.; Associate Professor; Medicine; Oregon Health & Science University Portland, or 972393098

Timing: Fiscal Year 2004; Project Start 01-AUG-1998; Project End 31-MAR-2009

Summary: (provided by applicant): Hypertension affects 25 million Americans, contributing importantly to stroke, myocardial infarction and **kidney failure.** Both environmental and genetic factors contribute to hypertension. The kidney plays a central role in blood pressure homeostasis by controlling salt excretion. An important part of the salt homeostatic system is the thiazide-sensitive Na-CI cotransplorter. Dysfunction of this transport protein leads to Gitelman's syndrome, an autosomal recessive disorder of salt wasting, hypokalemia and alkalosis. We have shown that many mutations causing Gitelman's syndrome create misfolded proteins, thus activating the quality control mechanism of the endoplasmic reticulum. Recently, a hypertensive disorder, pseudohypoaldosteronism type II, has been shown to result from mutations in WNK (without lysine) kinases. We show preliminary data indicating that WNK kinases regulate thiazide-sensitive Na-CI cotransporter activity. WNK4 suppresses thiazide-sensitive Na-CI cotransporter activity by more than 80%. WNK1 does not alter Na-CI cotransporter activity by itself, but instead inhibits WNK4 activity. WNK1 is known to be regulated by osmolality, as is the thiazide-sensitive Na-CI cotransporter. We postulate that the WNK kinase system regulates thiazide-sensitive Na-CI cotransport in response to changes in luminal osmolality. We will test the hypotheses that 1) WNK4 downregulates thiazide-sensitive Na-CI cotransporter activity by interacting with this transport protein and phosphorylating it, 2) WNK1 inhibits WNK4-mediated suppression of thiazide-sensitive Na-CI cotransporter activity by interacting with and phosphoryiating WNK4, 3) pseudohypoaldosteronism type II results from increased WNK1 activity leading to inhibited WNK4 mediated suppression of Na-CI reabsorption by the distal tubule, 4) specific threonine moieties on the Na-CI cotransporter are phosphorylated in response to WNK stimulation, 5) WNK4 is expressed at tight junctions along the distal tubule and regulates paracellular ion permeability, and 6) WNK kinases link paracellular to transcellular conductance. The results of experiments described in this proposal will illuminate molecular mechanisms of hypertension. Although Mendelian forms of hypertension are rare, they help to elucidate mechanisms of blood pressure regulation that almost certainly contribute to the more common essential variety.

Website: http://crisp.cit.nih.gov/crisp/Crisp_Query.Generate_Screen

- **Project Title: RENAL FAILURE GENES IN THE SOUTHEASTERN US**

Principal Investigator & Institution: Freedman, Barry I.; Professor and Chief; Internal Medicine; Wake Forest University Health Sciences Winston-Salem, Nc 27157

Timing: Fiscal Year 2002; Project Start 30-SEP-1999; Project End 31-AUG-2004

Summary: The purpose of this study is to identify the genes causing diabetic and non- diabetic **renal failure** (RF) in high risk black and white families residing in the southeastern United States.. Diabetes is the most common cause of end- stge renal disease (ESRD) in the U.S.. At most, 30% of diabetic patients are susceptible to RF with its progression to ESRD and high mortality rate. Selected diabetic families demonstrate multi-generational clustering of renal disease. An inherited basis for RF is also supported by reports that blacks are more likely than whites to develop RF. These racial differences are not fully explained by racial differences in prevalence or severity pf diabetes mellitus or hypertension, socioeconomic factors or access to healthcare. In order to identify genes causing RF we will continue to identify, clinically characterize, and collect DNA from 400 families (200 black, 200 white) with type 2 diabetic ESRD index cases and additional first degree relatives with type 2 diabetes mellitus. This phase of the project employs the unique "Family History orf relatives with type 2 diabetes mellitus. This phase of the project employs the unique "Family History of ESRD" database, independently compiled by the federally-funded ESRD Network 6 (Southeastern Kidney Council). This registry currently contains family history data from more than 20,00 incident patients with ESRD who started dialysis after September, 1993. Approximately 60% of patients are black and 40% have diabetic RF. Candidate genes will be screened for linkage to RF at the Wake Forest University Baptist Medical Center, and DNA and clinical data will also be supplied to the study's Genetic Analysis and Data Coordinating Center (GADCC) for a comprehensive genome wide survey to identify novel loci causing RF. The identification of RF genes would form a genetic basis for detection of high risk individuals and lead to the development of intervention and treatment strategies for prevention of kidney disease.

Website: http://crisp.cit.nih.gov/crisp/Crisp_Query.Generate_Screen

- **Project Title: RENIN ANGIOTENSIN SYSTEM BLOCKAGE-DN (RASS)**

Principal Investigator & Institution: Mauer, S Michael.; Professor; Pediatrics; University of Minnesota Twin Cities 200 Oak Street Se Minneapolis, Mn 554552070

Timing: Fiscal Year 2003; Project Start 16-MAR-1997; Project End 31-MAY-2008

Summary: (provided by applicant): Diabetes nephropathy (DN) is the most important cause of **kidney failure.** Patients (pts) with Type 1 diabetes mellitus (DM) who develop DN have a markedly increased death rate from **kidney failure,** coronary artery disease and stroke. Glycemia only partly explains why some pts develop these DM complications. Further, since tight blood sugar control is extremely difficult to maintain, other efforts need to be made to reduce risks of DM complications. Renin-angiotensin system (RAS) inhibitors slow the progress of established DN. The specific aim of this study is to determine whether treatment at the early stages of DM can slow or stop DN structural changes. The long-term objective is to prevent DN from developing. Two hundred eight five pts ages 16-59 with 2-29 yrs of Type 1 DM and no renal functional abnormalities have been randomized into a parallel, double-blind, placebo-controlled study involving 3 groups (95 pts/group). Each group receives an angiotensin-converting enzyme inhibitor (ACEI) (enalapril), or an angiotensin II receptor blocker (losartan), or placebo. All pts have their usual DM management. Baseline studies included measures of glomerular filtration rate (GFR), urinary albumin excretion rate (UAE), blood pressure (BP), and a percutaneous renal biopsy. Pts are followed by quarterly measures of BP, HbA1C, UAE, and drug compliance. There are annual measures of GFR and a repeat renal biopsy after 5 yrs in the study. The main endpoint is kidney structural changes over time, especially mesangial fractional volume [Vv(Mes/glom)]. Secondary endpoints will be other DN structural measures and measures of kidney function (UAE, GFR). These studies will determine whether RAS blockage in the early stages of DN can prevent the early kidney structural changes in this important disorder. Ancillary studies will evaluate the effects of treatment group on the development and progression of diabetic retinopathy and will develop predictors of study participants' compliance.

Website: http://crisp.cit.nih.gov/crisp/Crisp_Query.Generate_Screen

- **Project Title: RESISTANCE TRAINING DURING MAINTENANCE DIALYSIS**

Principal Investigator & Institution: Sceppa, Carmen C.; Nutrition Exercise Physiology Sarcopenla (Neps) Lab; Tufts University Boston Boston, Ma 02111

Timing: Fiscal Year 2003; Project Start 30-SEP-2003; Project End 31-MAR-2005

Summary: (provided by applicant): There is a rising incidence of **kidney failure** in the US, with poor outcomes and high cost. **End-stage renal disease** (ESRD) affects almost 375,000 individuals in the US at a cost of more than $14 billion per year. Despite advances in dialysis and transplantation therapies, **kidney failure** leads to poor outcomes, poor prognosis and high health care costs. Malnutrition and the underlying systemic inflammatory response developed during the course of chronic kidney disease, worsen during ESRD, and leads to adverse outcomes, increased morbidity and mortality. Muscle wasting, impaired functional capacity and poor quality of life are the most important factors associated with malnutrition and inflammation in **renal failure.** We have shown in pre-dialysis patients with moderate **chronic renal insufficiency** that the anabolic effects of resistance exercise training result in significant improvements in protein utilization, nutritional status and functional capacity even in the context of anorexia and prescribed low protein diets. Thus, we propose to develop, test and implement a progressive resistance exercise routine for ESRD patients during the hemodialysis session. Our hypotheses are that the addition of 30-45 min of resistance exercise training during the dialysis session will counteract the burden of renal disease and will result in: 1) A feasible and safe exercise modality for ESRD patients (6-wk feasibility phase tested in 10 patients); 2) Net anabolism as evidenced by: improved nutritional status (i.e. increased protein catabolic rate, muscle mass and muscle strength); and reduced systemic inflammatory response (i.e. reduced C-reactive protein and interleukin-6, and increased serum albumin levels) compared to a randomly assigned control group on hemodilaysis but not exercise training (6-mo efficacy phase tested in 20 patients/group); and that 3) Improved self-reported physical function (i.e. increased SF-36 physical component scale) observed with resistance training will be associated with the improvements in nutritional status and inflammatory response. The long-term goal is to implement resistance exercise training routines during hemodialysis to overcome the underlying malnutrition and inflammation of ESRD and to improve disease outcome and prognosis. By implementing such intervention, we hope to offer a therapeutic strategy that can be incorporated to the standard of care of ESRD patients by working in conjunction with the dialysis unit staff.

Website: http://crisp.cit.nih.gov/crisp/Crisp_Query.Generate_Screen

- **Project Title: ROLE OF KAP EXPRESSION IN THE DIABETIC KIDNEY**

Principal Investigator & Institution: Coschigano, Karen T.; None; Ohio University Athens 105 Research & Technology Center Athens, Oh 457012979

Timing: Fiscal Year 2002; Project Start 01-JUL-2002; Project End 30-JUN-2004

Summary: (provided by applicant): Kidney damage is a frequent complication of both type I and type II diabetes, often ending in **kidney failure,** or **end-stage renal disease** (ESRD). Diabetic nephropathy, the single most common cause of ESRD, is a progressive disease that takes several years to develop and often goes undiagnosed. The long-term goal of this project is to design specific, targeted markers and therapeutic approaches for the diagnosis, treatment, and prevention of human diabetic kidney disease. Toward this end, previous work identified a cDNA whose mRNA expression decreases markedly with increasing kidney damage, both in a diabetes-dependent and in a diabetes-independent mouse model of glomeruloscierosis. This cDNA encodes kidney androgen-regulated protein (KAP), a kidney-specific protein found only in renal proximal tubule cells. Since decreasing levels of KAP mRNA are associated with progressive kidney damage, it is proposed that maintenance of high levels of KAP mRNA expression will protect the kidney from glomerular hypertrophy and diabetic damage. This hypothesis will be tested by expressing KAP mRNA in the kidneys of mice under the direction of a heterologous promoter and then assessing the extent of kidney damage after induction of diabetes by streptozotocin injection. Acceptance of the hypothesis could lead to the development of KAP as a therapeutic drug for the prevention of kidney damage.

Website: http://crisp.cit.nih.gov/crisp/Crisp_Query.Generate_Screen

- **Project Title: S6K AND MTOR AS TARGETS FOR TUBEROUS SCLEROSIS**

Principal Investigator & Institution: Guan, Kun-Liang; Associate Professor; Oncoimmune Ltd Columbus, Oh 43210

Timing: Fiscal Year 2003; Project Start 01-JUL-2003; Project End 30-JUN-2004

Summary: (provided by applicant): Tuberous sclerosis (TSC) is a common autosomal dominant genetic disorder occurring in approximately 1/6000 of the population. TSC is characterized by the development of hamartomas in a wide range of human tissues. Common clinic symptoms include seizures, mental retardation, **kidney failure,** facial angiofibromas, and cardial rhabdomyomas. Mutation in either TSC1 or TSC2 gene is responsible for TSC. Recent genetic studies have indicated that TSC I/TSC2 are involved in cell growth control and function as tumor suppressors. The TSC1 and TSC2 proteins form a physical and functional complex in the cell. The long-tern objectives of this project are to identify critical cellular targets, which mediate the physiological functions of TSC I/TSC2 and to verify potential drug targets for TSC. The specific aims of this proposal are: 1. To demonstrate that TSC1 and TSC2 function through the mammalian target of rapamycin (mTOR); 2. To validate S6K as a key downstream effector of TSC1/ TSC2. Biochemical, molecular and cell biological approaches will be used to accomplish these specific aims.

Website: http://crisp.cit.nih.gov/crisp/Crisp_Query.Generate_Screen

- **Project Title: STEM CELL THERAPY IN ACUTE RENAL FAILURE**

Principal Investigator & Institution: Lin, Fangming; Pediatrics; University of Texas Sw Med Ctr/Dallas Dallas, Tx 753909105

Timing: Fiscal Year 2003; Project Start 01-MAY-2003; Project End 30-APR-2008

Summary: (provided by applicant): Current treatment options for acute **renal failure** are limited. The recovery from **renal failure** is incomplete if renal epithelial cells fail to regenerate. Since stem cells have diverse developmental potential, we propose to test the hypothesis that mouse hematopoietic stem cells (HSCs) and mouse embryonic stem cells (ES cells) can aid in the regeneration of renal tubules after acute **renal failure.** In our preliminary studies, we isolated HSCs from male Rosa 26 mice and injected them into female C57 BL mice that had renal ischemia/reperfusion injury. At 4 weeks after HSC transplantation, we detected Lac Z positive cells in the renal tubules of female recipient kidneys. The presence of the male specific SRY gene, and the cells with Y chromosome positive signals in female recipient kidneys confirmed that male donor HSC-derived cells had located to the kidneys. In the first aim of the proposal, we will examine whether exogenous HSCs can transdifferentiate to functional renal tubular cells by staining the kidney tissues with X-gal for the donor marker, and with antibodies to tubular transporters for renal cell markers. We will test the dose response to various numbers of HSCs injected and will examine the effect of HSCs in mice with bilateral renal ischemia/reperfusion injury. The number of donor-derived cells in the kidneys will be correlated with serum BUN and creatinine levels. We will also test whether mobilization of endogenous HSCs with stem cell factor (SCF) and G-CSF can accelerate the recovery of renal function after ischemic injury. In the second aim, we will examine if ES cells can be induced to differentiate to renal cells. Using a unique strain of transgenic mice that express GFP specifically in the epithelial cells of renal tubules and the developing GU tract, we will generate an ES cell line that will allow us to identify and isolate live tubular epithelial cells. ES cells will be induced to form embryoid bodies, and then further cultured with growth factors, conditions known to induce human ES cells to express renal cell markers. GFP positive cells will be isolated with FRCS sorting. The GFP expressing tubular epithelial cells will be injected under the capsule of the kidneys after ischemia/reperfusion injury. The kidney sections will be stained with antibodies to GFP and tubular transporters to test the functional role of transplanted ES cell-derived tubular epithelial cells. The results of this proposal will permit novel understanding of plasticity of HSCs and renal tubular development from ES cells and open up the possibility of treating renal diseases, such as acute **renal failure,** with stem cell replacement therapy.

Website: http://crisp.cit.nih.gov/crisp/Crisp_Query.Generate_Screen

- **Project Title: TISSUE PRODUCTS AND KITS FROM RENAL DISEASE**

Principal Investigator & Institution: Barnes, Veronique L.; Probetex, Inc. 12000 Network Blvd, Ste B-200 San Antonio, Tx 78249

Timing: Fiscal Year 2004; Project Start 14-MAY-2004; Project End 30-APR-2005

Summary: (provided by applicant): **Kidney failure** due to **end-stage renal disease** is escalating at an alarming rate, motivating renal investigators and clinicians to identify research priorities and impediments in the search for better ways to prevent and treat renal disease. There is a crucial need for increases in resources and manpower in research in kidney disease. An impediment to renal research has been dwindling resources and loss of protected time to devote to their research in the face of an ever-increasing demand for further exploration of research ideas. There is a significant need and market potential for readily available reagents and tissue products from established models and human cases of renal disease. To address this deficit, Probetex was founded as a "Renal Research Resource Company" to create a repository of" off-the-shelf' tissue products from renal disease to provide readily available samples and help investigators to quickly and efficiently explore their research ideas on established and standardized models or identified cases of human renal disease. This Phase I application focuses on a line of sheep antibodies produced by Probetex that induce three classical immune models of human renal disease in the rat that have been widely used by the research community and represent salient pathological features observed in human renal disease: Mesangial Proliferative Glomeruonephritis (anti-Thy-1), Immune-mediated Crescentic Glomernlonephritis and Interstitial Nephritis (anti-GBM), and Membranous Nephropathy (anti-FxlA). This grant allows the company to verify the histopathological characteristics of each model and to produce and validate tissue products (tissue sections, protein lysates, purified RNA, and prefabricated Western and Northern blots) for potential commercialization. Probetex will develop a strategy for the manufacture of multiple tissue arrays of these products for comparison analysis of samples of different diseases in the same application. As part of the long-range goal, a plan for Phase II will be developed to expand the scope of products available in the repository by large-scale development, tissue procurement and out-sourcing strategies.

Website: http://crisp.cit.nih.gov/crisp/Crisp_Query.Generate_Screen

- **Project Title: TISSUE SPECIFIC NUTRITIONAL ADAPTATIONS IN RENAL FAILURE**

Principal Investigator & Institution: Price, S Russ.; Associate Professor; Medicine; Emory University 1784 North Decatur Road Atlanta, Ga 30322

Timing: Fiscal Year 2002; Project Start 01-AUG-1996; Project End 31-MAY-2004

Summary: The essential branched-chain amino acids (BCAA) play critical roles in maintaining normal protein homeostasis and they influence critical intracellular signaling pathways that regulate metabolic functions. In normal individuals, nutritional adaptations to a reduced dietary protein intake (e.g., fasting, a low protein diet prescription) decrease the irreversible degradation of BCAA. Catabolic conditions like chronic **renal failure** (CRF) or acute diabetes impair these adaptive responses that preserve protein mass, thus contributing to the loss of lean body mass. The goals of Dr. Price and colleagues are to understand the mechanisms that regulate the activity of branched-chain alpha-ketoacid dehydrogenase (BCKAD), the rate-limiting enzyme in BCAA degradation, in the major tissues where BCAA are catabolized, and to determine if there are common signals in different catabolic states that regulate BCKAD activity, and hence, BCAA levels. To address these goals, the investigators will evaluate three hypotheses: 1) Acidification and glucocorticoids influence transcription of BCKAD subunit genes through specific cis-acting response elements. The investigators will identify specific DNA promoter elements in the BCKAD E2 gene that confer responses to acidification and glucocorticoids. 2) Abnormalities in BCAA utilization in rats with CRF result from tissue-specific alterations in BCKAD activity at both genetic and biochemical levels. The investigators will define how CRF influences the activities of BCKAD and BCKAD kinase, a unique kinase that inhibits BCKAD activity, in muscle, liver and kidney in a well-established rat model. They will measure BCKAD activity, BCKAD subunit and kinase proteins and amounts of subunit and kinase mRNAs 3) Insulin modulates BCKAD and/or BCKAD activities in different tissues by a mechanism requiring the critical signaling enzyme phosphatidylinositol 3-kinase. The investigators will determine the biochemical mechanism(s) that increase BCKAD activity in rat muscle, liver and kidney in response to acute diabetes mellitus (i.e., insulin insufficiency) and then examine the signaling mechanisms by which insulin regulates BCKAD and BCKAD kinase in cultured L6 muscle cells. The investigators findings will define cellular mechanisms regulating BCAA degradation in **uremia,** acute diabetes and other catabolic conditions.

Website: http://crisp.cit.nih.gov/crisp/Crisp_Query.Generate_Screen

- **Project Title: TRAINING ON HEMODYNAMIC & GAS EXCHANGE DURING SUBMAXIMAL EXERCISE**

  Principal Investigator & Institution: Joyner, Michael J.; Professor; Mayo Clinic Coll of Medicine, Rochester D/B/A/ Mayo Clinic College of Medicine Rochester, Mn 55905

  Timing: Fiscal Year 2002

  Summary: Nephropathic cystinosis is an inherited disease with multiple clinical manifestations including Fanconi's syndrome and progressive **kidney failure.** Within the past decade, cysteamine and phosphocysteamine were developed as orphan drugs. These compounds have now been found to be effective in reducing the rate of progression of cystinosis. However, multiple daily doses of medication and regular monitoring of white blood cell cystine levels are essential to optimal outcomes.

  Website: http://crisp.cit.nih.gov/crisp/Crisp_Query.Generate_Screen

## E-Journals: PubMed Central[16]

PubMed Central (PMC) is a digital archive of life sciences journal literature developed and managed by the National Center for Biotechnology Information (NCBI) at the U.S. National Library of Medicine (NLM).[17] Access to this growing archive of e-journals is free and unrestricted.[18] To search, go to **http://www.pubmedcentral.nih.gov/index.html#search**, and type "kidney failure" (or synonyms) into the search box. This search gives you access to full-text articles. The following is a sample of items found for kidney failure in the PubMed Central database:

- **31P-magnetic resonance spectroscopy assessment of subnormal oxidative metabolism in skeletal muscle of renal failure patients..** by Moore GE, Bertocci LA, Painter PL.; 1993 Feb;

  http://www.pubmedcentral.gov/picrender.fcgi?tool=pmcentrez&action =stream&blobtype=pdf&artid=287944

---

[16] Adapted from the National Library of Medicine:
**http://www.pubmedcentral.nih.gov/about/intro.html**.
[17] With PubMed Central, NCBI is taking the lead in preservation and maintenance of open access to electronic literature, just as NLM has done for decades with printed biomedical literature. PubMed Central aims to become a world-class library of the digital age.
[18] The value of PubMed Central, in addition to its role as an archive, lies the availability of data from diverse sources stored in a common format in a single repository. Many journals already have online publishing operations, and there is a growing tendency to publish material online only, to the exclusion of print.

- **A micropuncture study of renal phosphate transport in rats with chronic renal failure and secondary hyperparathyroidism..** by Bank N, Su WS, Aynedjian HS.; 1978 Apr;
  http://www.pubmedcentral.gov/picrender.fcgi?tool=pmcentrez&action
  =stream&blobtype=pdf&artid=372607

- **Abnormal Carbohydrate Metabolism in Chronic Renal Failure THE POTENTIAL ROLE OF ACCELERATED GLUCOSE PRODUCTION, INCREASED GLUCONEOGENESIS, AND IMPAIRED GLUCOSE DISPOSAL.** by Rubenfeld S, Garber AJ.; 1978 Jul;
  http://www.pubmedcentral.gov/picrender.fcgi?tool=pmcentrez&action
  =stream&blobtype=pdf&artid=371732

- **Acute Renal Failure in an Infant Associated with Cytotoxic Aeromonas sobria Isolated from Patient's Stool and from Aquarium Water as Suspected Source of Infection.** by Filler G.; 2000 Jan;
  http://www.pubmedcentral.gov/articlerender.fcgi?tool=pmcentrez&arti
  d=88758

- **Acute renal failure induced by topical ketoprofen.** by Krummel T, Dimitrov Y, Moulin B, Hannedouche T.; 2000 Jan 8;
  http://www.pubmedcentral.gov/articlerender.fcgi?tool=pmcentrez&arti
  d=27256

- **Acute renal failure with selective medullary injury in the rat..** by Heyman SN, Brezis M, Reubinoff CA, Greenfeld Z, Lechene C, Epstein FH, Rosen S.; 1988 Aug;
  http://www.pubmedcentral.gov/picrender.fcgi?tool=pmcentrez&action
  =stream&blobtype=pdf&artid=303528

- **Acute, rapidly progressive renal failure with simultaneous use of amphotericin B and pentamidine..** by Antoniskis D, Larsen RA.; 1990 Mar;
  http://www.pubmedcentral.gov/picrender.fcgi?tool=pmcentrez&action
  =stream&blobtype=pdf&artid=171617

- **Atrial natriuretic peptide protects against acute ischemic renal failure in the rat..** by Shaw SG, Weidmann P, Hodler J, Zimmermann A, Paternostro A.; 1987 Nov;
  http://www.pubmedcentral.gov/picrender.fcgi?tool=pmcentrez&action
  =stream&blobtype=pdf&artid=442375

- **Defective Cellular Immunity in Renal Failure: Depression of Reactivity of Lymphocytes to Phytohemagglutinin by Renal Failure Serum.** by Newberry WM, Sanford JP.; 1971 Jun;
  http://www.pubmedcentral.gov/picrender.fcgi?tool=pmcentrez&action
  =stream&blobtype=pdf&artid=292056

- **Effect of chronic renal failure and hemodialysis on carbohydrate metabolism..** by Hampers CL, Soeldner JS, Doak PB, Merrill JP.; 1966 Nov;
  http://www.pubmedcentral.gov/picrender.fcgi?tool=pmcentrez&action=stream&blobtype=pdf&artid=292856

- **Effect of chronic renal failure on Na,K-ATPase alpha 1 and alpha 2 mRNA transcription in rat skeletal muscle..** by Bonilla S, Goecke IA, Bozzo S, Alvo M, Michea L, Marusic ET.; 1991 Dec;
  http://www.pubmedcentral.gov/picrender.fcgi?tool=pmcentrez&action=stream&blobtype=pdf&artid=295823

- **Effect of Experimental Chronic Renal Insufficiency on Bone Mineral and Collagen Maturation.** by Russell JE, Avioli LV.; 1972 Dec;
  http://www.pubmedcentral.gov/picrender.fcgi?tool=pmcentrez&action=stream&blobtype=pdf&artid=332989

- **Effect of Hemodialysis and Renal Failure on Serum and Urine Concentrations of Cephapirin Sodium.** by McCloskey RV, Terry EE, McCracken AW, Sweeney MJ, Forland MF.; 1972 Feb;
  http://www.pubmedcentral.gov/picrender.fcgi?tool=pmcentrez&action=stream&blobtype=pdf&artid=444174

- **Effect of Renal Failure and Dialysis on the Serum Concentration of the Aminoglycoside Amikacin.** by Madhavan T, Yaremchuk K, Levin N, Pohlod D, Burch K, Fisher E, Cox F, Quinn EL.; 1976 Sep;
  http://www.pubmedcentral.gov/picrender.fcgi?tool=pmcentrez&action=stream&blobtype=pdf&artid=429772

- **Effects of chronic renal failure on protein synthesis and albumin messenger ribonucleic acid in rat liver..** by Zern MA, Yap SH, Strair RK, Kaysen GA, Shafritz DA.; 1984 Apr;
  http://www.pubmedcentral.gov/picrender.fcgi?tool=pmcentrez&action=stream&blobtype=pdf&artid=425130

- **Effects of Renal Failure and Dialysis on Cefazolin Pharmacokinetics.** by Madhavan T, Yaremchuk K, Levin N, Fisher E, Cox F, Burch K, Haas E, Pohlod D, Quinn EL.; 1975 Jul;
  http://www.pubmedcentral.gov/picrender.fcgi?tool=pmcentrez&action=stream&blobtype=pdf&artid=429262

- **Elevated plasma concentrations of lipoprotein(a) in patients with end-stage renal disease are not related to the size polymorphism of apolipoprotein(a)..** by Dieplinger H, Lackner C, Kronenberg F, Sandholzer C, Lhotta K, Hoppichler F, Graf H, Konig P.; 1993 Feb;
  http://www.pubmedcentral.gov/picrender.fcgi?tool=pmcentrez&action=stream&blobtype=pdf&artid=287937

- **Evidence suggesting a role for hydroxyl radical in gentamicin-induced acute renal failure in rats..** by Walker PD, Shah SV.; 1988 Feb; http://www.pubmedcentral.gov/picrender.fcgi?tool=pmcentrez&action =stream&blobtype=pdf&artid=329575

- **Glomerular Endothelial Cells in Uranyl Nitrate-induced Acute Renal Failure in Rats.** by Avasthi PS, Evan AP, Hay D.; 1980 Jan; http://www.pubmedcentral.gov/picrender.fcgi?tool=pmcentrez&action =stream&blobtype=pdf&artid=371346

- **Glomerular hemodynamics in established glycerol-induced acute renal failure in the rat..** by Wolfert AI, Oken DE.; 1989 Dec; http://www.pubmedcentral.gov/picrender.fcgi?tool=pmcentrez&action =stream&blobtype=pdf&artid=304079

- **Glycerol-induced hemoglobinuric acute renal failure in the rat. I. Micropuncture study of the development of oliguria..** by Oken DE, Arce ML, Wilson DR.; 1966 May; http://www.pubmedcentral.gov/picrender.fcgi?tool=pmcentrez&action =stream&blobtype=pdf&artid=292749

- **Hepatocyte growth factor prevents acute renal failure and accelerates renal regeneration in mice..** by Kawaida K, Matsumoto K, Shimazu H, Nakamura T.; 1994 May 10; http://www.pubmedcentral.gov/picrender.fcgi?tool=pmcentrez&action =stream&blobtype=pdf&artid=43784

- **Increased levels of circulating islet amyloid polypeptide in patients with chronic renal failure have no effect on insulin secretion..** by Ludvik B, Clodi M, Kautzky-Willer A, Schuller M, Graf H, Hartter E, Pacini G, Prager R.; 1994 Nov; http://www.pubmedcentral.gov/picrender.fcgi?tool=pmcentrez&action =stream&blobtype=pdf&artid=294639

- **Increased nitric oxide synthase activity despite lack of response to endothelium-dependent vasodilators in postischemic acute renal failure in rats..** by Conger J, Robinette J, Villar A, Raij L, Shultz P.; 1995 Jul; http://www.pubmedcentral.gov/picrender.fcgi?tool=pmcentrez&action =stream&blobtype=pdf&artid=185238

- **Increased plasma phenylacetic acid in patients with end-stage renal failure inhibits iNOS expression.** by Jankowski J, van der Giet M, Jankowski V, Schmidt S, Hemeier M, Mahn B, Giebing G, Tolle M, Luftmann H, Schluter H, Zidek W, Tepel M.; 2003 Jul 15; http://www.pubmedcentral.gov/articlerender.fcgi?tool=pmcentrez&arti d=164281

- **Influence of chronic renal failure on protein synthesis and albumin metabolism in rat liver..** by Grossman SB, Yap SH, Shafritz DA.; 1977 May;
  http://www.pubmedcentral.gov/picrender.fcgi?tool=pmcentrez&action=stream&blobtype=pdf&artid=372295

- **Influence of Renal Failure on Ciprofloxacin Pharmacokinetics in Rats.** by Nouaille-Degorce B, Veau C, Dautrey S, Tod M, Laouari D, Carbon C, Farinotti R.; 1998 Feb;
  http://www.pubmedcentral.gov/articlerender.fcgi?tool=pmcentrez&artid=105402

- **Influence of Renal Failure on Intestinal Clearance of Ciprofloxacin in Rats.** by Dautrey S, Rabbaa L, Laouari D, Lacour B, Carbon C, Farinotti R.; 1999 Mar;
  http://www.pubmedcentral.gov/articlerender.fcgi?tool=pmcentrez&artid=89180

- **Ischemic acute renal failure and antioxidant therapy in the rat. The relation between glomerular and tubular dysfunction..** by Bird JE, Milhoan K, Wilson CB, Young SG, Mundy CA, Parthasarathy S, Blantz RC.; 1988 May;
  http://www.pubmedcentral.gov/picrender.fcgi?tool=pmcentrez&action=stream&blobtype=pdf&artid=442599

- **Kinetic disposition of intravenous ceftriaxone in normal subjects and patients with renal failure on hemodialysis or peritoneal dialysis..** by Ti TY, Fortin L, Kreeft JH, East DS, Ogilvie RI, Somerville PJ.; 1984 Jan;
  http://www.pubmedcentral.gov/picrender.fcgi?tool=pmcentrez&action=stream&blobtype=pdf&artid=185440

- **Micropuncture Studies of the Recovery Phase of Myohemoglobinuric Acute Renal Failure in the Rat.** by Oken DE, DiBona GF, McDonald FD.; 1970 Apr;
  http://www.pubmedcentral.gov/picrender.fcgi?tool=pmcentrez&action=stream&blobtype=pdf&artid=322528

- **Monoclonality of parathyroid tumors in chronic renal failure and in primary parathyroid hyperplasia..** by Arnold A, Brown MF, Urena P, Gaz RD, Sarfati E, Drueke TB.; 1995 May;
  http://www.pubmedcentral.gov/picrender.fcgi?tool=pmcentrez&action=stream&blobtype=pdf&artid=295791

- **Neurodiagnostic Abnormalities in Patients with Acute Renal Failure EVIDENCE FOR NEUROTOXICITY OF PARATHYROID HORMONE.** by Cooper JD, Lazarowitz VC, Arieff AI.; 1978 Jun; http://www.pubmedcentral.gov/picrender.fcgi?tool=pmcentrez&action =stream&blobtype=pdf&artid=372670

- **Oxygen free radicals in ischemic acute renal failure in the rat..** by Paller MS, Hoidal JR, Ferris TF.; 1984 Oct; http://www.pubmedcentral.gov/picrender.fcgi?tool=pmcentrez&action =stream&blobtype=pdf&artid=425281

- **Parathyroid cell proliferation in normal and chronic renal failure rats. The effects of calcium, phosphate, and vitamin D..** by Naveh-Many T, Rahamimov R, Livni N, Silver J.; 1995 Oct; http://www.pubmedcentral.gov/picrender.fcgi?tool=pmcentrez&action =stream&blobtype=pdf&artid=185815

- **Pathophysiology of protracted acute renal failure in man..** by Moran SM, Myers BD.; 1985 Oct; http://www.pubmedcentral.gov/picrender.fcgi?tool=pmcentrez&action =stream&blobtype=pdf&artid=424096

- **Pharmacokinetics of ampicillin (2.0 grams) and sulbactam (1.0 gram) coadministered to subjects with normal and abnormal renal function and with end-stage renal disease on hemodialysis..** by Blum RA, Kohli RK, Harrison NJ, Schentag JJ.; 1989 Sep; http://www.pubmedcentral.gov/picrender.fcgi?tool=pmcentrez&action =stream&blobtype=pdf&artid=172685

- **Pharmacokinetics of Cefamandole in the Presence of Renal Failure and in Patients Undergoing Hemodialysis.** by Appel GB, Neu HC, Parry MF, Goldberger MJ, Jacob GB.; 1976 Oct; http://www.pubmedcentral.gov/picrender.fcgi?tool=pmcentrez&action =stream&blobtype=pdf&artid=429804

- **Pharmacokinetics of cefoperazone (2.0 g) and sulbactam (1.0 g) coadministered to subjects with normal renal function, patients with decreased renal function, and patients with end-stage renal disease on hemodialysis..** by Reitberg DP, Marble DA, Schultz RW, Whall TJ, Schentag JJ.; 1988 Apr; http://www.pubmedcentral.gov/picrender.fcgi?tool=pmcentrez&action =stream&blobtype=pdf&artid=172210

- **Pharmacokinetics of ceforanide in patients with end stage renal disease on hemodialysis..** by Hess JR, Berman SJ, Boughton WH, Sugihara JG, Musgrave JE, Wong EG, Siemsen AM.; 1980 Feb; http://www.pubmedcentral.gov/picrender.fcgi?tool=pmcentrez&action =stream&blobtype=pdf&artid=283766

- **Pharmacokinetics of ceftriaxone in patients with renal failure and in those undergoing hemodialysis..** by Cohen D, Appel GB, Scully B, Neu HC.; 1983 Oct;
  http://www.pubmedcentral.gov/picrender.fcgi?tool=pmcentrez&action=stream&blobtype=pdf&artid=185368

- **Pharmacokinetics of Meropenem in Critically Ill Patients with Acute Renal Failure Treated by Continuous Hemodiafiltration.** by Krueger WA, Schroeder TH, Hutchison M, Hoffmann E, Dieterich HJ, Heininger A, Erley C, Wehrle A, Unertl K.; 1998 Sep;
  http://www.pubmedcentral.gov/articlerender.fcgi?tool=pmcentrez&artid=105844

- **Pharmacokinetics of moxalactam in patients with renal failure and during hemodialysis..** by Srinivasan S, Neu HC.; 1981 Sep;
  http://www.pubmedcentral.gov/picrender.fcgi?tool=pmcentrez&action=stream&blobtype=pdf&artid=181708

- **Pharmacokinetics of piperacillin in patients with moderate renal failure and in patients undergoing hemodialysis..** by Giron JA, Meyers BR, Hirschman SZ, Srulevitch E.; 1981 Feb;
  http://www.pubmedcentral.gov/picrender.fcgi?tool=pmcentrez&action=stream&blobtype=pdf&artid=181409

- **Pharmacokinetics, protein binding, and predicted extravascular distribution of moxalactam in normal and renal failure subjects..** by Peterson LR, Bean B, Fasching CE, Korchik WP, Gerding DN.; 1981 Sep;
  http://www.pubmedcentral.gov/picrender.fcgi?tool=pmcentrez&action=stream&blobtype=pdf&artid=181704

- **Renal Distribution Volumes of Indocyanine Green, [51Cr]EDTA, and 24Na in Man during Acute Renal Failure after Shock. IMPLICATIONS FOR THE PATHOGENESIS OF ANURIA.** by Reubi FC, Vorburger C, Tuckman J.; 1973 Feb;
  http://www.pubmedcentral.gov/picrender.fcgi?tool=pmcentrez&action=stream&blobtype=pdf&artid=302252

- **Renal Handling of Phosphorus in Oliguric and Nonoliguric Mercury-Induced Acute Renal Failure in Rats.** by Popovtzer MM, Massry SG, Villamil M, Kleeman CR.; 1971 Nov;
  http://www.pubmedcentral.gov/picrender.fcgi?tool=pmcentrez&action=stream&blobtype=pdf&artid=292177

- **Reversal of end-stage renal disease after aortic dissection using renal artery stent: a case report.** by Weiss AS, Ludkowski M, Parikh CR.; 2004;
  http://www.pubmedcentral.gov/articlerender.fcgi?tool=pmcentrez&artid=416478

- **Reversal of postischemic acute renal failure with a selective endothelinA receptor antagonist in the rat..** by Gellai M, Jugus M, Fletcher T, DeWolf R, Nambi P.; 1994 Feb;
  http://www.pubmedcentral.gov/picrender.fcgi?tool=pmcentrez&action=stream&blobtype=pdf&artid=293964

- **Shiga Toxin-Producing Escherichia coli-Associated Kidney Failure in a 40-Year-Old Patient and Late Diagnosis by Novel Bacteriologic and Toxin Detection Methods.** by Teel LD, Steinberg BR, Aronson NE, O'Brien AD.; 2003 Jul;
  http://www.pubmedcentral.gov/articlerender.fcgi?tool=pmcentrez&artid=165378

- **Steady-State Pharmacokinetics of Lamivudine in Human Immunodeficiency Virus-Infected Patients with End-Stage Renal Disease Receiving Chronic Dialysis.** by Bohjanen PR, Johnson MD, Szczech LA, Wray DW, Petros WP, Miller CR, Hicks CB.; 2002 Aug;
  http://www.pubmedcentral.gov/articlerender.fcgi?tool=pmcentrez&artid=127386

- **The anemia of chronic renal failure in sheep. Response to erythropoietin-rich plasma in vivo..** by Eschbach JW, Mladenovic J, Garcia JF, Wahl PW, Adamson JW.; 1984 Aug;
  http://www.pubmedcentral.gov/picrender.fcgi?tool=pmcentrez&action=stream&blobtype=pdf&artid=370494

- **The mechanism of acute renal failure after uranyl nitrate..** by Blantz RC.; 1975 Mar;
  http://www.pubmedcentral.gov/picrender.fcgi?tool=pmcentrez&action=stream&blobtype=pdf&artid=301791

- **Thyroid Dysfunction in Chronic Renal Failure A STUDY OF THE PITUITARY-THYROID AXIS AND PERIPHERAL TURNOVER KINETICS OF THYROXINE AND TRIIODOTHYRONINE.** by Lim VS, Fang VS, Katz AI, Refetoff S.; 1977 Sep;
  http://www.pubmedcentral.gov/picrender.fcgi?tool=pmcentrez&action=stream&blobtype=pdf&artid=372397

## The National Library of Medicine: PubMed

One of the quickest and most comprehensive ways to find academic studies in both English and other languages is to use PubMed, maintained by the National Library of Medicine. The advantage of PubMed over previously mentioned sources is that it covers a greater number of domestic and foreign references. It is also free to the public.[19] If the publisher has a Web site that offers full text of its journals, PubMed will provide links to that site, as well as to sites offering other related data. User registration, a subscription fee, or some other type of fee may be required to access the full text of articles in some journals.

To generate your own bibliography of studies dealing with kidney failure, simply go to the PubMed Web site at **www.ncbi.nlm.nih.gov/pubmed**. Type "kidney failure" (or synonyms) into the search box, and click "Go." The following is the type of output you can expect from PubMed for "kidney failure" (hyperlinks lead to article summaries):

- **A patient's guide to kidney failure.**
  Author(s): Carson A, Isles C.
  Source: Edtna Erca J. 1996 July-September; 22(3): 43-5.
  http://www.ncbi.nlm.nih.gov/entrez/query.fcgi?cmd=Retrieve&db=pubmed&dopt=Abstract&list_uids=10723335

- **Acute kidney failure: a pediatric experience over 20 years.**
  Author(s): Williams DM, Sreedhar SS, Mickell JJ, Chan JC.
  Source: Archives of Pediatrics & Adolescent Medicine. 2002 September; 156(9): 893-900. Review.
  http://www.ncbi.nlm.nih.gov/entrez/query.fcgi?cmd=Retrieve&db=pubmed&dopt=Abstract&list_uids=12197796

- **Acute kidney failure: prerenal, renal, or postrenal?**
  Author(s): Levinsky NG.
  Source: Hosp Pract (Off Ed). 1985 March 15; 20(3): 68G-68J, 68N, 68Q Passim. No Abstract Available.
  http://www.ncbi.nlm.nih.gov/entrez/query.fcgi?cmd=Retrieve&db=pubmed&dopt=Abstract&list_uids=3932406

---

[19] PubMed was developed by the National Center for Biotechnology Information (NCBI) at the National Library of Medicine (NLM) at the National Institutes of Health (NIH). The PubMed database was developed in conjunction with publishers of biomedical literature as a search tool for accessing literature citations and linking to full-text journal articles at Web sites of participating publishers. Publishers that participate in PubMed supply NLM with their citations electronically prior to or at the time of publication.

- **Adult type 1 primary hyperoxaluria: diagnosis by liver biopsy in a patient with end-stage kidney failure.**
  Author(s): Schillinger F, Montagnac R, Milcent T, Bressieux JM.
  Source: Journal of the American Academy of Dermatology. 1991 March; 24(3): 514-5.
  http://www.ncbi.nlm.nih.gov/entrez/query.fcgi?cmd=Retrieve&db=pubmed&dopt=Abstract&list_uids=2061463

- **Aggressive peritoneal dialysis for treatment of acute kidney failure after neonatal heart transplantation.**
  Author(s): Vricella LA, de Begona JA, Gundry SR, Vigesaa RE, Kawauchi M, Bailey LL.
  Source: The Journal of Heart and Lung Transplantation: the Official Publication of the International Society for Heart Transplantation. 1992 March-April; 11(2 Pt 1): 320-9.
  http://www.ncbi.nlm.nih.gov/entrez/query.fcgi?cmd=Retrieve&db=pubmed&dopt=Abstract&list_uids=1576138

- **An 8-year old boy with recurrent macroscopic hematuria, weight loss, and kidney failure.**
  Author(s): Kemper MJ, Bergstrasser E, Pawlik H, Gaspert A, Neuhaus TJ.
  Source: The Journal of Pediatrics. 2003 March; 142(3): 342-5.
  http://www.ncbi.nlm.nih.gov/entrez/query.fcgi?cmd=Retrieve&db=pubmed&dopt=Abstract&list_uids=12640387

- **Antithymocyte gamma globulin, low-dosage cyclosporine, and tapering steroids as an immunosuppressive regimen to avoid early kidney failure in heart transplantation.**
  Author(s): Deeb GM, Kolff J, McClurken JB, Dunn J, Balsara R, Ochs R, Badellino M, Hollander T, Eldridge C, Clancey M, et al.
  Source: J Heart Transplant. 1987 March-April; 6(2): 79-83.
  http://www.ncbi.nlm.nih.gov/entrez/query.fcgi?cmd=Retrieve&db=pubmed&dopt=Abstract&list_uids=3305833

- **Attitudes of Canadian nephrologists, family physicians and patients with kidney failure toward primary care delivery for chronic dialysis patients.**
  Author(s): Zimmerman DL, Selick A, Singh R, Mendelssohn DC.
  Source: Nephrology, Dialysis, Transplantation: Official Publication of the European Dialysis and Transplant Association - European Renal Association. 2003 February; 18(2): 305-9.
  http://www.ncbi.nlm.nih.gov/entrez/query.fcgi?cmd=Retrieve&db=pubmed&dopt=Abstract&list_uids=12543885

- **Bile composition in patients with chronic renal insufficiency.**
  Author(s): Mareckova O, Skala I, Marecek Z, Maly J, Kocandrle V, Schuck O, Blaha J, Prat V.
  Source: Nephrology, Dialysis, Transplantation: Official Publication of the European Dialysis and Transplant Association - European Renal Association. 1990; 5(6): 423-5.
  http://www.ncbi.nlm.nih.gov/entrez/query.fcgi?cmd=Retrieve&db=pubmed&dopt=Abstract&list_uids=2122317

- **Calcifying panniculitis and kidney failure. Considerations on pathogenesis and treatment of calciphylaxis.**
  Author(s): Grob JJ, Legre R, Bertocchio P, Payan MJ, Andrac L, Bonerandi JJ.
  Source: International Journal of Dermatology. 1989 March; 28(2): 129-31.
  http://www.ncbi.nlm.nih.gov/entrez/query.fcgi?cmd=Retrieve&db=pubmed&dopt=Abstract&list_uids=2737810

- **Cancer screening and life expectancy of Canadian patients with kidney failure.**
  Author(s): Kajbaf S, Nichol G, Zimmerman D.
  Source: Nephrology, Dialysis, Transplantation: Official Publication of the European Dialysis and Transplant Association - European Renal Association. 2002 October; 17(10): 1786-9.
  http://www.ncbi.nlm.nih.gov/entrez/query.fcgi?cmd=Retrieve&db=pubmed&dopt=Abstract&list_uids=12270985

- **Carbamoylation of glomerular and tubular proteins in patients with kidney failure: a potential mechanism of ongoing renal damage.**
  Author(s): Kraus LM, Gaber L, Handorf CR, Marti HP, Kraus AP Jr.
  Source: Swiss Medical Weekly: Official Journal of the Swiss Society of Infectious Diseases, the Swiss Society of Internal Medicine, the Swiss Society of Pneumology. 2001 March 24; 131(11-12): 139-4.
  http://www.ncbi.nlm.nih.gov/entrez/query.fcgi?cmd=Retrieve&db=pubmed&dopt=Abstract&list_uids=11416886

- **Cardiology patient page. Kidney failure and cardiovascular disease.**
  Author(s): Abbott KC, Bakris GL.
  Source: Circulation. 2003 October 21; 108(16): E114-5.
  http://www.ncbi.nlm.nih.gov/entrez/query.fcgi?cmd=Retrieve&db=pubmed&dopt=Abstract&list_uids=14568888

- **Care of the older person with kidney failure.**
  Author(s): Celis Villagomez MM.
  Source: Edtna Erca J. 1998 January-March; 24(1): 22-4.
  http://www.ncbi.nlm.nih.gov/entrez/query.fcgi?cmd=Retrieve&db=pubmed&dopt=Abstract&list_uids=9873280

- **Combined peritoneal and haemodialysis therapy for chronic renal insufficiency.**
  Author(s): Karatson A, Mako J, Szollosi G, Boros G, Solt I, Mehes M, Brasch H, Samik J.
  Source: International Urology and Nephrology. 1990; 22(4): 379-87.
  http://www.ncbi.nlm.nih.gov/entrez/query.fcgi?cmd=Retrieve&db=pubmed&dopt=Abstract&list_uids=2228501

- **Current status of prevention, diagnosis, and management of coronary artery disease in patients with kidney failure.**
  Author(s): Vaitkus PT.
  Source: American Heart Journal. 2000 June; 139(6): 1000-8. Review.
  http://www.ncbi.nlm.nih.gov/entrez/query.fcgi?cmd=Retrieve&db=pubmed&dopt=Abstract&list_uids=10827380

- **Death attributed to kidney failure in communities with endemic urinary schistosomiasis.**
  Author(s): Forsyth DM, Bradley DJ, McMahon J.
  Source: Lancet. 1970 August 29; 2(7670): 472-3.
  http://www.ncbi.nlm.nih.gov/entrez/query.fcgi?cmd=Retrieve&db=pubmed&dopt=Abstract&list_uids=4195155

- **Delayed nephrologist referral and inadequate vascular access in patients with advanced chronic kidney failure.**
  Author(s): Avorn J, Winkelmayer WC, Bohn RL, Levin R, Glynn RJ, Levy E, Owen W Jr.
  Source: Journal of Clinical Epidemiology. 2002 July; 55(7): 711-6.
  http://www.ncbi.nlm.nih.gov/entrez/query.fcgi?cmd=Retrieve&db=pubmed&dopt=Abstract&list_uids=12160919

- **Development of an instrument to measure knowledge about kidney function, kidney failure, and treatment options.**
  Author(s): Chambers JK, Boggs DL.
  Source: Anna J. 1993 December; 20(6): 637-42, 650; Discussion 643.
  http://www.ncbi.nlm.nih.gov/entrez/query.fcgi?cmd=Retrieve&db=pubmed&dopt=Abstract&list_uids=8267407

- **Diabetes with kidney failure.**
  Author(s): Friedman EA.
  Source: Lancet. 1986 November 29; 2(8518): 1285.
  http://www.ncbi.nlm.nih.gov/entrez/query.fcgi?cmd=Retrieve&db=pubmed&dopt=Abstract&list_uids=2878168

- **Diagnosis of functional kidney failure of cirrhosis with Doppler sonography: prognostic value of resistive index.**
  Author(s): Maroto A, Gines A, Salo J, Claria J, Gines P, Anibarro L, Jimenez W, Arroyo V, Rodes J.
  Source: Hepatology (Baltimore, Md.). 1994 October; 20(4 Pt 1): 839-44.
  http://www.ncbi.nlm.nih.gov/entrez/query.fcgi?cmd=Retrieve&db=pubmed&dopt=Abstract&list_uids=7927224

- **Digoxin, hyperkalemia, and kidney failure.**
  Author(s): Jain A, Lin ST.
  Source: Annals of Emergency Medicine. 1997 May; 29(5): 696; Author Reply 696-7.
  http://www.ncbi.nlm.nih.gov/entrez/query.fcgi?cmd=Retrieve&db=pubmed&dopt=Abstract&list_uids=9140262

- **Digoxin, hyperkalemia, and kidney failure.**
  Author(s): Kuhn M.
  Source: Annals of Emergency Medicine. 1997 May; 29(5): 695-6; Author Reply 696-7.
  http://www.ncbi.nlm.nih.gov/entrez/query.fcgi?cmd=Retrieve&db=pubmed&dopt=Abstract&list_uids=9140261

- **Digoxin, hyperkalemia, and kidney failure.**
  Author(s): Rees SM, Nelson L.
  Source: Annals of Emergency Medicine. 1997 May; 29(5): 694-5; Author Reply 696-7.
  http://www.ncbi.nlm.nih.gov/entrez/query.fcgi?cmd=Retrieve&db=pubmed&dopt=Abstract&list_uids=9140260

- **Disease management for Medicaid's kidney failure patients: the Florida initiative.**
  Author(s): Bozikis JP.
  Source: Nephrol News Issues. 2001 April; 15(5): 31-2, 38-40. No Abstract Available.
  http://www.ncbi.nlm.nih.gov/entrez/query.fcgi?cmd=Retrieve&db=pubmed&dopt=Abstract&list_uids=12108961

- **Disposition of digoxin immune Fab in patients with kidney failure.**
  Author(s): Ujhelyi MR, Robert S, Cummings DM, Colucci RD, Sailstad JM, Vlasses PH, Findlay JW, Zarowitz BJ.
  Source: Clinical Pharmacology and Therapeutics. 1993 October; 54(4): 388-94.
  http://www.ncbi.nlm.nih.gov/entrez/query.fcgi?cmd=Retrieve&db=pubmed&dopt=Abstract&list_uids=8222481

- **Does chronic kidney failure lead to mental failure? A neuropsychologic survey of self-sufficient outpatients.**
  Author(s): Brancaccio D, Damasso R, Spinnler H, Sterzi R, Vallar G.
  Source: Archives of Neurology. 1981 December; 38(12): 757-8.
  http://www.ncbi.nlm.nih.gov/entrez/query.fcgi?cmd=Retrieve&db=pubmed&dopt=Abstract&list_uids=6797387

- **Does end-stage kidney failure influence hepatitis C progression in hemodialysis patients?**
  Author(s): Luzar B, Ferlan-Marolt V, Brinovec V, Lesnicar G, Klopcic U, Poljak M.
  Source: Hepatogastroenterology. 2003 January-February; 50(49): 157-60.
  http://www.ncbi.nlm.nih.gov/entrez/query.fcgi?cmd=Retrieve&db=pubmed&dopt=Abstract&list_uids=12630013

- **Dramatic reduction in sandimmune (CyA) dosage may be effective in reversal of severe hyperbilirubinemia and post-transplant acute kidney failure linked to CyA toxicity.**
  Author(s): Szewczyk Z, Hruby Z, Uzar J, Skora K, Szydlowski Z, Witkiewicz W, Patrzalek D.
  Source: Transplantation Proceedings. 1987 October; 19(5): 4021-4.
  http://www.ncbi.nlm.nih.gov/entrez/query.fcgi?cmd=Retrieve&db=pubmed&dopt=Abstract&list_uids=3313989

- **Elevated blood concentrations of cyclosporine and kidney failure after bezafibrate in renal graft recipient.**
  Author(s): Hirai M, Tatuso E, Sakurai M, Ichikawa M, Matsuya F, Saito Y.
  Source: The Annals of Pharmacotherapy. 1996 July-August; 30(7-8): 883-4.
  http://www.ncbi.nlm.nih.gov/entrez/query.fcgi?cmd=Retrieve&db=pubmed&dopt=Abstract&list_uids=8826580

- **End-stage kidney failure in children: a brief commentary on hemodialysis and transplantation.**
  Author(s): Chan JC.
  Source: Clinical Pediatrics. 1976 November; 15(11): 991-5.
  http://www.ncbi.nlm.nih.gov/entrez/query.fcgi?cmd=Retrieve&db=pubmed&dopt=Abstract&list_uids=788987

- **Extraskeletal calcification in patients with chronic kidney failure.**
  Author(s): Drueke TB, Touam M, Thornley-Brown D, Rostand SG.
  Source: Adv Nephrol Necker Hosp. 2000; 30: 333-56. Review. No Abstract Available.
  http://www.ncbi.nlm.nih.gov/entrez/query.fcgi?cmd=Retrieve&db=pubmed&dopt=Abstract&list_uids=11068650

- **Fibrosis causes progressive kidney failure.**
  Author(s): Cohen EP.
  Source: Medical Hypotheses. 1995 November; 45(5): 459-62. Review.
  http://www.ncbi.nlm.nih.gov/entrez/query.fcgi?cmd=Retrieve&db=pubmed&dopt=Abstract&list_uids=8748086

- **Fluid balance modelling in patients with kidney failure.**
  Author(s): Chamney PW, Johner C, Aldridge C, Kramer M, Valasco N, Tattersall JE, Aukaidey T, Gordon R, Greenwood RN.
  Source: Journal of Medical Engineering & Technology. 1999 March-April; 23(2): 45-52.
  http://www.ncbi.nlm.nih.gov/entrez/query.fcgi?cmd=Retrieve&db=pubmed&dopt=Abstract&list_uids=10356673

- **Gastric intramucosal acidosis in patients with chronic kidney failure.**
  Author(s): Diebel L, Kozol R, Wilson RF, Mahajan S, Abu-Hamdan D, Thomas D.
  Source: Surgery. 1993 May; 113(5): 520-6.
  http://www.ncbi.nlm.nih.gov/entrez/query.fcgi?cmd=Retrieve&db=pubmed&dopt=Abstract&list_uids=8488469

- **Granulomatous interstitial nephritis, hypercalcemia and rapidly progressive kidney failure secondary to sarcoidosis with exclusive renal involvement.**
  Author(s): Fernandez Giron F, Fernandez Mora F, Conde-Garcia J, Benitez Sanchez M, Merino Perez MJ, Cruz Munoz S, Gonzalez Martinez J.
  Source: American Journal of Nephrology. 2001 November-December; 21(6): 514-6.
  http://www.ncbi.nlm.nih.gov/entrez/query.fcgi?cmd=Retrieve&db=pubmed&dopt=Abstract&list_uids=11799273

- **Growth factors in the treatment of wasting in kidney failure.**
  Author(s): Chen Y, Fervenza FC, Rabkin R.
  Source: Journal of Renal Nutrition: the Official Journal of the Council on Renal Nutrition of the National Kidney Foundation. 2001 April; 11(2): 62-6. Review.
  http://www.ncbi.nlm.nih.gov/entrez/query.fcgi?cmd=Retrieve&db=pubmed&dopt=Abstract&list_uids=11295025

- **Home dialysis for kidney failure.**
  Author(s): Blagg CR, Sawyer TK.
  Source: The New England Journal of Medicine. 1973 September 6; 289(10): 537.
  http://www.ncbi.nlm.nih.gov/entrez/query.fcgi?cmd=Retrieve&db=pubmed&dopt=Abstract&list_uids=4723579

- **Hyperkalemia and digoxin toxicity in a patient with kidney failure.**
  Author(s): Fenton F, Smally AJ, Laut J.
  Source: Annals of Emergency Medicine. 1996 October; 28(4): 440-1.
  http://www.ncbi.nlm.nih.gov/entrez/query.fcgi?cmd=Retrieve&db=pubmed&dopt=Abstract&list_uids=8839532

- **Hyperosmolar nonketotic syndrome associated with rhabdomyolysis and acute kidney failure.**
  Author(s): Lustman CC, Guerin JM, Barbotin-Larrieu FE.
  Source: Diabetes Care. 1991 February; 14(2): 146-7.
  http://www.ncbi.nlm.nih.gov/entrez/query.fcgi?cmd=Retrieve&db=pubmed&dopt=Abstract&list_uids=2060421

- **Intestinal dialysis for kidney failure. Personal experience.**
  Author(s): Schloerb PR.
  Source: Asaio Trans. 1990 January-March; 36(1): 4-7. No Abstract Available.
  http://www.ncbi.nlm.nih.gov/entrez/query.fcgi?cmd=Retrieve&db=pubmed&dopt=Abstract&list_uids=2407279

- **Introduction: diabetes and kidney failure.**
  Author(s): Friedman EA.
  Source: Adv Ren Replace Ther. 2001 January; 8(1): 1-3. Review. No Abstract Available.
  http://www.ncbi.nlm.nih.gov/entrez/query.fcgi?cmd=Retrieve&db=pubmed&dopt=Abstract&list_uids=11172322

- **Kidney failure after treatment with 90Y-DOTATOC.**
  Author(s): Schumacher T, Waldherr C, Mueller-Brand J, Maecke H.
  Source: European Journal of Nuclear Medicine and Molecular Imaging. 2002 March; 29(3): 435.
  http://www.ncbi.nlm.nih.gov/entrez/query.fcgi?cmd=Retrieve&db=pubmed&dopt=Abstract&list_uids=12002721

- **Kidney failure and analgesic drugs.**
  Author(s): Horowitz RS, Wilson VL, Dart RC.
  Source: The New England Journal of Medicine. 1995 June 1; 332(22): 1515;
  Author Reply 1515-6.
  http://www.ncbi.nlm.nih.gov/entrez/query.fcgi?cmd=Retrieve&db=pu
  bmed&dopt=Abstract&list_uids=7739694

- **Kidney failure and analgesic drugs.**
  Author(s): Faich G.
  Source: The New England Journal of Medicine. 1995 June 1; 332(22): 1514;
  Author Reply 1515-6.
  http://www.ncbi.nlm.nih.gov/entrez/query.fcgi?cmd=Retrieve&db=pu
  bmed&dopt=Abstract&list_uids=7739693

- **Kidney failure and analgesic drugs.**
  Author(s): Nelson EB.
  Source: The New England Journal of Medicine. 1995 June 1; 332(22): 1514-
  5; Author Reply 1515-6.
  http://www.ncbi.nlm.nih.gov/entrez/query.fcgi?cmd=Retrieve&db=pu
  bmed&dopt=Abstract&list_uids=7619128

- **Kidney failure and transplantation in China.**
  Author(s): Ikels C.
  Source: Social Science & Medicine (1982). 1997 May; 44(9): 1271-83.
  http://www.ncbi.nlm.nih.gov/entrez/query.fcgi?cmd=Retrieve&db=pu
  bmed&dopt=Abstract&list_uids=9141161

- **Kidney failure due to methoxyflurane.**
  Author(s): Mazzia VD.
  Source: Leg Med. 1982;: 59-71. No Abstract Available.
  http://www.ncbi.nlm.nih.gov/entrez/query.fcgi?cmd=Retrieve&db=pu
  bmed&dopt=Abstract&list_uids=7121187

- **Kidney failure in infants and children.**
  Author(s): Chan JC, Williams DM, Roth KS.
  Source: Pediatrics in Review / American Academy of Pediatrics. 2002
  February; 23(2): 47-60. Review.
  http://www.ncbi.nlm.nih.gov/entrez/query.fcgi?cmd=Retrieve&db=pu
  bmed&dopt=Abstract&list_uids=11826257

- **Kidney failure in liver disease.**
  Author(s): Wardle EN.
  Source: British Medical Journal. 1978 July 1; 2(6129): 56.
  http://www.ncbi.nlm.nih.gov/entrez/query.fcgi?cmd=Retrieve&db=pubmed&dopt=Abstract&list_uids=678813

- **Kidney failure or cancer. Should immunosuppression be continued in a transplant patient with malignant melanoma?**
  Author(s): Cuchural GJ Jr, Levey AS, Pauker SG.
  Source: Medical Decision Making: an International Journal of the Society for Medical Decision Making. 1984; 4(1): 82-107.
  http://www.ncbi.nlm.nih.gov/entrez/query.fcgi?cmd=Retrieve&db=pubmed&dopt=Abstract&list_uids=6374354

- **Laragh's lessons in pathophysiology and clinical pearls for treating hypertension. Lesson XXIV: on the major roles of the renin system in the pathogenesis of hypertension and of its sequelae, heart attack, heart failure, kidney failure, and stroke: replies to commonly asked questions.**
  Author(s): Laragh J.
  Source: American Journal of Hypertension: Journal of the American Society of Hypertension. 2001 August; 14(8 Pt 1): 733-42. Review.
  http://www.ncbi.nlm.nih.gov/entrez/query.fcgi?cmd=Retrieve&db=pubmed&dopt=Abstract&list_uids=11497187

- **Leukemia and kidney failure: case presentation and review of the literature.**
  Author(s): Reed AM, Silberman T, Blau E.
  Source: Wmj. 1998 September; 97(8): 56-7. Review. No Abstract Available.
  http://www.ncbi.nlm.nih.gov/entrez/query.fcgi?cmd=Retrieve&db=pubmed&dopt=Abstract&list_uids=9775756

- **Lipoproteins and vascular changes in chronic kidney failure.**
  Author(s): Wanner C.
  Source: Adv Nephrol Necker Hosp. 2000; 30: 215-20. Review. No Abstract Available.
  http://www.ncbi.nlm.nih.gov/entrez/query.fcgi?cmd=Retrieve&db=pubmed&dopt=Abstract&list_uids=11068644

- **Medical nutrition therapy in chronic kidney failure: integrating clinical practice guidelines.**
  Author(s): Beto JA, Bansal VK.
  Source: Journal of the American Dietetic Association. 2004 March; 104(3): 404-9. Review.
  http://www.ncbi.nlm.nih.gov/entrez/query.fcgi?cmd=Retrieve&db=pubmed&dopt=Abstract&list_uids=14993863

- **Metabolic consequences of feeding a high-carbohydrate, high-fiber diet to diabetic patients with chronic kidney failure.**
  Author(s): Parillo M, Riccardi G, Pacioni D, Iovine C, Contaldo F, Isernia C, De Marco F, Perrotti N, Rivellese A.
  Source: The American Journal of Clinical Nutrition. 1988 August; 48(2): 255-9.
  http://www.ncbi.nlm.nih.gov/entrez/query.fcgi?cmd=Retrieve&db=pubmed&dopt=Abstract&list_uids=2841839

- **Morphine in kidney failure.**
  Author(s): Berkovitch M, Ito S, Shear NH, Koren G.
  Source: Clinical Pharmacology and Therapeutics. 1994 July; 56(1): 114.
  http://www.ncbi.nlm.nih.gov/entrez/query.fcgi?cmd=Retrieve&db=pubmed&dopt=Abstract&list_uids=8033489

- **Mucocele of the appendix: an unusual cause of obstructive kidney failure.**
  Author(s): Parada R, Rosales A, Algaba F, Lluis F, Villavicencio H.
  Source: British Journal of Urology. 1998 September; 82(3): 444-5.
  http://www.ncbi.nlm.nih.gov/entrez/query.fcgi?cmd=Retrieve&db=pubmed&dopt=Abstract&list_uids=9772888

- **Mutation of BSND causes Bartter syndrome with sensorineural deafness and kidney failure.**
  Author(s): Birkenhager R, Otto E, Schurmann MJ, Vollmer M, Ruf EM, Maier-Lutz I, Beekmann F, Fekete A, Omran H, Feldmann D, Milford DV, Jeck N, Konrad M, Landau D, Knoers NV, Antignac C, Sudbrak R, Kispert A, Hildebrandt F.
  Source: Nature Genetics. 2001 November; 29(3): 310-4.
  http://www.ncbi.nlm.nih.gov/entrez/query.fcgi?cmd=Retrieve&db=pubmed&dopt=Abstract&list_uids=11687798

- **My kidney failure experiences.**
  Author(s): Lindsay M.
  Source: Adv Ren Replace Ther. 1997 October; 4(4): 400-1. No Abstract Available.
  http://www.ncbi.nlm.nih.gov/entrez/query.fcgi?cmd=Retrieve&db=pubmed&dopt=Abstract&list_uids=9356693

- **Normal response to anti-HBV vaccination in children with chronic renal insufficiency.**
  Author(s): La Manna A, Polito C, Foglia AC, Opallo A, Cafaro MR, Di Toro R.
  Source: Child Nephrol Urol. 1991; 11(4): 203-5.
  http://www.ncbi.nlm.nih.gov/entrez/query.fcgi?cmd=Retrieve&db=pubmed&dopt=Abstract&list_uids=1838031

- **Nutritional status of patients with different levels of chronic renal insufficiency. Modification of Diet in Renal Disease (MDRD) Study Group.**
  Author(s): Kopple JD, Berg R, Houser H, Steinman TI, Teschan P.
  Source: Kidney International. Supplement. 1989 November; 27: S184-94.
  http://www.ncbi.nlm.nih.gov/entrez/query.fcgi?cmd=Retrieve&db=pubmed&dopt=Abstract&list_uids=2636655

- **Nutritional therapy in kidney failure.**
  Author(s): Kopple JD.
  Source: Nutrition Reviews. 1981 May; 39(5): 193-206. Review.
  http://www.ncbi.nlm.nih.gov/entrez/query.fcgi?cmd=Retrieve&db=pubmed&dopt=Abstract&list_uids=6796915

- **Oral pharmacokinetics of pirenzepine in patients with chronic renal insufficiency, failure, and maintenance haemodialysis.**
  Author(s): MacGregor T, Matzek K, Keirns J, Vinocur M, Chonko A.
  Source: European Journal of Clinical Pharmacology. 1990; 38(4): 405-6.
  http://www.ncbi.nlm.nih.gov/entrez/query.fcgi?cmd=Retrieve&db=pubmed&dopt=Abstract&list_uids=2344866

- **Pharmacokinetics of nicotine in kidney failure.**
  Author(s): Molander L, Hansson A, Lunell E, Alainentalo L, Hoffmann M, Larsson R.
  Source: Clinical Pharmacology and Therapeutics. 2000 September; 68(3): 250-60.
  http://www.ncbi.nlm.nih.gov/entrez/query.fcgi?cmd=Retrieve&db=pubmed&dopt=Abstract&list_uids=11014406

- **Phosphate binder usage in kidney failure patients.**
  Author(s): Bleyer AJ.
  Source: Expert Opinion on Pharmacotherapy. 2003 June; 4(6): 941-7. Review.
  http://www.ncbi.nlm.nih.gov/entrez/query.fcgi?cmd=Retrieve&db=pubmed&dopt=Abstract&list_uids=12783590

- **Plasma and urinary growth hormone and insulin-like growth factor I in children with chronic renal insufficiency.**
  Author(s): Perrone L, Sinisi AA, Criscuolo T, Manzo T, Maresca G, Bellastella A, del Gado R.
  Source: Child Nephrol Urol. 1990; 10(2): 72-5.
  http://www.ncbi.nlm.nih.gov/entrez/query.fcgi?cmd=Retrieve&db=pubmed&dopt=Abstract&list_uids=2253254

- **Plasma levels of 5-hydroxyindole-acetic acid in chronic renal insufficiency and their effect on platelet aggregation.**
  Author(s): Sebekova K, Opatrny K, Dzurik R.
  Source: Nephron. 1991; 58(2): 253-4.
  http://www.ncbi.nlm.nih.gov/entrez/query.fcgi?cmd=Retrieve&db=pubmed&dopt=Abstract&list_uids=1714044

- **Praying for the power of patience (POP)--life is great, even with kidney failure!**
  Author(s): DeCuir JR.
  Source: Adv Ren Replace Ther. 1998 July; 5(3): 252-3. No Abstract Available.
  http://www.ncbi.nlm.nih.gov/entrez/query.fcgi?cmd=Retrieve&db=pubmed&dopt=Abstract&list_uids=9686636

- **Prevalence of anemia and correlations with mild and chronic renal insufficiency.**
  Author(s): Boineau FG, Lewy JE, Roy S, Baluarte G, Pomrantz A, Waldo B.
  Source: The Journal of Pediatrics. 1990 February; 116(2): S60-2.
  http://www.ncbi.nlm.nih.gov/entrez/query.fcgi?cmd=Retrieve&db=pubmed&dopt=Abstract&list_uids=2299484

- **Prevalence of chronic renal insufficiency in the course of idiopathic recurrent calcium stone disease: risk factors and patterns of progression.**
  Author(s): Marangella M, Bruno M, Cosseddu D, Manganaro M, Tricerri A, Vitale C, Linari F.
  Source: Nephron. 1990; 54(4): 302-6.
  http://www.ncbi.nlm.nih.gov/entrez/query.fcgi?cmd=Retrieve&db=pubmed&dopt=Abstract&list_uids=2325794

- **Preventing acute renal failure in patients with chronic renal insufficiency: nursing implications.**
  Author(s): Zorzanello MM.
  Source: Anna J. 1989 October; 16(6): 433-8.
  http://www.ncbi.nlm.nih.gov/entrez/query.fcgi?cmd=Retrieve&db=pubmed&dopt=Abstract&list_uids=2818012

- **Preventing kidney failure: primary care physicians must intervene earlier.**
  Author(s): Hebert CJ.
  Source: Cleve Clin J Med. 2003 April; 70(4): 337-44. Erratum In: Cleve Clin J Med. 2003 June; 70(6): 501.
  http://www.ncbi.nlm.nih.gov/entrez/query.fcgi?cmd=Retrieve&db=pubmed&dopt=Abstract&list_uids=12701988

- **Prevention of end-stage kidney failure.**
  Author(s): Asscher AW.
  Source: Verh Dtsch Ges Inn Med. 1974; 80: 594-7. No Abstract Available.
  http://www.ncbi.nlm.nih.gov/entrez/query.fcgi?cmd=Retrieve&db=pubmed&dopt=Abstract&list_uids=4454628

- **Relation between pediatric experience and treatment recommendations for children and adolescents with kidney failure.**
  Author(s): Furth SL, Hwang W, Yang C, Neu AM, Fivush BA, Powe NR.
  Source: Jama: the Journal of the American Medical Association. 2001 February 28; 285(8): 1027-33.
  http://www.ncbi.nlm.nih.gov/entrez/query.fcgi?cmd=Retrieve&db=pubmed&dopt=Abstract&list_uids=11209173

- **Renal dialysis for kidney failure in North Carolina: history, practice, and lessons.**
  Author(s): Gutman RA.
  Source: N C Med J. 1984 June; 45(6): 359-63. No Abstract Available.
  http://www.ncbi.nlm.nih.gov/entrez/query.fcgi?cmd=Retrieve&db=pubmed&dopt=Abstract&list_uids=6377092

- **Renal functional response to dopamine during and after arteriography in patients with chronic renal insufficiency.**
  Author(s): Hans B, Hans SS, Mittal VK, Khan TA, Patel N, Dahn MS.
  Source: Radiology. 1990 September; 176(3): 651-4.
  http://www.ncbi.nlm.nih.gov/entrez/query.fcgi?cmd=Retrieve&db=pubmed&dopt=Abstract&list_uids=2202010

- **Renal osteodystrophy in children with end-stage kidney failure.**
  Author(s): Chan JC.
  Source: Va Med. 1979 May; 106(5): 384-90.
  http://www.ncbi.nlm.nih.gov/entrez/query.fcgi?cmd=Retrieve&db=pubmed&dopt=Abstract&list_uids=463255

- **Respiratory distress and kidney failure in a 9-month-old infant.**
  Author(s): Toomey DA, Landier W.
  Source: Journal of Pediatric Health Care: Official Publication of National Association of Pediatric Nurse Associates & Practitioners. 1998 September-October; 12(5): 271-2, 283-4.
  http://www.ncbi.nlm.nih.gov/entrez/query.fcgi?cmd=Retrieve&db=pubmed&dopt=Abstract&list_uids=9987260

- **Reversal of end-stage kidney failure in two scleroderma patients treated with anticoagulation.**
  Author(s): Kohorst WR, Bay WH.
  Source: American Journal of Kidney Diseases: the Official Journal of the National Kidney Foundation. 1982 November; 2(3): 347-8.
  http://www.ncbi.nlm.nih.gov/entrez/query.fcgi?cmd=Retrieve&db=pubmed&dopt=Abstract&list_uids=7148825

- **Risk of kidney failure associated with the use of acetaminophen, aspirin, and nonsteroidal antiinflammatory drugs.**
  Author(s): Perneger TV, Whelton PK, Klag MJ.
  Source: The New England Journal of Medicine. 1994 December 22; 331(25): 1675-9.
  http://www.ncbi.nlm.nih.gov/entrez/query.fcgi?cmd=Retrieve&db=pubmed&dopt=Abstract&list_uids=7969358

- **Serum cysteine proteinase inhibitors with special reference to kidney failure.**
  Author(s): Hopsu-Havu VK, Joronen I, Havu S, Rinne A, Jarvinen M, Forsstrom J.
  Source: Scandinavian Journal of Clinical and Laboratory Investigation. 1985 February; 45(1): 11-6.
  http://www.ncbi.nlm.nih.gov/entrez/query.fcgi?cmd=Retrieve&db=pubmed&dopt=Abstract&list_uids=3919439

- **Serum osteocalcin concentrations in children with chronic renal insufficiency who are not undergoing dialysis. Growth Failure in Children with Renal Diseases Study.**
  Author(s): Friedman AL, Heiliczer JD, Gundberg CM, Mak RH, Boineau FG, McEnery PT, Chan JC.
  Source: The Journal of Pediatrics. 1990 February; 116(2): S55-9.
  http://www.ncbi.nlm.nih.gov/entrez/query.fcgi?cmd=Retrieve&db=pubmed&dopt=Abstract&list_uids=2405137

- **Serum soluble Fas (CD95) and Fas ligand profiles in chronic kidney failure.**
  Author(s): Perianayagam MC, Murray SL, Balakrishnan VS, Guo D, King AJ, Pereira BJ, Jaber BL.
  Source: The Journal of Laboratory and Clinical Medicine. 2000 October; 136(4): 320-7.
  http://www.ncbi.nlm.nih.gov/entrez/query.fcgi?cmd=Retrieve&db=pubmed&dopt=Abstract&list_uids=11039853

- **Shiga toxin-producing Escherichia coli-associated kidney failure in a 40-year-old patient and late diagnosis by novel bacteriologic and toxin detection methods.**
  Author(s): Teel LD, Steinberg BR, Aronson NE, O'Brien AD.
  Source: Journal of Clinical Microbiology. 2003 July; 41(7): 3438-40.
  http://www.ncbi.nlm.nih.gov/entrez/query.fcgi?cmd=Retrieve&db=pubmed&dopt=Abstract&list_uids=12843115

- **Should kidney failure patients be treated for kidney function or urenic syndrome?**
  Author(s): Nose Y.
  Source: Artificial Organs. 1996 February; 20(2): 99-100.
  http://www.ncbi.nlm.nih.gov/entrez/query.fcgi?cmd=Retrieve&db=pubmed&dopt=Abstract&list_uids=8712968

- **Simultaneous heart and kidney transplantation as treatment for end-stage heart and kidney failure.**
  Author(s): Laufer G, Kocher A, Grabenwoger M, Berlakovich GA, Zuckermann A, Ofner P, Grimm M, Steininger R, Muhlbacher F.
  Source: Transplantation. 1997 October 27; 64(8): 1129-34.
  http://www.ncbi.nlm.nih.gov/entrez/query.fcgi?cmd=Retrieve&db=pubmed&dopt=Abstract&list_uids=9355828

- **Southwestern Internal Medicine Conference: bone disease in kidney failure: diagnosis and management.**
  Author(s): Cronin RE.
  Source: The American Journal of the Medical Sciences. 1993 September; 306(3): 192-205. Review.
  http://www.ncbi.nlm.nih.gov/entrez/query.fcgi?cmd=Retrieve&db=pubmed&dopt=Abstract&list_uids=8128983

- **The impact of transplantation on survival with kidney failure.**
  Author(s): Kasiske BL, Snyder J, Matas A, Collins A.
  Source: Clin Transpl. 2000;: 135-43.
  http://www.ncbi.nlm.nih.gov/entrez/query.fcgi?cmd=Retrieve&db=pubmed&dopt=Abstract&list_uids=11512307

- **The pharmacokinetics of morphine and morphine glucuronides in kidney failure.**
  Author(s): Osborne R, Joel S, Grebenik K, Trew D, Slevin M.
  Source: Clinical Pharmacology and Therapeutics. 1993 August; 54(2): 158-67.
  http://www.ncbi.nlm.nih.gov/entrez/query.fcgi?cmd=Retrieve&db=pubmed&dopt=Abstract&list_uids=8354025

- **The social contract and the treatment of permanent kidney failure.**
  Author(s): Rettig RA.
  Source: Jama: the Journal of the American Medical Association. 1996 April 10; 275(14): 1123-6.
  http://www.ncbi.nlm.nih.gov/entrez/query.fcgi?cmd=Retrieve&db=pubmed&dopt=Abstract&list_uids=8601933

- **Twenty-four-hour plasma growth hormone (GH) profiles, urinary GH excretion, and plasma insulin-like growth factor-I and -II levels in prepubertal children with chronic renal insufficiency and severe growth retardation.**
  Author(s): Hokken-Koelega AC, Hackeng WH, Stijnen T, Wit JM, de Muinck Keizer-Schrama SM, Drop SL.
  Source: The Journal of Clinical Endocrinology and Metabolism. 1990 September; 71(3): 688-95.
  http://www.ncbi.nlm.nih.gov/entrez/query.fcgi?cmd=Retrieve&db=pubmed&dopt=Abstract&list_uids=2394775

- **Urodilatin, a new therapy to prevent kidney failure after heart transplantation.**
  Author(s): Hummel M, Kuhn M, Bub A, Mann B, Schneider B, von Eickstedt KW, Forssmann WG, Hetzer R.
  Source: The Journal of Heart and Lung Transplantation: the Official Publication of the International Society for Heart Transplantation. 1993 March-April; 12(2): 209-17; Discussion 217-8.
  http://www.ncbi.nlm.nih.gov/entrez/query.fcgi?cmd=Retrieve&db=pubmed&dopt=Abstract&list_uids=8476893

- **Use of psychotropics in patients with kidney failure.**
  Author(s): Levy NB.
  Source: Psychosomatics. 1985 September; 26(9): 699-701, 705, 709.
  http://www.ncbi.nlm.nih.gov/entrez/query.fcgi?cmd=Retrieve&db=pubmed&dopt=Abstract&list_uids=4048374

- **Utility of radioisotopic filtration markers in chronic renal insufficiency: simultaneous comparison of 125I-iothalamate, 169Yb-DTPA, 99mTc-DTPA, and inulin. The Modification of Diet in Renal Disease Study.**
  Author(s): Perrone RD, Steinman TI, Beck GJ, Skibinski CI, Royal HD, Lawlor M, Hunsicker LG.
  Source: American Journal of Kidney Diseases: the Official Journal of the National Kidney Foundation. 1990 September; 16(3): 224-35.
  http://www.ncbi.nlm.nih.gov/entrez/query.fcgi?cmd=Retrieve&db=pubmed&dopt=Abstract&list_uids=2205098

- **Vasculitis with acute kidney failure and torasemide.**
  Author(s): Palop-Larrea V, Sancho-Calabuig A, Gorriz-Teruel JL, Martinez-Mir I, Pallardo-Mateu LM.
  Source: Lancet. 1998 December 12; 352(9144): 1909-10.
  http://www.ncbi.nlm.nih.gov/entrez/query.fcgi?cmd=Retrieve&db=pubmed&dopt=Abstract&list_uids=9863798

- **Vitamin E may slow kidney failure owing to oxidative stress.**
  Author(s): Fryer MJ.
  Source: Redox Report: Communications in Free Radical Research. 1997 October-December; 3(5-6): 259-61. Review.
  http://www.ncbi.nlm.nih.gov/entrez/query.fcgi?cmd=Retrieve&db=pubmed&dopt=Abstract&list_uids=9754323

- **Why are homocysteine levels increased in kidney failure? A metabolic approach.**
  Author(s): Blom HJ, De Vriese AS, De Vriese S.
  Source: The Journal of Laboratory and Clinical Medicine. 2002 May; 139(5): 262-8. Review. Erratum In: J Lab Clin Med 2002 September; 140(3): 210. De Vriese S [corrected to De Vriese an S].
  http://www.ncbi.nlm.nih.gov/entrez/query.fcgi?cmd=Retrieve&db=pubmed&dopt=Abstract&list_uids=12032486

- **Why don't the British treat more patients with kidney failure?**
  Author(s): Wing AJ.
  Source: British Medical Journal (Clinical Research Ed.). 1983 October 22; 287(6400): 1157-8.
  http://www.ncbi.nlm.nih.gov/entrez/query.fcgi?cmd=Retrieve&db=pubmed&dopt=Abstract&list_uids=6414608

# Vocabulary Builder

The following vocabulary builder provides definitions of words used in this chapter that have not been defined in previous chapters:

**Anorexia:** Lack or loss of appetite for food. Appetite is psychologic, dependent on memory and associations. Anorexia can be brought about by unattractive food, surroundings, or company. [NIH]

**ATP:** ATP an abbreviation for adenosine triphosphate, a compound which serves as a carrier of energy for cells. [NIH]

**Biophysics:** The science of physical phenomena and processes in living organisms. [NIH]

**Blot:** To transfer DNA, RNA, or proteins to an immobilizing matrix such as nitrocellulose. [NIH]

**CDNA:** Synthetic DNA reverse transcribed from a specific RNA through the action of the enzyme reverse transcriptase. DNA synthesized by reverse transcriptase using RNA as a template. [NIH]

**Chickenpox:** A mild, highly contagious virus characterized by itchy blisters all over the body. [NIH]

**Clamp:** A u-shaped steel rod used with a pin or wire for skeletal traction in the treatment of certain fractures. [NIH]

**Cloning:** The production of a number of genetically identical individuals; in genetic engineering, a process for the efficient replication of a great number of identical DNA molecules. [NIH]

**Cyclin:** Molecule that regulates the cell cycle. [NIH]

**Cytokine:** Small but highly potent protein that modulates the activity of many cell types, including T and B cells. [NIH]

**Deletion:** A genetic rearrangement through loss of segments of DNA (chromosomes), bringing sequences, which are normally separated, into close proximity. [NIH]

**Diaphragm:** Contraceptive intra-uterine device. [NIH]

**Dissection:** Cutting up of an organism for study. [NIH]

**Effector:** It is often an enzyme that converts an inactive precursor molecule into an active second messenger. [NIH]

**Embryogenesis:** The process of embryo or embryoid formation, whether by sexual (zygotic) or asexual means. In asexual embryogenesis embryoids arise directly from the explant or on intermediary callus tissue. In some cases they arise from individual cells (somatic cell embryoge). [NIH]

**Enamel:** A very hard whitish substance which covers the dentine of the anatomical crown of a tooth. [NIH]

**Fold:** A plication or doubling of various parts of the body. [NIH]

**FRC:** The functional residual capacity is the volume of gas remaining in the lungs at the end-expiratory level; the FRC has to be measured indirectly because the residual volume, RV, which is a subdivision of the FRC, cannot be removed from the lung; the techniques. [NIH]

**Heterogeneity:** The property of one or more samples or populations which implies that they are not identical in respect of some or all of their parameters, e. g. heterogeneity of variance. [NIH]

**Immunologic:** The ability of the antibody-forming system to recall a previous experience with an antigen and to respond to a second exposure with the prompt production of large amounts of antibody. [NIH]

**Initiation:** Mutation induced by a chemical reactive substance causing cell changes; being a step in a carcinogenic process. [NIH]

**Insight:** The capacity to understand one's own motives, to be aware of one's own psychodynamics, to appreciate the meaning of symbolic behavior. [NIH]

**Islet:** Cell producing insulin in pancreas. [NIH]

**Kb:** A measure of the length of DNA fragments, 1 Kb = 1000 base pairs. The largest DNA fragments are up to 50 kilobases long. [NIH]

**Linkage:** The tendency of two or more genes in the same chromosome to remain together from one generation to the next more frequently than expected according to the law of independent assortment. [NIH]

**Lod:** The lowest analyte content which, if actually present, will be detected with reasonable statistical certainty and can be identified according to the identification criteria of the method. If both accuracy and precision are constant over a concentration range. [NIH]

**Lymphoma:** Tumor of lymphatic tissue. [NIH]

**Modification:** A change in an organism, or in a process in an organism, that is acquired from its own activity or environment. [NIH]

**MRNA:** The RNA molecule that conveys from the DNA the information that is to be translated into the structure of a particular polypeptide molecule. [NIH]

**Neutrophil:** A motile, short-lived polymorphonuclear leucocyte with a multilobed nucleus and a cytoplasm filled with numerous minute granules, which is primarily responsible for maintaining normal host defenses against invading microorganisms. [NIH]

**Orf:** A specific disease of sheep and goats caused by a pox-virus that is transmissible to man and characterized by vesiculation and ulceration of the lips. [NIH]

**Patch:**  A piece of material used to cover or protect a wound, an injured part, etc.: a patch over the eye. [NIH]

**Pediatrics:**  The branch of medical science concerned with children and their diseases. [NIH]

**Pharmacokinetic:**  The mathematical analysis of the time courses of absorption, distribution, and elimination of drugs. [NIH]

**Phosphorylated:**  Attached to a phosphate group. [NIH]

**Phosphorylating:**  Attached to a phosphate group. [NIH]

**Plaque:**  A clear zone in a bacterial culture grown on an agar plate caused by localized destruction of bacterial cells by a bacteriophage. The concentration of infective virus in a fluid can be estimated by applying the fluid to a culture and counting the number of. [NIH]

**Plasticity:**  In an individual or a population, the capacity for adaptation: a) through gene changes (genetic plasticity) or b) through internal physiological modifications in response to changes of environment (physiological plasticity). [NIH]

**Pneumology:**  The study of disease of the air passages. [NIH]

**Polymorphism:**  The occurrence together of two or more distinct forms in the same population. [NIH]

**Promoter:**  A chemical substance that increases the activity of a carcinogenic process. [NIH]

**Protocol:**  The detailed plan for a clinical trial that states the trial's rationale, purpose, drug or vaccine dosages, length of study, routes of administration, who may participate, and other aspects of trial design. [NIH]

**Recombination:**  The formation of new combinations of genes as a result of segregation in crosses between genetically different parents; also the rearrangement of linked genes due to crossing-over. [NIH]

**Salivary:**  The duct that convey saliva to the mouth. [NIH]

**Segmental:**  Describing or pertaining to a structure which is repeated in similar form in successive segments of an organism, or which is undergoing segmentation. [NIH]

**Streptococcal:**  Caused by infection due to any species of streptococcus. [NIH]

**Therapeutics:**  The branch of medicine which is concerned with the treatment of diseases, palliative or curative. [NIH]

**Ulcer:**  A localized necrotic lesion of the skin or a mucous surface. [NIH]

**Vasodilators:**  Any nerve or agent which induces dilatation of the blood vessels. [NIH]

**Vector:** Plasmid or other self-replicating DNA molecule that transfers DNA between cells in nature or in recombinant DNA technology. [NIH]

**Vitro:** Descriptive of an event or enzyme reaction under experimental investigation occurring outside a living organism. Parts of an organism or microorganism are used together with artificial substrates and/or conditions. [NIH]

**Zoster:** A virus infection of the Gasserian ganglion and its nerve branches, characterized by discrete areas of vesiculation of the epithelium of the forehead, the nose, the eyelids, and the cornea together with subepithelial infiltration. [NIH]

# CHAPTER 4. PATENTS ON KIDNEY FAILURE

## Overview

You can learn about innovations relating to kidney failure by reading recent patents and patent applications. Patents can be physical innovations (e.g. chemicals, pharmaceuticals, medical equipment) or processes (e.g. treatments or diagnostic procedures). The United States Patent and Trademark Office defines a patent as a grant of a property right to the inventor, issued by the Patent and Trademark Office.[20] Patents, therefore, are intellectual property. For the United States, the term of a new patent is 20 years from the date when the patent application was filed. If the inventor wishes to receive economic benefits, it is likely that the invention will become commercially available to patients with kidney failure within 20 years of the initial filing. It is important to understand, therefore, that an inventor's patent does not indicate that a product or service is or will be commercially available to patients with kidney failure. The patent implies only that the inventor has "the right to exclude others from making, using, offering for sale, or selling" the invention in the United States. While this relates to U.S. patents, similar rules govern foreign patents.

In this chapter, we show you how to locate information on patents and their inventors. If you find a patent that is particularly interesting to you, contact the inventor or the assignee for further information.

---

[20]Adapted from The U. S. Patent and Trademark Office:
http://www.uspto.gov/web/offices/pac/doc/general/whatis.htm.

## Patents on Kidney Failure

By performing a patent search focusing on kidney failure, you can obtain information such as the title of the invention, the names of the inventor(s), the assignee(s) or the company that owns or controls the patent, a short abstract that summarizes the patent, and a few excerpts from the description of the patent. The abstract of a patent tends to be more technical in nature, while the description is often written for the public. Full patent descriptions contain much more information than is presented here (e.g. claims, references, figures, diagrams, etc.). We will tell you how to obtain this information later in the chapter. The following is an example of the type of information that you can expect to obtain from a patent search on kidney failure:

- **Agent for protecting against renal failure**

  Inventor(s): Inouye; Shigeharu (Yokohama, JP), Koeda; Takemi (Yokohama, JP), Niida; Taro (Yokohama, JP), Niizato; Tetsutaro (Kawasaki, JP), Tsuruoka; Takashi (Kawasaki, JP)

  Assignee(s): Neiji Seika Kaisha, Ltd. (Tokyo, JP)

  Patent Number: 4,122,171

  Date filed: April 11, 1977

  Abstract: D-glucaro-1,5-lactam and its pharmaceutically acceptable salts are useful as an agent of protecting against **renal failure** or damage induced by administration of aminoglycosidic antibiotics.

  Excerpt(s): This invention relates to an agent for protecting against **renal failure** or insufficiency which comprises as the active ingredient D-glucaro-1,5-lactam or a pharmaceutically acceptable salt thereof. More particularly, this invention relates to a drug for protecting against **renal failure** or insufficiency induced by a chemotherapeutic agent which is more or less nephrotoxic to the kidney, and especially this invention is directed to a drug for preventing **renal failure** induced by an aminoglycosidic antibiotic such as the kanamycins and 3',4'-dideoxykanamycin B. This invention further relates to a process for protecting against **renal failure** or insufficiency in animals or humans which is induced by oral or parenteral administration of aminoglycosidic antibiotic.... Aminoglycosidic antibiotics such as kanamycin A, kanamycin B, 3',4'-dideoxykanamycin B and gentamicin are widely used as antibacterial agents which are remarkably effective for therapeutic treatment of the infections caused by gram-negative and gram-positive bacteria and acid-fast bacteria. However, it has been stated that administration of aminoglycosidic antibiotic such as neomycins, kanamycins, streptomycin and gentamicin may frequently induce **renal failure** or insufficiency in humans as a main side-effect. It is known that various indicators of the degree of renal dysfunction become worse as the amount of aminoglycosidic antibiotic given to patients increase. It is also known that precaution must be taken when an aminoglycosidic antibiotic is given to such a patient suffering from **renal failure**.... To protect against or reduce **renal failure** or insufficiency induced by aminoglycosidic antibiotics is very beneficial in clinical practice. For instance, the "Journal of Antibiotics" Vol. 29, No. 2, pages 187-194 (February 1976) describes some tests where aceglactone (namely, 2,5-di-O-acetyl-D-glucaro-1,4;3,6-dilactone) and its related compounds such as D-glucaro-1,4;3,6-dilactone, sodium D-glucaro-1,4-lactone and sodium D-glucaro-3,6-lactone are administered to rats in an attempt to prevent against or reduce **renal failure** induced by aminoglycosidic antibiotics.

Web site: http://www.delphion.com/details?pn=US04122171__

- **Anipamil for the treatment of chronic renal failure**

  Inventor(s): Chan; Laurence (Auroro, CO), Kretzschmar; Rolf (Gruenstadt, DE), Lehmann; Hans D. (Hirschberg, DE), Schrier; Robert W. (Denver, CO)

  Assignee(s): BASF Aktiengesellschaft (Ludwigshafen, DE)

  Patent Number: 5,039,709

  Date filed: November 30, 1989

  Abstract: The use of anipamil and its salts with physiologically tolerated acids for the treatment of chronic **renal failure** is described.

  Excerpt(s): The present invention relates to a new use of 1,7-bis(3-methoxyphenyl)-7-cyano-3-methylazanonadecane (anipamil).... The object of the present invention was to find novel compounds for the treatment of chronic **renal failure**.... In accordance with this we have now found that anipamil and its physiologically tolerated salts can be used for the treatment of chronic **renal failure**.

  Web site: http://www.delphion.com/details?pn=US05039709__

- **Composition for alleviating symptoms of uremia in patients**

Inventor(s): Dickstein; Jack (Huntingdon Valley, PA), Ranganathan; Natarajan (Broomall, PA)

Assignee(s): Kibow Biotech Inc. (Philadelphia, PA)

Patent Number: 6,706,263

Date filed: April 20, 2000

Abstract: Microencapsulated and/or enteric coated compositions containing a mixture of sorbents with specific adsorption affinities for uremic toxins including ammonia, urea, creatinine, phenols, indoles, and middle molecular weight molecules and a bacterial source which metabolizes urea and ammonia are provided. Also provided are methods of using these compositions to alleviate symptoms of **uremia** in patients.

Excerpt(s): Kidney disease is ranked fourth among the major diseases in the United States afflicting over 20 million Americans. More than 90,000 patients die each year because of kidney diseases. In recent years the number of **chronic kidney failure** patients has increased about 11 percent annually. About 80,000 Americans on dialysis die of various complications each year and more than 27,000 are on waiting lists for kidney transplants each year with only about 11,000 of these patients receiving transplants.... Nearly 250,000 Americans suffer from **end stage renal disease** (ESRD), which is the final stage in chronic **renal failure.** Currently hemo- or peritoneal-dialysis and renal transplant are the only treatment modalities. However, the economic costs of these treatment modalities is extremely high. For example, in 1996 in the United States alone, the annual cost of ESRD treatment was over 14 billion dollars. In developing and underdeveloped countries with low health care budgets, ESRD patients are deprived access to such treatments due to their high costs. Accordingly, there is a need for alternative modalities of treatment for **uremia**..... A number of treatment attempts have been based on the use of the bowel as a substitute for kidney function. During a normal digestive process the gastrointestinal tract delivers nutrients and water to the bloodstream and eliminates waste products and undigested materials through the bowel. The intestinal wall regulates absorption of nutrients, electrolytes, water and certain digestive aiding substances such as bile acids. The intestinal wall also acts as a semipermeable membrane allowing small molecules to pass from the intestinal tract into the bloodstream and preventing larger molecules from entering the circulation.

Web site: http://www.delphion.com/details?pn=US06706263__

- **CRFG-1a, a target and marker for chronic renal failure**

  Inventor(s): Laping; Nicholas J (West Chester, PA), Olson; Barbara (Norristown, PA), Zhu; Yuan (Blue Bell, PA)

  Assignee(s): Smithkline Beecham Corporation (Philadelphia, PA)

  Patent Number: 5,879,908

  Date filed: February 9, 1998

  Abstract: CRFG-1a polypeptides and polynucleotides and methods for producing such polypeptides by recombinant techniques are disclosed. Also disclosed are methods for utilizing CRFG-1a polypeptides and polynucleotides in the design of protocols for the treatment of chronic renal disease, renal ischemia, diabetic nephropathy, acute **renal failure,** Neurodegenerative disease, and Alzheimer's disease, among others, and diagnostic assays for such conditions.

  Excerpt(s): This application claims the benefit of U.S. provisional application Ser. No. 60/045,203, filed Apr. 30, 1997, which is herein incorporated by reference in its entirety.... This invention relates to newly identified polynucleotides, polypeptides encoded by them and to the use of such polynucleotides and polypeptides, and to their production. More particularly, the polynucleotides and polypeptides of the present invention relate to GTP binding protein family, hereinafter referred to as chronic **renal failure** gene-1a (CRFG-1a). The invention also relates to inhibiting or activating the action of such polynucleotides and polypeptides.... The sequence of CRFG-1a is similar to uncharacterized putative GTP binding proteins of yeast (YPL093w), Halobacterium cutirubrum and GTP1/OBG family of GTP binding proteins from Methanobacterium thermoautotrophicum. GTP binding proteins play important roles in intracellular transport, protein targeting and vesicle fusion.

  Web site: http://www.delphion.com/details?pn=US05879908__

- **CRFG-1b, a target and marker for chronic renal failure**

  Inventor(s): Laping; Nicholas J (West Chester, PA), Olson; Barbara (Norristown, PA), Zhu; Yuan (Blue Bell, PA)

  Assignee(s): SmithKline Beecham Corporation (Philadelphia, PA)

  Patent Number: 6,255,471

  Date filed: February 9, 1998

Abstract: CRFG-1b polypeptides and polynucleotides and methods for producing such polypeptides by recombinant techniques are disclosed. Also disclosed are methods for utilizing CRFG-1b polypeptides and polynucleotides in the design of protocols for the treatment of chronic renal disease, renal ischemia, diabetic nephropathy, acute **renal failure,** neurodegenerative disease, and Alzheimer's disease, among others, and diagnostic assays for such conditions.

Excerpt(s): This invention relates to newly identified polynucleotides, polypeptides encoded by them and to the use of such polynucleotides and polypeptides, and to their production. More particularly, the polynucleotides and polypeptides of the present invention relate to GTP binding protein family, hereinafter referred to as chronic **renal failure** gene-1b (CRFG-1b). The invention also relates to inhibiting or activating the action of such polynucleotides and polypeptides.... The sequence of CRFG-1b is similar to uncharacterized putative GTP binding proteins of yeast (YPL093w), Halobacterium cutirubrum and GTP1/OBG family of GTP binding proteins from Methanobacterium thermoautotrophicum. GTP binding proteins play important roles in intracellular transport, protein targeting and vesicle fusion.... This indicates that the GTP binding proteins fainly has an established, proven history as therapeutic targets. Clearly there is a need for identification and characterization of fiuter members of GTP binding protein family which can play a role in preventing, ameliorating or correcting dysfunctions or diseases, including, but not limited to, chronic renal disease, renal ischemia, diabetic nephropathy, acute **renal failure,** Neurodegenerative disease, and Alzheimer's disease.

Web site: http://www.delphion.com/details?pn=US06255471__

- **Method and compositions for the treatment of renal failure**

Inventor(s): Bergstrom; Jonas (Stockholm, SE)

Assignee(s): Baxter International Inc. (Deerfield, IL)

Patent Number: 5,968,966

Date filed: October 9, 1997

Abstract: Methods and compositions for treating **renal failure** patients are provided. Pursuant to the present invention, a **renal failure** patient is provided with an intravenous or dialysis solution that includes a therapeutically effective amount of L-carnosine. In part, the L-carnosine will prevent the **renal failure** patient from developing L-carnosine deficiency.

Excerpt(s): The present invention relates generally to the treatment of diseases. More specifically the present invention relates to methods and compositions for the treatment of renal disease.... Of course, due to a variety of diseases and insults **renal failure** can occur in a patient. Acute **renal failure** can result from: direct renal tubular injury; renal ischemic; and intra-tubular obstruction. **Renal failure** results in diminished glomerular filtration and reduced secretion of metabolic waste products, water and electrolytes. Resultant fluid overload, electrolyte imbalances, and uremic syndrome can result in organ dysfunction ultimately resulting in death.... It is known to use dialysis to support a patient whose renal function is decreased to a point where the kidneys no longer sufficiently function. Dialysis provides a method for supplementing and replacing renal function in certain patients. Two principal dialysis methods are utilized: hemodialysis dialysis; and peritoneal dialysis.

Web site: http://www.delphion.com/details?pn=US05968966___

- **Method and formulations for the therapy of acute renal failure**

Inventor(s): Humes; H. David (Ann Arbor, MI)

Assignee(s): The Regents of the University of Michigan (Ann Arbor, MI)

Patent Number: 5,360,790

Date filed: August 23, 1993

Abstract: The therapy of patients with nephrotoxic or ischemic acute **renal failure** with epidermal growth factor and/or transforming growth factor-.alpha. is disclosed.

Excerpt(s): This invention relates to phamaceutical compositions containing epidermal growth factor (EGF) and/or transforming growth factor (TGF)-.alpha. and to the use of such compositions in treating acute **renal failure**.... Acute **renal failure** (ARF) is a common clinical syndrome. It is defined as an abrupt decline in renal function. Most clinicians accept the definition of ARF as a rise in serum creatinine of greater than 0.2 to 0.5 mg/dL per day and a rise in blood urea nitrogen (BUN) of greater than 5 to 10 mg/dL per day over several days.... It may occur in a patient with previously normal renal function but may also be superimposed on stable but impaired renal function. The clinical manifestations of this disorder arise from the decline in glomerular filtration rate (GFR) and the inability of the kidney to excrete the toxic metabolic wastes produced by the body. It is recognized clinically by rising levels of blood urea nitrogen (BUN) and serum creatinine concentration and may present dramatically with a patient progressing from normal renal function to symptomatic **uremia** within a week.

Web site: http://www.delphion.com/details?pn=US05360790__

- **Method for dialysis**

Inventor(s): Chen; Wei-Tzuoh (Downers Grove, IL)

Assignee(s): The United States of America as represented by the Administrator of (Washington, DC)

Patent Number: 4,601,830

Date filed: October 28, 1981

Abstract: A method and apparatus for the hemodialysis of the blood of **kidney failure** patients. The concentration of the dialysis solution is initially selected so that the solution osmolality approximates the osmolality of the patient's blood. The dialysis solution concentration is then reduced linearly as a function of time as the dialysis is carried out. The conductivity of the dialysis solution is measured and compared with high and low limit references. If the conductivity is outside the limits, an alarm is given and the concentration of the dialysis solution is held constant. A timer controls a proportional pumping means to reduce the concentration of the dialysis solution and concurrently reduces the conductivity reference limits for the alarm.

Excerpt(s): This invention relates to a method and apparatus for dialysis in which the concentration of the dialysis solution is varied as a function of time during the treatment.... A patient undergoing dialysis often suffers uncomfortable and debilitating side effects as nausea, vomiting, headaches, hypotension and the like. It is theorized that these side effects are caused by the disequilibrium or substantial difference between the osmolality level of the patient's blood and that of the dialysis solution during the dialysis procedure. The flow of blood through the dialyzer is changed markedly by removing osmotic particles and other substances. This kind of treatment causes a disequilibrium in the patient's body system precipitating the side effects noted above.... In accordance with this invention, I provide a dialysis method and an apparatus for carrying out the method in which the dialysis solution concentration is initially established with an osmolality at a level comparable with the osmolality of the patient's blood. During the course of the dialysis treatment, the concentration of the dialysis solution is reduced at a rate corresponding generally with the reduction of osmolality of the blood, as impurities are removed. Thus, the disequilibrium in the patient's system is minimized.

Web site: http://www.delphion.com/details?pn=US04601830__

- **Method for producing low potassium juice with improved taste and product thereof**

Inventor(s): Goto; Takushi (Urawa, JP), Katamune; Koji (Sakado, JP), Kinoshita; Toshio (Tokyo, JP), Kinoshita; Yuko (Tokyo, JP), Takizawa; Toshio (Odawara, JP)

Assignee(s): Meiji Seika Kaisha Ltd. (Tokyo, JP)

Patent Number: 6,387,425

Date filed: January 24, 2000

Abstract: A method for producing low potassium juice with improved taste. The process includes the steps of treating potassium-containing juice with a cation exchange resin to remove 90% or more of the potassium content in the juice and adding a calcium compound which is calcium carbonate in the form of solid. The juice produced has improved taste and nutritional balance. It is also good for patients suffering from **kidney failure.**

Excerpt(s): The present invention relates to a method for producing a low potassium juice with improved taste and more particularly to a method for producing a juice with improved taste by decreasing the concentration of potassium in the juice and adding a calcium compound thereto. Further, the present invention relates to a juice suitable for patients suffering from **kidney failure** who are allowed to take up limited amounts of potassium and to whom administration of calcium carbonate is necessary.... In cells of animals inclusive of humans, potassium mainly exists in an intracellular liquid and in a pair with sodium which exists mainly in an extracellular liquid and plays an important role in maintaining the homeostasis of a living organism as one of major factor in the acid base equilibrium. However, since patients suffering from **kidney failure** have decreased functions of excreting potassium and of maintaining blood ion balance so that they tend to be suffered from hyperkalemia, hyperphosphatemia, or hypocalcemia. An extreme increase in serum potassium level may cause the stop of the heart function and, in the worst cases, fatal situation.... Therefore, patients with **kidney failure** are subjected to strict restriction on the uptake of potassium and, in particular, they cannot freely take fruit or vegetables containing potassium in large amounts. As described above, patients with **kidney failure** tend to be suffered from hyperphosphatemia or hypocalcemia, and hence administration of calcium carbonate to such patients is necessary. Further, in the case of those patients who are subjected to the restriction on the uptake of fruit and vegetables, there arises a new problem that the contents of meal are unbalanced and it is difficult to maintain a nutritional balance.

Web site: http://www.delphion.com/details?pn=US06387425__

- **Method for treatment of acute renal failure**

  Inventor(s): Greenwald; James E. (100 N. Euclid Ave., Ste. 902, St. Louis, MO 63108)

  Assignee(s): none reported

  Patent Number: 5,486,519

  Date filed: August 22, 1994

  Abstract: A method is disclosed for treatment of acute **renal failure** which comprises administering to a warm-blooded mammal manifesting acute **renal failure** a small but effective amount of zaprinast sufficient to effect acceleration of recovery from said acute **renal failure.**

  Excerpt(s): Acute **renal failure** (ARF) is a major problem in contemporary medicine.... Five percent (5%) of all hospitalized patients are affected by some degree of acute renal dysfunction (1).... Fifty percent (50%) of all patients diagnosed with ARF will die, thus demonstrating the morbidity and mortality associated with this disease (2).

  Web site: http://www.delphion.com/details?pn=US05486519__

- **Method of prophylaxis of acute renal failure**

  Inventor(s): Clark; Ross G. (Pacifica, CA)

  Assignee(s): Genentech, Inc. (South San Francisco, CA)

  Patent Number: 5,273,961

  Date filed: September 22, 1992

  Abstract: A method is disclosed for the prophylactic treatment of mammals at risk for acute **renal failure,** whether due to renal ischemia or nephrotoxic damage. This method involves administering to the mammal, before or at the time that the acute **renal failure** is expected to occur or is occurring, an effective amount of IGF-I. Preferably, the IGF-I is native-sequence, mature human IGF-I.

  Excerpt(s): This invention relates to a method of preventing or ameliorating acute **renal failure** in mammals The acute **renal failure** may be due to reduced renal blood flow or nephrotoxins leading to cell necrosis and reduced kidney function.... Insulin-like growth factor I (IGF-I) is a polypeptide naturally occurring in human body fluids, for example, blood and human cerebral spinal fluid. Most tissues, including the kidney, produce IGF-I together with specific IGF-binding proteins. IGF-I production is under the dominant stimulatory influence of growth hormone (GH), and some of the IGF-I binding proteins are also influenced by GH. See Tanner et al., Acta Endocrinol., 84: 681-696 (1977); Uthne et al., J. Clin. Endocrinol. Metab., 39: 548-554 (1974). IGF-I has been isolated from human serum and produced recombinantly. See, e.g., EP 123,228 and 128,733.... Human growth hormone (hGH) is a single-chain polypeptide consisting of 191 amino acids (molecular weight 21,500). Disulfide bonds link positions 53 and 165 and positions 182 and 189. Niall, Nature, New Biology. 230: 90 (1971). hGH is a potent anabolic agent, especially due to retention of nitrogen, phosphorus, potassium, and calcium. Treatment of hypophysectomized rats with GH can restore at least a portion of the growth rate of the rats. Moore et al., Endocrinology, 122: 2920.2926 (1988). Among its most striking effects in hypopituitary (GH-deficient) subjects is accelerated linear growth of bone growth plate cartilage resulting in increased stature. Kaplan, Growth Disorders in Children and Adolescents (Springfield, Ill.: Charles C. Thomas, 1964).

Web site: http://www.delphion.com/details?pn=US05273961__

## Method of retarding the progression of chronic renal failure

Inventor(s): Walser; Mackenzie (Ruxton, MD)

Assignee(s): The Johns Hopkins University (Baltimore, MD)

Patent Number: 5,175,144

Date filed: November 29, 1988

Abstract: Progression of chronic **renal failure** can be retarded (slowed or arrested) by administering to humans suffering from such disorder an agent which suppresses the production of glucocorticoids in the human. The agents may be administered alone or in combination with a protein restricted and/or phosphorus restricted diet. Examples of suitable agents which either suppress production of glucocorticoids or block binding to their receptors include sodium valproate, enkephalins, opioids, clonidine, ketoconazole, oxytocin, and mifepristone.

Excerpt(s): Since the first anecdotal evidence that nutritional therapy may slow the progression of chronic **renal failure** (see Walser M., "Ketoacids in the Treatment of **Uremia**," Clinical Nephrology, 3:180-7 (1975)), there has been growing interest in two possibilities: (1) that a common mechanism causes progression of many types of chronic **renal failure,** and (2) that this process can be slowed or arrested by diet or drugs.... Many mechanisms have been postulated, based on experiments in animals and/or clinical observations. Factors proposed to contribute to progression include arterial pressure, and more specifically, glomerular capillary pressure which is reduced by angiotensin-converting enzyme inhibitors; serum calcium times phosphorus product; urinary phosphorus excretion; protein intake itself; hyperuricemia; hypertriglyceridemia; hypercholesterolemia; and hyperoxalemia. As yet, no studies have examined the influence of such factors acting in concert on progression of chronic **renal failure**.... Ketoacid mixtures, administered in conjunction with a low protein, low phosphate diet, have been reported to slow progression in several studies, see Mitch, W. E., et al., "The Effect of a Keto Acid-Amino Acid Supplement to a Restricted Diet on the Progression of Chronic **Renal Failure**," New England Journal of Medicine, 311:623-9 (1984); Gretz, N., et al., "Low-Protein Diet Supplemented by Ketoacids in Chronic Renal Failure: A Prospective Study," Kidney International, 24, Suppl. 16:S263-7 (1983); and Barsotti, G., et al., "Effects on Renal Function of a Low-Nitrogen Diet Supplemented with Essential Amino Acids and Keto Analogs and of Hemodialysis and Free Protein Supply in Patients with Chronic **Renal Failure**," Nephron, 27:113-7 (1981), but see Burns, J., et al., "Comparison of the Effects of Ketoacid Analogs and Essential Amino Acids on Nitrogen Homeostasis in Uremic Patients on Moderately Protein-Restricted Diets," American Journal of Clinical Nutrition, 31:1767-1775 (1978).

Web site: http://www.delphion.com/details?pn=US05175144__

- **Method of retarding the progression of chronic renal failure**

Inventor(s): Walser; Mackenzie (Ruxton, MD)

Assignee(s): The Johns Hopkins University (Baltimore, MD)

Patent Number: 5,591,736

Date filed: July 3, 1995

Abstract: The progression of chronic **renal failure** in humans may be retarded by administration of dehydroepiandrosterone (DHEA) in effective amounts. The administration of DHEA is preferably oral at a dose of about 400 to 1600 mg/day. Patients suffering from severe chronic **renal failure** are also preferably maintained on a protein-restricted diet during DHEA administration.

Excerpt(s): The present invention relates to a treatment method for retarding the progression of chronic **renal failure** in humans.... Advanced chronic renal disease in humans is typically associated with multiple endocrine and metabolic abnormalities. Conventional therapy for treating chronic **renal failure** has focused on protein-restricted diets in conjunction with administration of ketoacid analogs of amino acids; see U.S. Pat. Nos. 4,100,160, 4,228,099 and 4,352,814, all of Walser, and U.S. Pat. No. 4,752,619 of Walser et al.... Another technique for slowing the progression of chronic **renal failure** is described by Walser in U.S. Pat. No. 5,175,144 and in U.S. application Ser. No. 07/996,757, where the treatment involves administration of ketoconazole or other agent that suppresses glucocorticoid production.

Web site: http://www.delphion.com/details?pn=US05591736__

- **Method of treating acute renal failure**

  Inventor(s): Hausheer; Frederick Herman (Boerne, TX)

  Assignee(s): BioNumerik Pharmaceuticals, Inc. (San Antonio, TX)

  Patent Number: 6,172,119

  Date filed: February 9, 1999

Abstract: This invention relates to a method of treating patients afflicted with acute **renal failure.** The method includes administering to a patient in need of treatment an effective amount of a thiol or reducible disulfide compound according to the formula set forth in the specification.

  Excerpt(s): This invention relates to a method for treating a patient suffering from acute **renal failure.** The method involves administering an effective amount of a disulfide or thiol-containing compound to a patient suffering from acute **renal failure....** Acute **renal failure** (ARF) is a severe, and often imminently life-threatening condition. There are many mechanisms which may be responsible for the pathogenesis of ARF. These include occlusions of the renal arteries, glomerular disease (glomerulonephritis, for one), infection (sepsis), disseminated intravascular coagulation (usually with cortical necrosis of the kidney), obstruction of urine flow due to tumors or other obstruction, acute tubular nephritis (ischemic or toxic), and others.... Methods of treating acute **renal failure** vary, depending on the cause. In the case of sepsis-induced ARF, the mechanism is generally similar to shock, and the treatment methods include the infusion of antibiotics in efforts to kill the bacteria and/or endotoxins. Coagulation is treated with anti-coagulant agents and supportive measures such as catheterization. Toxic nephritis is generally treated with antidotal therapy, depending upon the type of poison.

  Web site: http://www.delphion.com/details?pn=US06172119__

- **Methods for treating renal failure**

Inventor(s): Hsu; Chen Hsing (3720 Tremont Dt., Ann Harbor, MI 48105)

Assignee(s): none reported

Patent Number: 5,753,706

Date filed: February 3, 1997

Abstract: Methods of controlling phosphate metabolism and metabolic acidosis in patients suffering from **renal failure** and associated hyperphosphatemia or patients predisposed to development of a hyperphosphatemic condition are provided. The method in accordance with this invention comprises administering to a patient a ferric-containing compound selected from the group consisting of ferric citrate, ferric acetate, and combinations thereof. Therapeutic benefit can be realized in accordance with such method by administering the compound orally to a patient to contact and bind with ingested phosphate in the patient's digestive tract, and thereby prevent its intestinal absorption.

Excerpt(s): The present invention relates generally to the control of phosphate retention and particularly, to methods for treating patients suffering from **renal failure** and associated hyperphosphatemia.... Phosphate is primarily excreted through the kidney. Phosphate retention therefore inevitably occurs in **renal failure**. Phosphate restriction plays an important role in slowing down deterioration of renal function as well as soft tissue calcification in **renal failure**. A high intake of dietary phosphorus in experimental **renal failure** worsens renal function (Haut, L. L., Kidney Int 17:722-731 (1980); Karlinsky, D. et al., Kidney Int 17:293-302 (1980)) and a low phosphate intake arrests progression of chronic **renal failure.** Lumlertgul, D. et al., Kidney Int 29:658-666 (1986). Recent studies have demonstrated that phosphate restriction either increases plasma calcitriol (the most potent vitamin D metabolite) and suppresses secondary hyperparathyroidism (Portale, A. A. et al., J. Clin. Invest 73:1580-1589 (1989); Kilav, R. et al., J Clin. Invest 96:327-333 (1995); Lopez, H. et al., Am. J Physiol 259:F432-437 (1990)), or directly inhibits parathyroid cell proliferation. Naveh-Many, T. et al., Am. Soc. Nephrol 6:968 (1995). Taken together, maintaining a normal plasma concentration and tissue content of phosphate is an important means to prevent secondary hyperparathyroidism, renal osteodystrophy and soft tissue calcification in **renal failure**.... Dietary restriction of phosphate is difficult to achieve and thrice weekly dialysis alone can not remove daily absorbed phosphate. Therefore, phosphate binding agents have generally been employed to control phosphate metabolism in **renal failure.** For the last 30 years nephrologist have been using aluminum carbonate or aluminum hydroxide as phosphate binding agents. Concerns about aluminum toxicity in **renal failure** have prompted increased use of calcium carbonate and calcium acetate and a cessation in the use of aluminum compounds. However, calcium carbonate or other calcium preparations are not only inadequate to remove all the ingested dietary phosphate, but also provide too much calcium to **end stage renal disease (ESRD)** patients.

Web site: http://www.delphion.com/details?pn=US05753706__

- **Morphogen treatment for chronic renal failure**

Inventor(s): Cohen; Charles M. (Weston, MA), Sampath; Kuber T. (Holliston, MA)

Assignee(s): Curis, Inc. (Cambridge, MA)

Patent Number: 6,498,142

Date filed: May 6, 1996

Abstract: The present invention provides methods for the treatment, and pharmaceuticals for use in the treatment, of mammalian subjects at risk chronic **renal failure,** or at risk of a need for renal replacement therapy. The methods involve the administration of certain morphogens, inducers of those morphogens, or agonists of the corresponding morphogen receptors, or implantation of renal cells induced with those morphogens. The morphogens useful in the invention include osteogenic protein-1 (OP-1) and other members of the OP-1 subfamily of the TGF-.beta. superfamily of growth factors.

Excerpt(s): The present invention relates generally to methods of treatment for renal disease. In particular, the invention relates to methods of treatment for conditions which place mammals, including humans, at risk of chronic **renal failure.** The methods involve the administration of certain morphogens, inducers of those morphogens, or agonists of the corresponding morphogen receptors, or implantation of renal cells induced with those morphogens.... The mammalian renal system serves primary roles both in the removal of catabolic waste products from the bloodstream and in the maintenance of fluid and electrolyte balances in the body. Renal failures are, therefore, life-threatening conditions in which the build-up of catabolites and other toxins, and/or the development of significant imbalances in electrolytes or fluids, may lead to the failure of other major organs systems and death. As a general matter, **renal failure** is classified as "acute" or "chronic." As detailed below, the differences between these two conditions are not merely a matter of severity or rapidity but, rather, reflect differences in etiology, prognosis, and treatment.... Acute **renal failure** is defined as an abrupt cessation or substantial reduction of renal function and, in as many as 90-95% of cases, may be secondary to trauma, surgery or another acute medical condition. Acute **renal failure** may be due to pre-renal causes (e.g., decreased cardiac output, hypovolemia, altered vascular resistance) or to post-renal causes (e.g., obstructions or constrictions of the ureters, bladder or urethra) which do not directly involve the kidneys and which, if treated quickly, will not entail significant loss of nephrons or other damage to the kidneys. Alternatively, acute **renal failure** may be due to intrinsic renal causes which involve a more direct insult or injury to the kidneys, and which may entail permanent damage to the nephrons or other kidney structures. Intrinsic causes of acute **renal failure** include but are not limited to infectious diseases (e.g., various bacterial, viral or parasitic infections), inflammatory diseases (e.g., glomerulonephritis, systemic lupus erythematosus), ischemia (e.g., renal artery occlusion), toxic syndromes (e.g., heavy metal poisoning, side-effects of antimicrobial treatments or chemotherapy), and direct traumas.

Web site: http://www.delphion.com/details?pn=US06498142__

- **Nutritional composition for management of renal failure**

Inventor(s): Madsen; David C. (Libertyville, IL), Tucker; Hugh N. (Chicago, IL)

Assignee(s): Baxter Travenol Laboratories, Inc. (Deerfield, IL)

Patent Number: 4,357,343

Date filed: June 26, 1981

Abstract: A novel amino acid composition is provided for the nutritional maintenance of **renal failure** patients.

Excerpt(s): This invention relates to compositions and methods for nutritional management of **renal failure.** In particular it is directed at novel amino acid compositions for meeting the specialized nutritional requirements of patients suffering **renal failure** and the attendant derangements of normal amino acid metabolism and dialysis-induced losses in the body's amino acid complement.... Renal failure may be classified as acute or chronic. Acute **renal failure** is characterized by an abrupt, often reversible impairment (partial or total) of renal function, manifested by inadequate urine formation. Acute **renal failure** usually appears rapidly--on the order of one to several days--either with or without prior renal dysfunction. Urine output may range from total anuria through stages of oliguria, to polyuria in the diuretic (recovery) phase.... Acute **renal failure** follows from a diversity of possible causes, which are divided into two categories: nephrotoxic injury and renal ischemia. Nephrotoxic injury results from sensitivity response or excessive and/or continuous exposure to drugs, chemicals, heavy metals, etc., which prove toxic to the renal tubular cells, while renal ischemia results from clinical situations causing hypovolemia, hypotension, and/or acute dehydation. Some commonly encountered etiologic factors include: complications of anesthesia, major surgery, obstetrical complications and trauma.

Web site: http://www.delphion.com/details?pn=US04357343__

- **Nutritional supplement for treatment of uremia**

  Inventor(s): Bermudez; Henri (Boulonge Billancourt, FR), Bordat; Claude (Dordives, FR), Walser; Mackenzie (Ruxton, MD)

  Assignee(s): Synthelabo (Paris, FR), The Johns Hopkins University (Baltimore, MD)

  Patent Number: 4,752,619

  Date filed: December 23, 1985

  Abstract: Mixtures of mixed salts formed between branched-chain alpha keto-acids and basic L-amino acids are useful in the nutritional treatment of chronic **renal failure** (uremia). These compositions contain fewer component salts than other salt mixtures containing like proportions of basic amino acids and keto acids. The compositions can be used in conjunction with a 20-30 g/day mixed quality protein diet and a vitamin and mineral supplement.

  Excerpt(s): This invention relates to compositions for use in the nutritional treatment of chronic **renal failure** (uremia). More specifically, this invention relates to mixtures of mixed salts formed between branched-chain alpha-keto acids and basic L-amino acids. The compositions can be used in conjunction with a 20-30 g/day mixed quality protein diet, and a vitamin and mineral supplement.... Salts of basic L-amino acids, such as L-arginine and L-ornithine, and alpha-keto analogs of branched-chain essential amino acids, namely alpha-ketoisocaproate, alpha-ketoisovalerate and alpha-keto-beta-methylvalerate are disclosed in U.S. Pat. Nos. 4,228,099, 4,296,127 and 4,320,146, for use in the treatment of hepatic disorders characterized by hyperammonemia and portal systemic encephalopathy, and for treatment of **renal failure**.... Branched-chain keto acids, and alpha-ketoisocaproate in particular, are known to exhibit a nitrogen- or protein-sparing effect in patients with chronic **renal failure**. That is, branched-chain keto acids reduce urinary nitrogen loss. These keto acids have been used to improve the nitrogen balance in patients suffering from a number of different nitrogen wasting conditions.

Web site: http://www.delphion.com/details?pn=US04752619__

- **Preventing renal failure**

  Inventor(s): Edwards; K. David G. (427 Washington St., New York, NY 10013)

  Assignee(s): none reported

  Patent Number: 4,250,191

  Date filed: November 30, 1978

  Abstract: A method and substances are featured for reducing the risk of incurring renal damage or failure. Substances useful in the treatment of hyperlipidemia and closely-related vascular conditions have been found to reduce or prevent **renal failure.** The substances most generally utilized are derivatives of phenoxyacetic acid. These substances are administered from 0.01 to 0.25% by weight of the dietary materials ingested by the host which is equivalent to 0.2 to 6.0 grams per day in man.

  Excerpt(s): This invention relates to a method and substances for protecting against **renal failure** or damage.... In the past, elevated serum cholesterol and triglyceride concentrations were considered as high risk factors together with cigarette smoking and hypertension for coronary artery disease. This was especially so, when both lipid parameters were elevated simultaneously. Therefore, it was not surprising to find exaggerated incidence of atherosclerosis and coronary heart disease in the human nephrotic syndrome, the advanced stages of which were traditionally accompanied by high lipid levels.... As a countermeasure to coronary and vascular problems, it was suggested that antihyperlipidemic drugs be used. Indeed, recent studies indicate that the drug clofibrate (Atromid-S) gives significant protection against ischaemic heart disease and death in patients with angina pectoris.

  Web site: http://www.delphion.com/details?pn=US04250191__

- **Treatment of acute renal failure by administration of N-acetylcysteine**

  Inventor(s): Weinberg; Assa (344 N. Fairfax Ave., Los Angeles, CA 90036)

  Assignee(s): Weinberg; Assa (Los Angeles, CA)

  Patent Number: 6,355,682

  Date filed: May 11, 2001

Abstract: A method for treating the damages caused by an acute **renal failure** is disclosed. The method according to the present invention comprises the administration of a therapeutically effective dose of N-acetylcysteine.

Excerpt(s): The present invention relates to the field of treatment of patients who have been afflicted with acute **renal failure**.... Acute **renal failure** or a rapid deterioration of the renal function is a common disturbance during which the kidneys' filtering capacity is lost and, as a result, a rapid accumulation of waste material, mainly nitrogenous products, occurs in the body. One of the most common causes for such **renal failure** is due to the reduction or interruption of the blood supply to the kidneys. Such reduction or interruption of the blood supply to the kidneys could be generally described as renal ischemia.... There are multiple medical conditions that could cause the interruption of the renal circulation. Depending on the duration of an interruption, the outcome of an acute **renal failure** can be quite devastating. Every cardiovascular event associated with hypotension has a potential of causing a reduction in renal vascular supply. Other conditions, such as gastrointestinal hemorrage, extensive burn, trauma, surgery or anesthesia may also cause hypovolemia, i.e. a low blood volume. Hypovolemia may lead to a dramatic reduction in the blood circulating to the kidneys which may lead to a rapid deterioration in renal function.

Web site: http://www.delphion.com/details?pn=US06355682__

- **Treatment of chronic renal failure with imidazole angiotensin-II receptor antagonists**

Inventor(s): Carini; David J. (Wilmington, DE), Duncia; John Jonas V. (Newark, DE), Wong; Pancras C. (Wilmington, DE)

Assignee(s): E. I. Du Pont de Nemours and Company (Wilmington, DE)

Patent Number: 5,210,079

Date filed: February 7, 1992

Abstract: Substituted imidazoles such as 2-butyl-4-chloro-1-[(2'-(1H-tetrazol-5-yl)biphenyl-4-yl)methyl]-5-(hydroxy methyl)imidazole and 2-butyl-4-chloro-1-[(2'-carboxybiphenyl-4-yl)-methyl]-5-(hydroxymethyl)imi dazole and pharmaceutically acceptable salts thereof are useful for treating chronic **renal failure,** mediated by angiotensin-II.

Excerpt(s): This invention relates to a method of treating chronic **renal failure** and, in particular, to a method which utilizes imidazole angiotensin-II (AII) receptor antagonists to treat chronic **renal failure** mediated by angiotensin-II.... Angiotensin converting enzyme inhibitors may have beneficial effects over other antihypertensive agents in progressive renal disease of various origins including diabetic nephropathy, essential hypertension and other intrinsic renal diseases (See, e.g., Hypertension: Pathophysiology, Diagnosis, and Management, ed. by J. H. Laragh and B. M. Brenner, vol. 1, pp. 1163-1176, Raven Press, Ltd., New York, 1990; Hypertension: Pathophysiology, Diagnosis, and Management, ed. by J. H. Laragh and B. M. Brenner, vol. 2, pp. 1677-1687, Raven Press, Ltd., New York, 1990). For instance, in partially nephrectomized rats, glomerular capillary hypertension in the remnant kidney is associated with progressive proteinuria, focal glomerular sclerosis, and moderate hypertension. Angiotensin converting enzyme inhibitors, which lower systemic arterial pressure and glomerular capillary pressure, limit the progression of glomerular injury.... There are other antihypertensive agents which lower systemic arterial blood pressure to a similar extent, but fail to reduce glomerular capillary pressure. Such agents do not prevent the progression of glomerular injury. It is speculated that in these rats intrarenal generation of angiotensin-II constricts the renal efferent arteriole and causes an increase in glomerular hydraulic pressure. Glomerular hyperfiltration, hyperperfusion and/or hypertension may then initiate and induce glomerular lesions. Thus, blockade of the intrarenal formation of angiotensin-II by angiotensin converting enzyme inhibitors may retard the deterioration of **renal failure.**

Web site: http://www.delphion.com/details?pn=US05210079__

- **Use of oligosaccharides for the treatment of pruritus cutaneus associated with renal failure**

Inventor(s): Ando; Kunio (Kanagawa-ken, JP), Hosokawa; Tomoyoshi (Kanagawa-ken, JP), Nakamura; Tetsuo (Tokyo, JP), Shimaoka; Tatsuro (Tochigi-ken, JP)

Assignee(s): Institute of Immunology Co., Ltd. (Tokyo, JP)

Patent Number: 5,972,905

Date filed: February 20, 1998

Abstract: A pharmaceutical agent for improvement in pruritus cutaneus associated with **renal failure** and/or for the treatment of **renal failure** and/or its complications containing as an effective ingredient oligosaccharide or oligosaccharides such as, but not limited to fructo-oligosaccharide, galacto-oligosaccharide, isomalto-oligosaccharide, malto-oligosaccharide, lacto-sucrose and/or xylo-oligosaccharide, in particular, lactulose, rhamnose and lactitol.

Excerpt(s): This invention relates to a new pharmaceutical composition for alleviation of various syndromes, in particular pruritus cutaneus, characteristic to **renal failure** and hemodialysis patients.... Among the countries all over the world, the hemodialysis therapy is most widely practiced in Japan. This therapy over an extended time, however, induces various serious problems. The hemodialysis therapy for a long time, for example, causes the onset of complications such as cardiovascular disorder, anemia, abnormal bone metabolism, dysbolism, and/or immunodeficiency. In addition, it is said that 60-80% of the hemodialysis patients suffer from pruritus cutaneus. Although pruritus cutaneus itself does not impose direct threatening on the life of the patients, its persistent and chronic torment, night and day, is unbearable to the patients, both physically and mentally. From the view point of the maintenance and improvement in the quality of life, pruritus cutaneus is now a big problem in the treatment of the patients.... As a possible cause of pruritus cutaneus, 1. stimulation of the nerve ending by a certain substance accumulated in the blood by **renal failure,** 2. a decline in the pruritus threshold value due to change in the pH value, etc., or 3. abnormal secretion by the skin glands such as sebaceous glands and sweat glands, is suspected but it Is not yet clear what is responsible for it. For its treatment, antihistaminic agent is generally administered but it has limitation in its efficacy. Besides, due to its side effects like drowsiness, vertigo or generalized malaise, its administration must be discontinued in many cases. In addition, anti-allergic agent, adrenocortical agent or tranquilizer is administered but no agent alone can relieve the patients from the torment and establishment of an effective therapy has been expected.

Web site: http://www.delphion.com/details?pn=US05972905__

- **Use of prostaglandin (PGE2) receptor a (EP4) selective agonists for the treatment of acute and chronic renal failure**

Inventor(s): Paralkar; Vishwas M. (Madison, CT), Thompson; David D. (Gales Ferry, CT)

Assignee(s): Pfizer Inc. (New York, NY)

Patent Number: 6,610,719

Date filed: January 29, 2001

Abstract: This invention is directed to methods and compositions of treating acute or chronic **renal failure** or dysfunction, or conditions caused thereby, comprising administering prostaglandin agonists, which are EP.sub.4 receptor selective prostaglandin agonists.

Excerpt(s): The present invention relates to methods and pharmaceutical compositions comprising receptor selective prostaglandin (PGE.sub.2) agonists for the treatment of kidney diseases, such as chronic and acute **renal failure** or dysfunction, in animals, particularly mammals. More specifically, the present invention relates to such methods and pharmaceutical compositions comprising type 4 (EP.sub.4) receptor selective prostaglandin (PGE.sub.2) agonists.... The naturally occurring prostaglandins are comprised of several biological entities including PBD, PGE, PGF, PGG, PGH and PGI. It has been well documented that prostaglandins have effects on many of the organs and systems of the body.... In the kidney, the prostaglandins modulate renal blood flow and may serve to regulate urine formation by both renovascular and tubular effects. In clinical studies, PGE, has been used to improve creatinine clearance in patients with chronic renal disease, to prevent graft rejection and cyclosporine toxicity in renal transplant patients, to reduce the urinary albumin excretion rate and N-acetyl-beta-D-glucosaminidase levels in patients with diabetic nephropathy, and to improve urea clearance in healthy volunteers. PGE.sub.1 also has been administered intravenously during surgeries to prevent **renal failure.**

Web site: http://www.delphion.com/details?pn=US06610719__

- **Use of pyruvate to treat acute renal failure**

Inventor(s): Nath; Karl A. (St. Louis Park, MN)

Assignee(s): Regents of the University of Minnesota (Minneapolis, MN)

Patent Number: 5,210,098

Date filed: February 26, 1992

Abstract: A therapeutic method is provided to arrest or prevent **acute kidney failure** by administration of a non-toxic pyruvate salt to a patient in need of such treatment.

Excerpt(s): The classification of cessation of renal function into acute and chronic **renal failure** demarcates disease states that are distinct in etiology, pathogenesis, rate of loss of renal function, potential for recovery of renal function and therapeutic strategies applied in their management. Chronic **renal failure** is characterized by an inexorable loss of renal function, which can last for several years after the initial presentation of renal insufficiency, culminating in end-stage disease. The arrival of end-stage disease signifies irretrievable loss of renal function and necessitates replacement of renal function by dialysis or transplantation. The leading causes of chronic **renal failure** are assorted glomerulonephritides, diabetic nephropathy, chronic tubulointerstitial diseases and polycystic kidney diseases. See F. N. Ziyadeh, Textbook of Internal Medicine, Vol. 1, W. E. Kelley, ed., J. B. Lippincott Co., Philadelphia (1989) at pages 883-889; M. Walser, Kid. Int., 37, 1195 (1990).... Management of patients with chronic **renal failure** utilizes strategies that retard the rate of loss of renal function, thereby delaying the onset of end-stage disease. Such therapeutic strategies include treatment of systemic hypertension, correction of perturbed calcium/phosphate homeostasis and restriction in dietary protein intake (W. E. Mitch, Ann. Rev. Med., 35, 249 (1984)). Some studies have indicated that dietary supplementation with alpha-keto acids in conjunction with restricted protein and phosphate intake may be efficacious in retarding the progression of established renal disease (W. E. Mitch et al., N. Engl. J. Med., 311, 623 (1984)). The mechanism by which dietary supplementation with alpha-keto acids may act to alleviate progressive renal injury is unknown.... Acute **renal failure** is characterized by a relatively abrupt decline in renal function. Temporary replacement of renal function by dialysis may be indicated within days of the instigating insult and may be necessary for several weeks during the maintenance phase of acute **renal failure.** While recovery of renal function usually occurs, there is substantial morbidity and mortality during the initiation, maintenance and recovery phases of acute **renal failure.** The recovery phase of acute **renal failure,** once complete, usually allows the resumption of normal renal function. Conditions that predispose to acute **renal failure** include ineffective renal perfusion, systemic hypotension of any cause, sepsis, major trauma, nephrotoxic insults such as aminoglycoside antibiotics and radiographic contrast agents, and obstruction to the urinary tract (M. Brezis et al., The Kidney, B. M. Brenner et al., eds., W. B. Saunders (3rd ed. 1986) at pages 735-799). Less commonly, acute **renal failure** may arise from certain types of glomerulonephritis and vasculitis.

Web site: http://www.delphion.com/details?pn=US05210098__

## Patent Applications on Kidney Failure

As of December 2000, U.S. patent applications are open to public viewing.[21] Applications are patent requests which have yet to be granted (the process to

---

[21] This has been a common practice outside the United States prior to December 2000.

achieve a patent can take several years). The following patent applications have been filed since December 2000 relating to kidney failure:

- **Compositions and methods for alleviating symptoms of uremia in patients**

Inventor(s): Dickstein, Jack; (Huntingdon Valley, PA), Ranganathan, Natarajan; (Broomall, PA)

Correspondence: Jane Massey Licata; Law Offices of Jane Massey Licata; 66 E Main Street; Marlton; NJ; 08053; US

Patent Application Number: 20010051150

Date filed: April 20, 2000

Abstract: Microencapsulated and/or enteric coated compositions containing a mixture of sorbents with specific adsorption affinities for uremic toxins including ammonia, urea, creatinine, phenols, indoles, and middle molecular weight molecules and a bacterial source which metabolizes urea and ammonia are provided. Also provided are methods of using these compositions to alleviate symptoms of **uremia** in patients.

Excerpt(s): This application claims the benefit of provisional U.S. Application Ser. No. 60/131,774, filed Apr. 30, 1999.... Kidney disease is ranked fourth among the major diseases in the United States afflicting over 20 million Americans. More than 90,000 patients die each year because of kidney diseases. In recent years the number of **chronic kidney failure** patients has increased about 11 percent annually. About 80,000 Americans on dialysis die of various complications each year and more than 27,000 are on waiting lists for kidney transplants each year with only about 11,000 of these patients receiving transplants.... Nearly 250,000 Americans suffer from **end stage renal disease** (ESRD), which is the final stage in chronic **renal failure.** Currently hemo- or peritoneal-dialysis and renal transplant are the only treatment modalities. However, the economic costs of these treatment modalities is extremely high. For example, in 1996 in the United States alone, the annual cost of ESRD treatment was over 14 billion dollars. In developing and underdeveloped countries with low health care budgets, ESRD patients are deprived access to such treatments due to their high costs. Accordingly, there is a need for alternative modalities of treatment for **uremia.**.

Web site: http://appft1.uspto.gov/netahtml/PTO/search-bool.html

- **Device and method for preventing kidney failure**

  Inventor(s): Hussein, Hany M.; (Newport Coast, CA)

  Correspondence: JAMES G O'NEILL; 3151 AIRWAY AVE SUITE K105; COSTA MESA; CA; 926264613

  Patent Application Number: 20020107536

  Date filed: February 7, 2002

  Abstract: A method and devices for protecting kidneys from irreversible damage. The method is based on controlling or restricting blood flow through renal arteries in order to prevent **kidney failure.** The devices are delivered to a renal artery for restricting the flow of blood through the artery to the kidney. The devices may take the form of internal restrictors, such as an orifice, a venturi, a tapered coil, or a perforated sleeve that is inserted in a renal artery, or external devices such as an inflatable cuff or balloon, or a clamp that is placed around a renal artery. The improved method of the present invention includes means for delivering the internal devices to renal arteries by a percutaneous catheter system, or external devices by endoscopic devices or surgery.

  Excerpt(s): This application is a continuation of pending provisional application No. 60/267,255 filed on Feb. 7, 2001.... This invention relates generally to medical devices and methods, and more particularly, to an improved device for and method of preventing **kidney failure.**... Clinical observation indicates that diabetic kidneys that receive their blood supply from stenosed renal arteries tend to be spared from **renal failure** compared to kidneys that receive their blood supply from patent renal arteries. Kidney dialysis and kidney transplants are costly and traumatic alternatives for treatment of **kidney failure.** Therefore, there exists a need in the art for an easy-to-use, less invasive and less costly device and method for protecting kidneys from irreversible damage that leads to **renal failure.**

  Web site: http://appft1.uspto.gov/netahtml/PTO/search-bool.html

- **HGF FOR TREATING ACUTE RENAL FAILURE**

  Inventor(s): KUDO, IKUE; (OSAKA-SHI, JP), NAGANO, TOMOKAZU; (OSAKA-SHI, JP)

  Correspondence: BIRCH STEWART KOLASCH & BIRCH; PO BOX 747; FALLS CHURCH; VA; 22040-0747; US

  Patent Application Number: 20010047079

  Date filed: February 24, 2000

Abstract: The present invention provides a pharmaceutical composition for treating acute **renal failure** caused by rhabdomyolysis comprising an effective amount of HGF.The present invention provides a method of treating acute **renal failure** caused by rhabdomyolysis comprising administering an effective amount of HGF to a patient in need thereof.

Excerpt(s): Acute **renal failure** is defined as having symptoms of azotemia, electrolyte imbalance, **uremia** and the like caused by acute renal dysfunction. Acute **renal failure** is classified into prerenal acute **renal failure,** renal acute **renal failure** and postrenal acute **renal failure** caused by renal dysfunction. Renal acute **renal failure** is classified into (1) vasculitis, glomerular lesion, (2) acute interstitial nephritis, (3) tubule obstruction and (4) acute **renal failure** in a narrow sense. Acute **renal failure** in a narrow sense is caused by acute tubular necrosis. The acute **renal failure** in a narrow sense results from (1) ischemia, (2) nephrotoxic substance, or (3) myolytic substance (e.g. myoglobin) and so on.... Ischemic acute **renal failure** is caused by bleeding from surgery, shock, external injury, burn and the like. Experimental animal model for ischemic acute **renal failure** is exemplified by renal artery ligation. In the rat model, BUN (blood urea nitrogen) and serum creatinine are increased, HGF (Hepatocyte Growth Factor) mRNA expression is enhanced 6 to 12 hours after ischemia, and then HGF bioactivity in rat kidney and plasma is activated (American Journal of Physiology, 1993; 265; 61-69).... Acute **renal failure** is also caused by a nephrotoxic substance such as anti-biotic agent, antitumor agent, contrast medium. An experimental animal model of acute **renal failure** caused by a nephrotoxic substance is made by administration of a compound such as mercurous chloride, cisplatin, and contrast medium to rats. Mercurous chloride administered rats show an increase of BUN and creatinine, enhancement of HGF mRNA expression and activity of HGF (Nephron 1996; 73; 735), as reported on ischemia model. It is suggested that HGF be involved in restoring a patient from **renal failure.**

Web site: http://appft1.uspto.gov/netahtml/PTO/search-bool.html

- **Method & apparatus for mitigating renal failure using mechanical vibration including ultrasound and heat**

Inventor(s): Cho, Young; (Cherry Hill, NJ)

Correspondence: CAESAR, RIVISE, BERNSTEIN,; COHEN & POKOTILOW, LTD.; 12TH FLOOR, SEVEN PENN CENTER; 1635 MARKET STREET; PHILADELPHIA; PA; 19103-2212; US

Patent Application Number: 20020123702

Date filed: February 25, 2002

Abstract: A method and apparatus for preventing or at least mitigating **renal failure** due to the presence of contrast media agents administered to patients. The method and apparatus applies either mechanical vibration, including ultrasonic energy, or heat to the vicinity of the kidneys at the patient's back to reduce the blood viscosity of the blood in the microvessels of the kidney.

Excerpt(s): This application is an Application based on Provisional Application Serial No. 60/271,558 filed Feb. 26, 2001 entitled METHOD & APPARATUS FOR MITIGATING **RENAL FAILURE** USING MECHANICAL VIBRATION INCLUDING ULTRASOUND, and whose entire disclosure is incorporated by reference herein.... The invention pertains to methods and apparatus for reducing blood viscosity of living beings, and more particularly, to methods and apparatus for preventing **renal failure** due to the administration of contrast media agents to a living being's blood.... With the use of such devices as magnetic resonance imaging (MRI) apparatus, there is a need to administer contrast media (CM) agents (for example, Acetrizoate, Iothalamate, Metrizamide, Iopamidol, Iodixanol, oral cholecystographic agents such as Iopanoic acid, Ipodate sodium, GI contrast agents such as Diatrizoate sodium, parenteral agents such as Diatrizoate Meglumine and any salts or combinations thereof) to the patient undergoing the MRI. For example, if a brain scan is being conducted using the MRI apparatus, the presence of the CM agent in the patient's bloodstream permits good tracking results. However, it has been well-documented that in certain numbers of patients, the administering of the CM agent to the patient causes **renal failure** that could ultimately result in the loss of the kidney.

Web site: http://appft1.uspto.gov/netahtml/PTO/search-bool.html

- **Method and a device for determining the dry weight of a patient with kidney failure**

Inventor(s): Chamney, Paul; (Herts, GB)

Correspondence: JACOBSON HOLMAN PLLC; 400 SEVENTH STREET N.W.; SUITE 600; WASHINGTON; DC; 20004; US

Patent Application Number: 20040064063

Date filed: November 7, 2003

Abstract: The invention relates to a method and a device for monitoring the fluid status of a patient with **kidney failure.** In case of **renal failure** all forms of ingested fluid accumulate in body tissues causing increased stress on the circulatory system. This surplus fluid has to be removed during a dialysis treatment by ultrafiltration of the blood. The amount of this surplus fluid or the weight corrected for this surplus fluid, i.e. the dry weight, is an important parameter for managing the fluid status of a dialysis patient. According to the invention the dry weight Wgt.sub.dry(t) of a patient at a time t is determined by determining the extracellular water volume ECV(t) of the patient at the time t, by determining the weight Wgt(t) of the patient at the time t and by deriving the dry weight Wgt.sub.dry(t) of the patient from an intersection of a function derived from the determined ECV(t) and Wgt(t) values with a previously established extracellular water volume (ECV) against dry weight (Wgt.sub.dry) reference relation representing healthy subjects. To obtain more accurate results it is also proposed to take into account a compartimental mass correction.DELTA.m(t). The invention also relates to a device for deriving the dry weight Wgt.sub.dry(t).

Excerpt(s): The invention relates to a method and a device for monitoring the fluid status of a patient according to the preamble of claims 1 and 12, respectively.... The kidneys carry out several functions for maintaining the health of a human body. First, they control the fluid balance by separating any excess fluid from the patient's blood volume. Second, they serve to purify the blood from any waste substances like urea or creatinine. Last not least they also control the levels of certain substances in the blood like electrolytes in order to ensure a healthy and necessary concentration level.... In case of **renal failure** all forms of ingested fluid accumulate in body tissues causing increased stress on the circulatory system. This surplus fluid has to be removed during a dialysis treatment by ultrafiltration of the blood. If insufficient fluid is removed the long term consequenses can be severe, leading to high blood pressure and cardiac failure. Cardiac failure itself is many times more likely to occur in dialysis patients and it is thought that states of fluid overload are one of the major contributing factors. Removal of too much fluid is also dangerous since the dialysis patient becomes dehydrated and this invariably leads to hypotension.

Web site: http://appft1.uspto.gov/netahtml/PTO/search-bool.html

- **Method and system for determining kidney failure**

Inventor(s): Van Hove, Jos W.J.; (Schiedam, NL), Oort, Geeske Van; (Rosmalen, NL)

Correspondence: MEDTRONIC, INC.; 710 MEDTRONIC PARKWAY NE; MS-LC340; MINNEAPOLIS; MN; 55432-5604; US

Patent Application Number: 20030083585

Date filed: October 26, 2001

Abstract: A method of determining **kidney failure** in a patient using an implantable medical device is described. In one embodiment, a first magnitude of a first polarization signal is measured. An additional magnitude of an additional polarization signal is measured after a first interval. A deflection differential between the first magnitude and the additional magnitude is determined and **kidney failure** in the patient is determined when the deflection differential is greater than an established threshold.

Excerpt(s): The present invention relates to the field of implantable medical devices. More particularly, the present invention relates to cardiac pacing systems that are capable of measure and compare polarization signals to thereby determine an occurrence of a **kidney failure**.... Implantable pulse generators (or IPGS) are well known in the prior art. After a stimulus in the heart, a charge builds up at the electrode tip, which results in a polarization signal that decays over time. While an initial magnitude of the polarization signal is dependent upon the configuration of the electrode as well as any fibrosis around the electrode tip, ionic concentration in the blood ambient the heart is a major factor in the generation of the initial magnitude. For a patient having a significant risk of experiencing **kidney failure**, the ionic concentration may increase with each succeeding dialysis of the patient. However, the medical arts have failed to utilize various measurements of the polarization signal to ascertain any increases in the ionic concentration with each succeeding dialysis of the patient.... Thus, prior to the present invention, a need existed in the medical arts for facilitating a determination of a **kidney failure** by a patient.

Web site: http://appft1.uspto.gov/netahtml/PTO/search-bool.html

- ## Method for preventing acute renal failure

Inventor(s): Warren, Howland Shaw JR.; (Cambridge, MA), Fink, Mitchell P.; (Pittsburgh, PA)

Correspondence: HAMILTON, BROOK, SMITH & REYNOLDS, P.C.; 530 VIRGINIA ROAD; P.O. BOX 9133; CONCORD; MA; 01742-9133; US

Patent Application Number: 20040068006

Date filed: October 3, 2003

Abstract: Disclosed is a method of treating acute **renal failure** in a subject. The method comprises the step of administering to the subject an effective amount of a composition comprising a 2-ketoalkanoic acid, a pharmaceutically acceptable salt of a 2-ketoalkanoic acid, an ester of a 2-ketoalkanoic acid, or an amide of a 2-ketoalkanoic acid. Preferably, the composition comprises an enolization agent and an alkyl aralkyl, alkoxyalkyl or carboxyalkyl ester of a 2-ketoalkanoic acid dissolved in a pharmaceutically acceptable vehicle.

Excerpt(s): This application is a continuation-in-part of International Application No. PCT/US02/10539, which designated the United States and was filed Apr. 3, 2002, published in English, which claims the benefit of U.S. Provisional Application No. 60/281,363, filed on Apr. 4, 2001. The entire teachings of these applications are incorporated herein by reference.... Renal failure is a major cause of long-term hospitalization and death. It is characterized by acute or chronic deterioration of kidney function that initially occurs in an individual who previously had normal kidney function or that progresses further in an individual already suffering from kidney disease and/or dysfunction. There are a number of factors which are predictive of whether a patient is likely to experience acute **renal failure.** Risk factors include pre-existing diseases or conditions such as diabetes, renal disease/dysfunction, hypotension, hemorrhagic shock, systemic inflammation, sepsis, temporary interruption of blood flow to the kidneys, liver disease or heart disease. Other risk factors include treatment with nephrotoxic drugs and contrast imaging agents. Subjects with two or more risk factors are said to be "at risk" for acute **renal failure.**... Although it is now possible to identify patients who are at risk for developing acute **renal failure,** treatments for preventing the condition are still inadequate. Thus, there is an urgent need for new methods of preventing and/or ameliorating the effects of acute **renal failure.**

Web site: http://appft1.uspto.gov/netahtml/PTO/search-bool.html

- **Method of measuring lipid components and method of examining of renal failure**

Inventor(s): Hiura, Hisahide; (Kakogawa, JP), Hotta, Osamu; (Sendai, JP), Shirahase, Yasushi; (Kobe, JP)

Correspondence: SUGHRUE MION, PLLC; 2100 PENNSYLVANIA AVENUE, N.W.; WASHINGTON; DC; 20037; US

Patent Application Number: 20030017523

Date filed: August 7, 2002

Abstract: The problems of the present invention are to provide a simple and convenient means for the examination of **renal failure** and to provide a method for the measurement of a lipid component in urine utilizing the said examining means.Means for solving the problems according to the present invention is a method for the measurement of a lipid component contained in urine and it provides a method for measurement of a lipid component in urine which is characterized in using a surface-active agent in a sufficient amount for solubilizing the insoluble fat in urine and in using an enzyme acting the lipid component. It also provides a simple and convenient means for the examination of **renal failure** by the measurement of a lipid component contained in urine, by the measurement of lipoproteins in urine and/or apoproteins in urine in addition to the above measurement and by a combination of measurement of surface antigen of leukocyte contained in urine therewith.

Excerpt(s): The present invention relates to a method for the measurement of lipid component in urine and to a reagent for the measurement. The present invention further relates to a examination means for **renal failure** utilizing the said method for the measurement.... Components contained in urinary sediment are diversified such as components derived from kidney, components mingled from urinary tract and crystalline components separated out in urine. Checking the type and the amount of the sediment is very important in judging the diseases of kidney and urinary tract and in knowing their degree. They are usually carried out by an observation under a microscope by a dyeing method. There are also shown that pathological diagnosis of IgA nephropathy is possible by checking the surface antigen of macrophage in urine (Rinsho Kensa, volume 42, 588.about.590, 1998) and that examination of **renal failure** is possible by judging the fat particle and oviform fat body (hereinafter, sometimes referred to as just "fat body") in urine by means of dyeing off at in the urinary sediment (Kensa to Gijutsu, volume 26, 441-446, 1998).... Further, in macrophage in a big size appeared in urine, surface antigen CD14 of leukocyte is negative while

25F9 is positive and that is greatly different from the usual macrophage where CD14 is positive while 25F9 is negative. In addition, it is shown that fat particle and oviform fat body belong to microphage in a big size and it is mentioned that measurement of them is useful as the examination for **renal failure** (Rinsho Byori, volume 47, Issue for General Meeting, 73, 1999).

Web site: http://appft1.uspto.gov/netahtml/PTO/search-bool.html

- **Method of use of erythropoietin to treat ischemic acute renal failure**

Inventor(s): Westenfelder, Christof; (Salt Lake City, UT)

Correspondence: Justin B. Rand; c/o BRINKS HOFER GILSON & LIONE; P.O. Box 10395; Chicago; IL; 60610; US

Patent Application Number: 20030083251

Date filed: November 1, 2001

Abstract: Recombinant erythropoietin is used in a method to prevent ischemic acute **renal failure** in patients at risk for developing ischemic acute **renal failure** and to treat fully-developed ischemic acute **renal failure.** The method is also used to prevent harmful cell apoptosis in renal tubular cells and to stimulate mitogenesis and motogenesis in renal tubular cells. The method comprises the administration of a composition of recombinant erythropoietin in a pharmacologically acceptable carrier to a patient for the purpose of preventing the development of ischemic acute **renal failure,** treating established acute **renal failure,** preventing harmful cell apoptosis in renal tubular cells.

Excerpt(s): This invention relates to a method of use of a composition of matter. More particularly, the invention relates to a novel method of using a pharmaceutical composition comprising erythropoietin for treating ischemic acute **renal failure** (ARF) and for preventing the onset of ischemic ARF.... Clinical acute **renal failure** (ARF) remains a common and serious complication associated with high morbidity and mortality. Moderately effective measures to prevent ARF include volume expansion, and in renal transplants, mannitol administration. The uremic state, volume and electrolyte disturbances can be readily corrected by hemodialysis, and outcomes are improved when more biocompatible dialysis membranes are used. In addition, administration of atrial natriuretic peptide has been found to speed the improvement of renal function in some patients with ARF.... In the induction phase of ARF, cell necrosis, apoptosis, and sub-lethal injury are observed [1,2,3,4,5,6]. These effects are thought to collectively contribute to the loss of renal function via pathological activation of tubuloglomerular feedback, back leak of ultrafiltrate, tubular obstruction and ineffective transport by partially depolarized tubular cells [1,2,3,4,5,6]. In the repair phase of ARF, reepithelialization of injured tubules is accomplished by migration of cells ("motogenesis") into deepithelialized nephron segments, cell proliferation ("mitogenesis"), and redifferentiation of newly generated and sublethally injured tubular cells [1,6,7]. Anabolic mechanisms and improvement of intrarenal hemodynamics are also critical to functional recovery [1,2,8,9,10].

Web site: http://appft1.uspto.gov/netahtml/PTO/search-bool.html

- **Therapeutic agent for renal failure**

  Inventor(s): Kurumatani, Hajimu; (Kanagawa, JP), Suzuki, Motohiro; (Kanagawa, JP)

  Correspondence: SCHNADER HARRISON SEGAL & LEWIS, LLP; 1600 MARKET STREET; SUITE 3600; PHILADELPHIA; PA; 19103

  Patent Application Number: 20030092760

  Date filed: November 7, 2002

  Abstract: The present invention relates to a therapeutic agent for **renal failure** comprising, as an active ingredient, a 4,8-inter-m-phenylene prostaglandin I.sub.2 derivative, and also relates to a method of treatment of **renal failure** using the same.

  Excerpt(s): The present invention relates to a therapeutic agent for **renal failure** comprising, as an active ingredient, a 4,8-inter-m-phenylene prostaglandin I.sub.2 derivative or a pharmacologically acceptable salt thereof.... Prostaglandins (PGs) are a class of naturally occurring compounds with a wide variety of physiological activities, which have a common prostanoic acid skeleton. Naturally occurring PGs are classified into PGAs, PGBs, PGCs, PGDs, PGEs, PGFs, PGGs, PGHs, PGIs and PGJs according to the structural characteristics of the 5-membered ring in the skeleton. It is and also classified into subclasses 1, 2, 3 and so on according to the ansaturation and oxidation. Various synthetic analogues of these PGs are known. Among these, PGI.sub.2, which is a typical PGI derivative, is called prostacycline (see Nature, vol. 268, p. 688, 1976). PGI.sub.2 is known as a substance having potent platelet aggregation inhibiting activity and peripheral vasodilator activity. Japanese Examined Patent Application Publication Nos. 2-12226, 2-57548 and 1-53672 have described 4,8-inter-m-phenylene PGI.sub.2 derivatives, in which the exo-enol ether moiety that is a structurally characteristic portion of PGI.sub.2 is converted to an inter-m-phenylene moiety to substantially improve the instability of PGI.sub.2. However, it has not yet recognized that such derivatives have therapeutic activities on **renal failure**.... Renal failure is a condition characterized by decreased number of functional nephrons, resulting in reduced excretion of nitrogenous metabolic products and eventually causing the failure to maintain homeostasis in the biological environment. Specifically, this can be said to be a condition in which blood urea nitrogen (BUN) and creatinine levels are continuously increased. **Renal failure** is categorized into two primary types: acute **renal failure** in which the onset is abrupt and recovery may occur; and chronic **renal failure** which is slowly progressive but irreversible.

Web site: http://appft1.uspto.gov/netahtml/PTO/search-bool.html

- **Therapies for chronic renal failure using one or more integrin antagonists**

Inventor(s): Allen, Andrew; (Lake Forest, IL), Lobb, Roy; (Westwood, MA), Pusey, Charles; (Ealing, GB)

Correspondence: Timothy P. Linkkila; BIOGEN, INC.; 14 Cambridge Center; Cambridge; MA; 02142; US

Patent Application Number: 20030007969

Date filed: March 12, 2002

Abstract: The present invention provides methods for the treatment, and pharmaceuticals for use in the treatment, of mammalian subjects in, or at risk of chronic **renal failure,** or at risk of a need for renal replacement therapy. The methods involve the administration of certain integrin antagonists.

Excerpt(s): This is a continuation of PCT/US00/25140, filed on Sep. 14, 2000, which claims priority from U.S. provisional application Serial No. 60/153,826 filed on Sep. 14, 1999.... The present invention relates generally to methods of treatment for renal disease. In particular, the invention relates to methods of treatment for conditions which place mammals, including humans, in, or at risk of, chronic **renal failure.** The methods involve the administration of certain integrin antagonists.... Many physiological processes require that cells come into close contact with other cells and/or extracellular matrix. Such adhesion events may be required for cell activation, migration (e.g., leukocyte migration), proliferation and differentiation. Cell-cell and cell-matrix interactions are mediated through several families of cell adhesion molecules, one family of which includes the integrins.

Web site: http://appft1.uspto.gov/netahtml/PTO/search-bool.html

- **Treatment or prevention of acute renal failure**

Inventor(s): Moskowitz, David W.; (St. Louis, MO)

Correspondence: PATREA L. PABST; HOLLAND & KNIGHT LLP; SUITE 2000, ONE ATLANTIC CENTER; 1201 WEST PEACHTREE STREET, N.E.; ATLANTA; GA; 30309-3400; US

Patent Application Number: 20030032650

Date filed: August 8, 2002

Abstract: Adenosine receptor antagonists, especially aminophyllline, are used to treat or prevent acute **renal failure.** In the preferred embodiment, aminophylline is administered by infusion so that it does not exceed a serum theophylline level of 15-20 micrograms/ml, most preferably the aminophylline is administered to achieve a serum theophylline concentration of 3-10 micrograms/ml, with an infusion rate of 0.1-0.6 mg/kg IBW/hour (IBW=ideal body weight). The adenosine receptor antagonist can also be used to help sustain a kidney for transplant purposes. Preferably, aminophylline is loaded while the kidney is still part of the donor. A dose of aminophylline of 5 mg/kg lean body weight is infused into the donor over a 30-60 min period, with cardiac monitoring. The infusion dose is decreased in the event of supraventricular or ventricular tachycardias. The kidney is removed and placed in the standard "cold" bath, but containing aminophylline at a dose of 5-10 micrograms/ml (5-10 mg/l). The kidney is then transported to the recipient. The recipient is similarly preloaded with 5 mg/kg lean body mass aminophylline intravenously over 30-60 min with cardiac monitoring, with a constant infusion of 0.1-0.3 mg/kg lean body mass/hr continuing during the next 24 hours after the kidney is transplanted into the recipient.

Excerpt(s): This application claims priority to U.S. S. No. 60/310,686 filed Aug. 8, 2001 and U.S. S. No. 60/352,075 filed Jan. 28, 2002.... This is generally in the field of treatment or prevention of acute **renal failure** due to prerenal causes by administration of an antagonist of adenosine signaling, such as aminophylline, and of treatment of kidney transplants (renal allografts) to prolong survival of the graft during cold ischemia and immediately after transplantation.... Acute **kidney failure** occurs when illness, infection, or injury damages the kidneys resulting in a rapid decline in the kidneys' ability to clear the blood of toxic substances. Temporarily, the kidneys cannot adequately remove fluids and wastes from the body or maintain the proper level of certain kidney-regulated chemicals leading to an accumulation of metabolic waste products, such as urea, in the blood.

Web site: http://appft1.uspto.gov/netahtml/PTO/search-bool.html

- **Use of des-Aspartate-angiotensin I as an agent for the treatment and prevention of glomerulosclerosis and renal failure**

Inventor(s): Sim, Meng Kwoon; (Singapore, SG), Tan, Chorh Chuan; (Singapore, SG)

Correspondence: KLARQUIST SPARKMAN, LLP; One World Trade Center, Suite 1600; 121 S.W. Salmon Street; Portland; OR; 97204; US

Patent Application Number: 20030086920

Date filed: October 11, 2002

Excerpt(s): The present invention relates generally to a method for the treatment and/or prophylaxis of renal-related disorders. More particularly, the present invention contemplates a method for the treatment and/or prophylaxis of glomerulosclerosis and/or end stage **renal failure** and/or related conditions. The method of the present invention is preferably practised by the administration of a derivative of angiotensin I. Generally, but not exclusively, the angiotensin I derivative exhibits anti-angiotensin II properties. In a preferred embodiment, the angiotensin I is des-Aspartate-angiotensin I or a derivative, homologue or analogue thereof. The present invention further contemplates compositions for use in the treatment and/or prophylaxis of renal-related disorders such as but not limited to glomerulosclerosis and/or end stage **renal failure**.... Renal failure and other renal related conditions contribute to significant morbidity and mortality in patients affected by such conditions. There is a need, therefore, to develop more efficacious pharmaceutical molecules useful in the treatment of renal conditions.... des-Aspartate angiotensin I (des-Asp-angiotensin I) is a nonapeptide produced from a decapeptide by the action of an aminopeptidase. The nonapeptide is produced from angiotensin I by enzymatic NH.sub.2-terminal degradation (1). des-Asp-angiotensin I is a substrate for plasma and pulmonary angiotensin converting enzyme (2). Furthermore, des-Asp-angiotensin I acts on a specific indomethacin-sensitive subtype of angiotensin receptor (3) and to antagonize the pressor (4) and hypertrophic (5) actions of angiotensin II. Angiotensin II is a key mediator of glomerulosclerosis in progressive kidney diseases (6-8). In work leading up to the present invention, the inventors determined that the anti-angiotensin II properties of des-Asp-angiotensin I can be exploited in the treatment and/or prophylaxis of renal-related disorders.

Web site: http://appft1.uspto.gov/netahtml/PTO/search-bool.html

- **Use of prostaglandin (PGE2) receptor 4 (EP4) selective agonists for the treatment of acute and chronic renal failure**

Inventor(s): Paralkar, Vishwas M.; (Madison, CT), Thompson, David D.; (Gales Ferry, CT)

Correspondence: Gregg C. Benson; Pfizer Inc.; Patent Department, MS 4159; Eastern Point Road; Groton; CT; 06340; US

Patent Application Number: 20010041729

Date filed: January 29, 2001

Abstract: This invention is directed to methods and compositions of treating acute or chronic **renal failure** or dysfunction, or conditions caused thereby, comprising administering prostaglandin agonists, which are EP.sub.4 receptor selective prostaglandin agonists.

Excerpt(s): This application claims the benefit of U.S. Provisional Application No. 60/178,968, filed Jan. 31, 2000.... The present invention relates to methods and pharmaceutical compositions comprising receptor selective prostaglandin (PGE.sub.2) agonists for the treatment of kidney diseases, such as chronic and acute **renal failure** or dysfunction, in animals, particularly mammals. More specifically, the present invention relates to such methods and pharmaceutical compositions comprising type 4 (EP.sub.4) receptor selective prostaglandin (PGE.sub.2) agonists.... The naturally occurring prostaglandins are comprised of several biological entities including PBD, PGE, PGF, PGG, PGH and PGI. It has been well documented that prostaglandins have effects on many of the organs and systems of the body.

Web site: http://appft1.uspto.gov/netahtml/PTO/search-bool.html

## Keeping Current

In order to stay informed about patents and patent applications dealing with kidney failure, you can access the U.S. Patent Office archive via the Internet at the following Web address: **http://www.uspto.gov/patft/index.html**. You will see two broad options: (1) Issued Patent, and (2) Published Applications. To see a list of issued patents, perform the following steps: Under "Issued Patents," click "Quick Search." Then, type "kidney failure" (or synonyms) into the "Term 1" box. After clicking on the search button, scroll down to see the various patents which have been granted to date on kidney failure.

You can also use this procedure to view pending patent applications concerning kidney failure. Simply go back to the following Web address:

**http://www.uspto.gov/patft/index.html**. Select "Quick Search" under "Published Applications." Then proceed with the steps listed above.

## Vocabulary Builder

The following vocabulary builder provides definitions of words used in this chapter that have not been defined in previous chapters:

**Airway:** A device for securing unobstructed passage of air into and out of the lungs during general anesthesia. [NIH]

**Allografts:** A graft of tissue obtained from the body of another animal of the same species but with genotype differing from that of the recipient; tissue graft from a donor of one genotype to a host of another genotype with host and donor being members of the same species. [NIH]

**Ameliorating:** A changeable condition which prevents the consequence of a failure or accident from becoming as bad as it otherwise would. [NIH]

**Aspartate:** A synthetic amino acid. [NIH]

**Benson:** Snowball-like bodies of calcium soaps occurring in a structurally intact vitreous body. [NIH]

**Bernstein:** A sensitive means of determining whether acid reflux is the cause of pain, but may be falsely negative in the patient receiving treatment. [NIH]

**Efferent:** Nerve fibers which conduct impulses from the central nervous system to muscles and glands. [NIH]

**Electrode:** Component of the pacing system which is at the distal end of the lead. It is the interface with living cardiac tissue across which the stimulus is transmitted. [NIH]

**Endoscopic:** A technique where a lateral-view endoscope is passed orally to the duodenum for visualization of the ampulla of Vater. [NIH]

**Enkephalin:** A natural opiate painkiller, in the hypothalamus. [NIH]

**Enzymatic:** Phase where enzyme cuts the precursor protein. [NIH]

**Generator:** Any system incorporating a fixed parent radionuclide from which is produced a daughter radionuclide which is to be removed by elution or by any other method and used in a radiopharmaceutical. [NIH]

**Imidazole:** $C_3H_4N_2$. The ring is present in polybenzimidazoles. [NIH]

**Impairment:** In the context of health experience, an impairment is any loss or abnormality of psychological, physiological, or anatomical structure or function. [NIH]

**Lactulose:** A mild laxative. [NIH]

**Migration:** The systematic movement of genes between populations of the same species, geographic race, or variety. [NIH]

**Sebaceous:** Gland that secretes sebum. [NIH]

**Segal:** The alternate presentation of two visual stimuli consisting of concentric circular spots of light of different size. [NIH]

**Sendai:** A virus that causes an important and widespread infection of laboratory mice; it belongs to the parainfluenza group of mixoviruses. The virus is widely used in cell fusion studies. [NIH]

**Stimulus:** That which can elicit or evoke action (response) in a muscle, nerve, gland or other excitable issue, or cause an augmenting action upon any function or metabolic process. [NIH]

**Threshold:** For a specified sensory modality (e. g. light, sound, vibration), the lowest level (absolute threshold) or smallest difference (difference threshold, difference limen) or intensity of the stimulus discernible in prescribed conditions of stimulation. [NIH]

**Trauma:** Any injury, wound, or shock, must frequently physical or structural shock, producing a disturbance. [NIH]

# CHAPTER 5. BOOKS ON KIDNEY FAILURE

## Overview

This chapter provides bibliographic book references relating to kidney failure. You have many options to locate books on kidney failure. The simplest method is to go to your local bookseller and inquire about titles that they have in stock or can special order for you. Some patients, however, feel uncomfortable approaching their local booksellers and prefer online sources (e.g. **www.amazon.com** and **www.bn.com**). In addition to online booksellers, excellent sources for book titles on kidney failure include the Combined Health Information Database and the National Library of Medicine. Once you have found a title that interests you, visit your local public or medical library to see if it is available for loan.

## Book Summaries: Federal Agencies

The Combined Health Information Database collects various book abstracts from a variety of healthcare institutions and federal agencies. To access these summaries, go to **http://chid.nih.gov/detail/detail.html**. You will need to use the "Detailed Search" option. To find book summaries, use the drop boxes at the bottom of the search page where "You may refine your search by." Select the dates and language you prefer. For the format option, select "Monograph/Book." Now type "kidney failure" (or synonyms) into the "For these words:" box. You will only receive results on books. You should check back periodically with this database which is updated every 3 months. The following is a typical result when searching for books on kidney failure:

- **Cardiac Dysfunction in Chronic Uremia**

  Source: Norwell, MA: Kluwer Academic Publishers. 1992. 231 p.

Contact: Available from Kluwer Academic Publishers. P.O. Box 358, Accord Station, Hingham, MA 02018-0358. (617) 871-6600. PRICE: $145 plus shipping and handling.

Summary: Cardiac disease is the major cause of death in dialysis patients, accounting for over one-third of deaths. This book focuses on myocardial function and dysfunction in chronic **uremia.**. It is written for practicing and training nephrologists, cardiologists, and internists, and for research workers in the field. The first section comprises five chapters that provide an overview of the burden of illness associated with cardiac disease in **end-stage renal disease** and a review of clinical epidemiological aspects of various cardiac diseases that occur in renal patients. The second section discusses abnormalities of left ventricular contractility and mass, and the factors that predispose to both systolic and diastolic disorders. The importance of hypertension, anemia, hyperparathyroidism, hyperlipidemia, and diabetes mellitus is reviewed. The final section concentrates on therapeutics. Data and opinion on management of congestive heart failure, cardiomyopathy, coronary artery disease, hypertension, and arrhythmias are provided. Each chapter includes numerous references and a subject index is appended to the volume. (AA-M).

- **Clinical Practice Guidelines for the Treatment of Anemia of Chronic Renal Failure**

Source: New York, NY: National Kidney Foundation. 1997. 174 p.

Contact: Available from National Kidney Foundation. 30 East 33rd Street, New York, NY 10016. (800) 622-9010. Fax (212) 689-9261. PRICE: $13.00. ISBN: 0962972177.

Summary: In March 1995, the National Kidney Foundation Dialysis Outcomes Quality Initiative (NKF-DOQI) was established, with the objective of improving patient outcomes and survival by providing recommendations for optimal clinical practices in four areas: hemodialysis adequacy, peritoneal dialysis adequacy, vascular access, and the treatment of anemia of chronic **renal failure** (CRF). This document presents 28 clinical practice guidelines for anemia. They are categorized in seven sections: anemia workup, target hematocrit and hemoglobin, iron support, administration of Epoetin (erythropoietin), inadequate epoetin response, the role of red blood cell transfusions, and possible adverse effects related to epoetin therapy. Each guideline is accompanied by a rationale, enabling dialysis caregivers to make informed decisions about the proper care plan for each individual patient. This document also includes a list of acronyms and abbreviations, a description of the guideline development methodology, endnotes, references, biographical sketches of the NKF-DOQI anemia work group members, and a complete listing of the articles reviewed by the anemia work group. 1 figure. 9 tables. 349 references. (AA-M).

- **Kidney Failure and the Federal Government**

Source: Washington, DC: National Academy Press. 1991. 426 p.

Contact: Available from National Academy Press. 2101 Constitution Avenue, NW, Washington, DC 20055. (800) 624-6242. PRICE: $39.96 plus shipping and handling. ISBN: 0309044324.

Summary: In the Social Security Amendments of 1972, Congress created an entitlement to Medicare for all persons with a diagnosis of permanent **kidney failure** who were fully or currently insured or eligible for benefits under Social Security, and for spouses or dependent children of such persons. The ESRD program is unique within Medicare in that it is the only case in which the diagnosis of a categorical disease provides the basis for an entitlement for persons of all ages. This book is the report of the Institute of Medicine (IOM), which was asked by Congress in 1987 to study the ESRD program with respect to the following issues: epidemiological and demographic factors that may affect access to treatment, quality of care, or the resource requirements of the program; access to treatment; quality of care; effect of reimbursement on quality of care; and the adequacy of existing data systems to monitor these factors. The book includes five sections. Part I is an overview of the study and the ESRD program. Part II deals with patients and providers, including the results of patient focus groups, ethical issues related to the initiation and termination of treatment and the problem patient, background information about the patient population, special ESRD groups (pediatric, elderly, diabetic, hypertensive, ethnic groups), and the nature and structure of dialysis and transplantation providers. Part III deals with access issues, including access to transplantation. Part IV addresses the relationship between reimbursement and quality, and Part V focuses on data and research. The conclusions and recommendations of the IOM committee are provided in each section. The book includes extensive appendices, including a glossary, a list of acronyms and initialisms, commissioned papers and contractor reports, survival analysis methods, IOM committee public hearings reports and workshop reports, and a list of the IOM patient focus group participants. A subject index concludes the volume. 17 figures. 64 tables.

- **Psychosocial Aspects of End-Stage Renal Disease: Issues of Our Times**

Source: Binghamton, NY: The Haworth Press. 1991. 218 p.

Contact: Haworth Press. 10 Alice Street, Binghamton, NY 13904-1580. (607) 722-2493. PRICE: $39.95 plus $3 shipping and handling. ISBN: 1560241497.

Summary: In this book, numerous specialists in the field of kidney disease offer insight into the psychosocial aspects of **end-stage renal disease.** Five sections explore renal disease and the family, the psychosocial dimensions of renal disease, ethical issues in the treatment of renal disease, staff/patient perspectives in the care of renal disease, and renal disease and special patient populations. Within these sections, 20 chapters cover topics including communication between the disciplines in health care provision, families coping with chronic illness, marital and family characteristics, hemodialysis, organ transplantation, dealing with death, illness intrusiveness, coping with the failure of a renal transplant, bioethics, dialysis staff attitudes, patient perceptions, AIDS and **end-stage renal disease,** and care of the geriatric nephrology patient.

- **Renal Failure: Blackwell's Basics of Medicine**

  Source: Oxford, England: Blackwell Science Ltd. 1995. 295 p.

  Contact: Available from Blackwell Science, Inc. 238 Main Street, Cambridge, MA 02142. (800) 215-1000 or (617) 876-7000. Fax (617) 492-5263. PRICE: $24.95. ISBN: 0865424306.

  Summary: This book for health professionals on **renal failure** is from a series that examines relevant topics in medicine using concepts that pertain to the basic sciences. In this series, readers learn to interpret clinical data based on pathophysiological concepts. Four sections in this book cover the following issues: essentials, pathophysiology, clinical picture, and management of **renal failure.** Each section offers questions, with answers of one or two paragraphs on relevant topics. The 555 questions are numbered for ease of access through the subject index. Specific topics covered include: the anatomy of the kidneys, the kidney function tests used for diagnosis and monitoring, electrolyte function, urine concentration and dilution, oral water load, the roles of aldosterone, the role of the kidney in acid base balance, potassium, dietary therapy, chronic **renal failure,** polyuria, water and salt homeostasis, metabolic acidosis, renal tubular acidosis, hyperkalemia, acute tubular necrosis, **uremia,** renal impairment associated with diabetes mellitus, etiology of **renal failure,** hepatorenal syndrome, obstructive uropathy, anemia and erythropoietin, osteodystrophy, dialysis, prognosis, cost factors, and kidney transplantation.

- **Pathogenetic and Therapeutic Aspects of Chronic Renal Failure**

  Source: New York, NY: Marcel Dekker, Inc. 1997. 242 p.

  Contact: Available from Marcel Dekker, Inc. 270 Madison Avenue, New York, NY 10016. (212) 696-9000. Fax (212) 685-4540. PRICE: $115.00. ISBN: 0824798945.

  Summary: This book is based on an international workshop, Chronic Renal Failure: Pathogenetic and Therapeutic Aspects, held in Berlin in May 1996. The first part of the book deals with arterial hypertension, hyperlipidemia, and metabolic acidosis as factors that accelerate the progression of chronic **renal failure** (CRF) and with the effect of dietary protein restriction as a measure to slow the advance of renal insufficiency. The second part addresses the etiology and pathophysiology of myocardial hypertrophy in general, and especially in **uremia,** and the influence of the dialysis regimen on the development of myocardial hypertrophy. The final section discusses the correction of renal anemia via treatment with recombinant human erythropoietin (rhEPO), with special emphasis on its effects on cardiac function and hypertrophy and on the function of parts of the endocrine system. Also included are an analysis of the use of rhEPO in renal transplant patients and an overview of the problems of iron supplementation in rhEPO treatment. The 17 chapters, each written by experts in the field, include reference lists; a subject index concludes the book.

- **Coping with Kidney Failure**

  Source: Garden City Park, NY: Avery Publishing Group. 1987. 309 p.

  Contact: Available from Avery Publishing Group. 120 Old Broadway, Garden City Park, NY 11040. (800) 548-5757 or (516) 741-2155. Fax (516) 742-1892. E-mail: info@averypublishing.com. Website: www.averypublishing.com. PRICE: $14.95 plus shipping and handling. ISBN: 0895293706.

  Summary: This book offers people with kidney disease a guide to adapting to life with **kidney failure.** The first part of the book presents background information on kidney failure: what it is, some of the causes of **kidney failure,** diagnostic considerations, symptoms and signs of **kidney failure,** and prevention and treatment strategies. The other main parts deal with different aspects of living with **kidney failure,** including kidney transplantation, dialysis (both hemodialysis and peritoneal dialysis), coping with emotions, changes in general lifestyle, and living with others. Specific chapters are offered on the child and adolescent with **kidney failure.** The author cautions that even if medical treatment is successful, both dialysis and transplantation can be psychologically debilitating and can cause considerable emotional difficulty. Suggestions for strategies and techniques to try are offered in the areas of diet, medications, dialysis equipment and supplies, physical changes, exercise, weight changes, nutritional needs, pain, financial problems, traveling, sexuality, dealing with family members, pregnancy, emotions, stress management. Throughout the book, the author offers vignettes of patients with **kidney failure** who have struggled with different issues and explains how they coped with their own situations. The book concludes with an appendix listing a few resources and a subject index.

- **Strength and Compassion in Kidney Failure**

Source: Norwell, MA: Kluwer Academic Publishers. 1998. 221 p.

Contact: Available from American Association of Kidney Patients (AAKP). 100 South Ashley Drive, Suite 280, Tampa, FL 3302. (800) 749-2257 or (813) 223-7099. Fax (813) 223-0001. E-mail: AAKPnat@aol.com. PRICE: $25.00 plus shipping and handling. ISBN: 079235236X.

Summary: This book presents a collection of medical columns, short stories, and letters written to offer hope, enthusiasm, and joy to people who have a chronic illness. The author, who was faced with the progressive loss of sight and ambulation from complications of diabetes, Addison's disease, and **renal failure,** demonstrates through her writing how she coped and prevailed despite her condition. Medical column topics include caring for diabetic feet and skin, eating, taking medications, traveling, coping with holidays, determining whether the findings of the Diabetes Control and Complications Trial are good or bad, and understanding the physical side of diabetes. Letters and commentary present personal messages about dealing with a chronic illness.

- **Kidney Failure: The Facts**

Source: Oxford, England: Oxford University Press. 1996. 235 p.

Contact: Available from Oxford University Press. Book Order Department, 2001 Evans Road, Cary, NC 27513. (800) 451-7556 or (919) 677-1303. PRICE: $18.95. ISBN: 0192626434.

Summary: This book provides people with kidney disease and their families with information about **kidney failure.** The author explains the causes and symptoms of **kidney failure** and focuses on the various treatment options, especially dialysis and transplantation. Eleven chapters are organized around questions that kidney patients commonly have, covering these topics: the role of the kidneys (anatomy and physiology); how to know if one has kidney disease (the symptoms); the potentially treatable causes of chronic **kidney failure;** the causes of

**kidney failure** for which there is as yet no treatment; what to expect when one's kidneys fail; artificial kidneys and dialysis; peritoneal dialysis; kidney transplantation; kidney patients with other special needs, including people with diabetes or paraplegia, children, and the elderly; a review of treatments for **kidney failure;** and the outlook for the future. The book includes two appendices: a list of commonly used abbreviations in nephrology and a list of organizations (United Kingdom, Australia, and United States) concerned with the welfare of kidney patients and information on kidney diseases. A subject index concludes the volume.

- **Kidney Failure: Coping and Feeling Your Best**

  Source: Atlanta, GA: Pritchett and Hull Associates, Inc. 1994. 48 p.

  Contact: Available from Pritchett and Hull Associates, Inc. 3440 Oakcliff Road NE, Suite 110, Atlanta, GA 30340-3079. (800) 241-4925. PRICE: $9.95 plus shipping; wholesale to health care professionals $5.50 plus shipping; quantity discounts available.

  Summary: This easy-to-read book supports patients during the difficult time of being diagnosed with **renal failure.** In the book, the author discusses **kidney failure** in general; explains peritoneal and hemodialysis; describes diet restrictions and medications for those with chronic **renal failure** (CRF); tells patients how to avoid problems, how to recognize them, and what to do if they occur; gives patients concrete ways to cope with a diagnosis of CRF; and contains interactive sections on meal planning, medication administration, weight monitoring, and using a support network. Weight and medicine charts are included, as is a brief resource list. The book is illustrated with cartoon line drawings, featuring a humorous personified kidney who leads the way.

- **Urea Kinetics in Nutritional Management of Pre-End-Stage Renal Disease, Including Hemodialysis Applications**

  Source: Morgan Hill, CA: Council on Renal Nutrition, Northern California-Northern Nevada. 1993. 30 p.

  Contact: Available from Council on Renal Nutrition, Northern California-Northern Nevada. c/o Elaine Rodgers, 560 Caprice Court, Morgan Hill, CA 95037. PRICE: $14.95 plus $2.50 postage (as of 1995). ISBN: 1883146518.

  Summary: This handbook describes the clinical use of urea kinetics in the nutritional management of the pre-ESRD patient. The handbook includes formulas and examples needed to calculate protein requirements and nitrogen balance in this patient population. Topics include the nutritional applications of protein catabolic rate; the calculation of protein catabolic rate; the calculation of creatinine clearance and creatinine generation rate; the use of creatinine data; spot urine; prediction of BUN on a prescribed level of protein intake and known renal function; the differences created by patient size; and practical guidelines for the use of urea kinetics. Also included are a summary of formulas and abbreviations; a clinical nutritional assessment summary; a urea kinetics summary worksheet; guidelines for determining lean body weight; and urine collection instructions. The booklet concludes with a brief glossary. 14 references.

- **Clinical Guide to Nutrition Care in End-Stage Renal Disease. 2nd ed**

Source: Chicago, IL: American Dietetic Association. 1994. 255 p.

Contact: Available from American Dietetic Association. 216 West Jackson Boulevard Chicago, IL 60606-6995. (312) 899-0040. PRICE: $24 for members; $28 for non-members; plus shipping and handling. ISBN: 0880911247.

Summary: This manual provides guidelines for the clinical nutrition care of patients with **end-stage renal disease** (ESRD). Designed for renal dietitians, the manual contains 14 chapters and 11 appendices covering topics including normal and diseased kidney anatomy and function; nutrition assessment in chronic **renal failure;** dietary treatment in the early stages of chronic **renal failure;** nutrition management of adult hemodialysis and peritoneal dialysis patients; the nutrition management of the adult renal transplant patient; nutrition management of the patient with diabetes and renal disease; nutrition recommendations for infants, children and adolescents with ESRD; enteral nutrition in **end-stage renal disease;** parenteral nutrition for the patient with **renal failure;** medications commonly prescribed in chronic **renal failure;** renal osteodystrophy; attaining nutrition goals for hyperlipidemic and obese renal patients; nutrition management of the patient with urolithiasis; nutrition care of the hospitalized patient with **renal failure;** helpful hints for common patient problems; the management of anemia in ESRD; pregnancy and dialysis; hyperdietism; forms and documents; disaster diet information for hemodialysis patients; guidelines for estimating renal dietitian staffing levels, and funding for ESRD nutrition services. One of the appendices lists professional organizations for renal dietitians and another provides a medication and manufacturer reference index. The volume concludes with a subject index.

- **Acute Renal Failure: Diagnosis, Treatment, and Prevention**

Source: New York, NY: Marcel Dekker, Inc. 1991. 519 p.

Contact: Available from Marcel Dekker, Inc. P.O. Box 5005, Monticello, NY 12701. (800) 228-1160 or (212) 696-9000. Fax (914) 796-1772. E-mail: bookorders@dekker.com. PRICE: $165.00. ISBN: 0824782259.

Summary: This medical text on the diagnosis, treatment, and prevention of acute **renal failure** (ARF) arose from the 1988 Symposium on Acute **Renal Failure.** The book presents 34 papers in 4 sections: background, pathogenesis, and diagnosis; nuclear magnetic resonance and the kidney; treatment of ARF; and prevention of ARF. Specific topics include the etiology of ARF; ARF in the tropics; ischemic ARF; animal studies of ARF; nephrotoxicity; magnetic resonance imaging (MRI); drug therapy; early transplant nonfunction; dialysis treatment of ARF in children; acquired resistance in ARF; ARF caused by ACE inhibitors; and ARF following use of radiocontrast agents. Each chapter, written by experts in the field, includes numerous charts and diagrams, as well as extensive references. A subject index concludes the volume.

- **Aluminum and Renal Failure**

  Source: Boston, MA: Kluwer Academic Publishers Group. 1990. 382 p.

  Contact: Available from Kluwer Academic Publishers. Order Department, P.O. Box 358, Accord Station, Hingham, MA 02018-0358. (617) 871-6600. Fax (617) 871-6528. E-mail: kluwer@world.std.com. PRICE: $205.50. ISBN: 0792303474.

  Summary: This monograph, part of the Development in Nephrology series, deals with the various aspects of and the most recent insights into aluminum accumulation, toxicity and **renal failure.** Besides providing a fundamental approach to the chemistry, the analysis and metabolism of aluminum are discussed, as well as the pathophysiological mechanisms of aluminum toxicity. Experimental models are proposed and the cellular and subcellular localization of the element is illustrated. Furthermore, the book focuses on the clinical consequences of aluminum accumulation and the current methods available for diagnosis and treatment. The monograph contains the most recent material on the pharmacokinetics of desferrioxamine and its chelates. Risk factors involved in the prevention of aluminum toxicity are also described. 38 figures, 35 tables, 1,491 references. (AA-M).

- **Atlas of Diseases of the Kidney. Volume 1: Disorders of Water, Electrolytes, and Acid-Base/Acute Renal Failure**

  Source: Philadelphia, PA: Current Medicine, Inc. 1999. [336 p.].

  Contact: Available from Blackwell Science, Inc. 350 Main Street, Malden, MA 02148. (800) 215-1000 or (781) 388-8250. Fax (781) 388-8270. E-mail:

csbooks@blacksci.com. PRICE: $75.00 plus shipping and handling. ISBN: 0632043857.

Summary: This volume is one in a series of five in the Atlas of Diseases of the Kidney, a set that offers educational images including colored photographs, schematics, tables, and algorithms. In Volume 1, the first section covers disorders of water and sodium balance; potassium, magnesium, phosphate, and calcium metabolism; and acid base balance. The second section addresses acute **renal failure** (ARF), including ischemic and nephrotoxic insults and the cellular and molecular mechanisms of renal injury and repair. Diagnostic evaluation, renal histology, nutrition and support therapies including intermittent hemodialysis, peritoneal dialysis, and continuous renal replacement therapies are illustrated. Other topics include ARF in the transplanted kidney; renal injury due to environmental toxins, drugs, and contrast agents; the pathophysiology of nephrotoxic ARF; and nutrition and metabolism in ARF. Each chapter features a detailed introduction and lengthy captions for each of the illustrations and diagrams offered. A subject index for Volume 1 and a section of full color plates concludes the book.

- **Atlas of Diseases of the Kidney. Volume 5: Dialysis as Treatment of End-Stage Renal Disease/Transplantation as Treatment of End-Stage Renal Disease**

Source: Philadelphia, PA: Current Medicine, Inc. 1999. [270 p.].

Contact: Available from Blackwell Science, Inc. 350 Main Street, Malden, MA 02148. (800) 215-1000 or (781) 388-8250. Fax (781) 388-8270. E-mail: csbooks@blacksci.com. PRICE: $75.00 plus shipping and handling. ISBN: 0632043911.

Summary: This volume is the last in a series of five that make up the Atlas of Diseases of the Kidney, a set that offers educational images including colored photographs, schematics, tables, and algorithms. In Volume 5, 7 chapters consider dialysis as treatment of **end stage renal disease** (ESRD), and 10 chapters cover transplantation as treatment of ESRD. The first section is organized to provide a systematic overview of dialytic procedures. The first chapter discusses the principles of dialysis and the mechanics of practical therapy. One essential feature of the dialysis procedure is the composition of dialysate, which is discussed in detail in the second chapter. Newer dialytic therapies such as high efficiency dialysis and continuous dialysis therapy techniques are discussed next; these treatments have resulted in shorter dialysis times in patients with chronic **renal failure** and have been useful in the management of complicated acute **renal failure** (ARF) patients. Other chapters cover peritoneal dialysis, problems with arteriovenous fistula access, dialysis prescription and methods of measuring urea, and several complications that afflict patients with **renal failure** who are on dialysis, including blood pressure regulation and chronic inflammation. The second section details transplantation, including several chapters on the evaluation of donors and recipients, including their posttransplant complications. One chapter addresses the technical aspects of transplantation, shows the operation, and provides the basis for making the diagnostic and therapeutic decisions necessary when a patient develops postoperative renal dysfunction. Other chapters cover combined kidney and pancreas transplantation, tissue typing and organ sharing, immunosuppressive drugs, and the management of renal transplant rejection. Finally, the special needs of pediatric transplantation and the intriguing area of recurrent disease are covered. Each chapter features a detailed introduction and lengthy captions for each of the illustrations and diagrams offered. A subject index for Volume 5 and a section of full color plates concludes the book.

- **Treatment Methods for Kidney Failure: Hemodialysis**

  Source: Bethesda, MD: National Kidney and Urologic Diseases Information Clearinghouse (NKUDIC). 2001. 14 p.

  Contact: Available from National Kidney and Urologic Diseases Information Clearinghouse (NKUDIC). 3 Information Way, Bethesda, MD 20892-3580. (800) 891-5390 or (301) 654-4415. Fax (301) 634-0716. E-mail: nkudic@info.niddk.nih.gov. Website: http://www.niddk.nih.gov/health/kidney/nkudic.htm. PRICE: Full-text available online at no charge; single copy free; bulk orders available. NIH Publication number: 01-4666.

  Summary: When the kidneys fail, harmful wastes build up in the body, the blood pressure may rise, and the body may retain excess fluid and not make enough red blood cells. When this happens, treatment is required to replace the work of the failed kidneys. Hemodialysis is the most common method used to treat advanced and permanent **kidney failure.** This booklet helps readers recently diagnosed with **kidney failure** understand hemodialysis. Topics include how hemodialysis works, adjusting to changes, getting the vascular access ready, equipment and procedures, tests to monitor how well the dialysis is working, conditions related to **kidney failure** and their treatments (anemia, renal osteodystrophy, itching, sleep disorders, amyloidosis), how diet can help, financial issues, and current research in this area. Medical or technical terms are defined in the text. The booklet concludes with a list of resources for additional information and a brief description of the activities of the National Kidney and Urologic Diseases Information Clearinghouse (NKUDIC), a service of the National Institute of Diabetes and Digestive and Kidney Diseases (NIDDK). 6 figures.

## Chapters on Kidney Failure

Frequently, kidney failure will be discussed within a book, perhaps within a specific chapter. In order to find chapters that are specifically dealing with kidney failure, an excellent source of abstracts is the Combined Health Information Database. You will need to limit your search to book chapters and kidney failure using the "Detailed Search" option. Go directly to the following hyperlink: **http://chid.nih.gov/detail/detail.html**. To find book chapters, use the drop boxes at the bottom of the search page where "You may refine your search by." Select the dates and language you prefer, and the format option "Book Chapter." By making these selections and typing in "kidney failure" (or synonyms) into the "For these words:" box, you will only receive results on chapters in books. The following is a typical result when searching for book chapters on kidney failure:

- **Management of Sequelae, Voiding Dysfunction and Renal Failure**

    Source: in Hamdy, F.C, et al. Management of Urologic Malignancies. New York, NY: Elsevier Science, Inc. 2002. p. 259-269.

    Contact: Available from Elsevier Science, Inc. Journal Information Center, 655 Avenue of the Americas, New York, NY 10010. (212) 633-3750. Fax (212) 633-3764. Website: www.elsevier.com. PRICE: $149.00. ISBN: 443054789.

    Summary: A small but significant percentage of men with prostate cancer present with or progress to a metastatic and terminal stage of the disease. After attempts to control the cancer with surgery, radiation, or hormonal therapy, the urologist must also know how to treat complications related to the progression of incurable cancer. Most commonly, these complications are bone pain and pathologic fractures related to bone metastases, urethral and ureteral obstruction with progression to renal (kidney) failure, and disseminated intravascular coagulation. Long-term complications of previous attempts at controlling the cancer through hormone therapy, radiation therapy, and surgery must also be addressed in providing care for these men. This chapter on the management of sequelae, voiding dysfunction, and **renal failure** associated with prostate cancer is from a reference guide to all urologic cancers; the textbook features a strong emphasis on best practice management choices. The authors of this chapter stress that because there is no known treatment capable of curing patients who are refractory to hormone therapy, treatment is aimed at preventing or minimizing they symptoms from these complications and prolonging survival where possible and desirable. A patient care algorithm is provided. 1 table. 81 references.

- **Acute and Chronic Renal Failure in Children**

  Source: in Gearhart, J.P.; Rink, R.C.; Mouriquand, P.D. Pediatric Urology. Philadelphia, PA: W.B. Saunders Company. 2001. p. 777-789.

  Contact: Available from Elsevier, Health Sciences Division. The Curtis Center, 625 Walnut Street, Philadelphia, PA 19106. (800) 523-1649. E-mail: custserv.ehs@elsevier.com. Website: www.us.elsevierhealth.com. PRICE: $239.00 plus shipping and handling. ISBN: 072168680X.

  Summary: Acute renal (kidney) failure (ARF) is characterized by a reversible increase in the blood concentration of creatinine and nitrogenous waste products and by the inability of the kidney to appropriately regulate fluid and electrolyte homeostasis. Chronic **renal failure** (CRF) results in similar alterations in fluid and electrolyte balance, but the metabolic derangements are irreversible. This chapter, from a comprehensive textbook on pediatric urology that emphasizes the pathophysiology of various disorders, reviews the common causes of ARF and CRF and the management of **renal failure,** including renal replacement therapy (dialysis and transplantation). The author notes that the purpose of renal replacement therapy is to remove endogenous and exogenous toxins and to maintain fluid, electrolyte, and acid-base balance until renal function improves (if the patient has ARF) or until transplantation can be achieved in children who have CRF. 2 figures. 3 tables. 108 references.

- **Anemia in Chronic Renal Failure**

  Source: in Johnson, R.J. and Feehally, J. Comprehensive Clinical Nephrology. 2nd ed. Orlando, FL: Mosby, Inc. 2003. p. 905-912.

  Contact: Available from Mosby, Inc. Order Fulfillment Department, 6277 Sea Harbor Drive, Orlando FL 32887. (800) 321-5068. Fax (800)874-6418. E-mail: custserv.ehs@elsevier.com Website: www.elsevierhealth.com. PRICE: $199.00. ISBN: 723432589.

  Summary: Anemia has been a known complication of renal (kidney) failure for over 160 years, but its etiology (cause) and management have been better elucidated over the past 20 years. This chapter on anemia in chronic **renal failure** (CRF) is from a comprehensive textbook that covers every clinical condition encountered in nephrology (the study of kidney disease). The author of this chapter discusses pathophysiology, clinical manifestations, diagnosis and differential diagnosis, treatment options, notably the use of erythropoietin (epoetin). The author concludes that the use of epoetin has been one of the most important advances in the management of the patient with CRF, yet its use is still not optimal. Not enough patients with progressive renal insufficiency are receiving epoetin for even partial correction of their anemia. The chapter is clinically focused and extensively illustrated in full color. 1 figure. 5 tables. 45 references.

- **Management of End-stage Renal Disease in Diabetes**

Source: in Johnson, R.J. and Feehally, J. Comprehensive Clinical Nephrology. 2nd ed. Orlando, FL: Mosby, Inc. 2003. p. 451-462.

Contact: Available from Mosby, Inc. Order Fulfillment Department, 6277 Sea Harbor Drive, Orlando FL 32887. (800) 321-5068. Fax (800)874-6418. E-mail: custserv.ehs@elsevier.com Website: www.elsevierhealth.com. PRICE: $199.00. ISBN: 723432589.

Summary: Diabetic nephropathy (kidney disease associated with diabetes mellitus) is the single largest cause of end stage renal (kidney) disease (ESRD) in American and European adults, accounting for over one third of all patients beginning renal replacement therapy (dialysis and transplantation). Diabetic nephropathy is a clinical syndrome characterized by persistent albuminuria (protein in the urine). Patients invariably develop associated hypertension (high blood pressure), a progressive increase in proteinuria, and a predictable and relentless decline in glomerular filtration rate (GFR, a measure of kidney function). This chapter on the management of ESRD in diabetes is from a comprehensive textbook that covers every clinical condition encountered in nephrology (the study of kidney disease). The author of this chapter covers the incidence of ESRD resulting from diabetic nephropathy, predialysis care for the person with diabetes, microvascular complications, macrovascular complications, blood pressure control, infection, metabolic complications, psychological and social care, peritoneal dialysis versus hemodialysis, survival and causes of death in people with diabetes and ESRD, the outcome of dialysis, hospitalization and technique survival, and kidney transplantation in patients with diabetes. The chapter is clinically focused and extensively illustrated in full color. 10 figures. 1 table. 34 references.

- **Acute Renal Failure and Dialysis**

Source: in Gutch, C.F.; Stoner, M.H.; Corea, A.L. Review of Hemodialysis for Nurses and Dialysis Personnel. 6th ed. St. Louis, MO: Mosby. 1999. p. 173-191.

Contact: Available from Harcourt Publishers. Foots Cray High Street, Sidcup, Kent DA14 5HP UK. 02083085700. Fax 02083085702. E-mail: cservice@harcourt.com. Website: www.harcourt-international.com. PRICE: $37.95 plus shipping and handling. ISBN: 0815120990.

Summary: Dialysis is often necessary for the treatment of acute kidney (renal) failure. The most common indications include **uremia,** hyperkalemia, acidosis, fluid overload, and drug overdose. This chapter on acute **renal failure** and dialysis is from a nursing text that poses questions and then answers those questions with the aim of giving a good understanding of the basic principles, basic diseases, and basic problems in the treatment of kidney patients by dialysis. The authors of the chapter define acute **renal failure** (ARF) as the rapid deterioration of kidney function and note that ARF is usually reversible if diagnosed and treated early. ARF is divided into three categories: prerenal, intrarenal, and postrenal. The most common indications for acute dialysis include **uremia,** pulmonary edema (fluid overload in the lungs), hyperkalemia (high amounts of potassium in the blood), acidosis, neurologic changes, and drug overdoses and poisonings. Treatment options for ARF include hemodialysis, isolated ultrafiltration, peritoneal dialysis, continuous renal replacement therapy (CRRT), and charcoal hemoperfusion. The chapter concludes with a brief section discussing the use of dialysis for patients undergoing rejection of a transplanted kidney. 4 figures.

- **Nutrition in Chronic Renal Failure**

Source: in Johnson, R.J. and Feehally, J. Comprehensive Clinical Nephrology. 2nd ed. Orlando, FL: Mosby, Inc. 2003. p. 935-943.

Contact: Available from Mosby, Inc. Order Fulfillment Department, 6277 Sea Harbor Drive, Orlando FL 32887. (800) 321-5068. Fax (800)874-6418. E-mail: custserv.ehs@elsevier.com Website: www.elsevierhealth.com. PRICE: $199.00. ISBN: 723432589.

Summary: Diet and nutrition play an integral role in the management of individuals with renal (kidney) disease. Abnormalities associated with chronic renal disease include retention of nitrogenous metabolites, a decreased ability to regulate levels of electrolytes and water, and certain vitamin deficiencies. Dietary intake can play a crucial role in managing these abnormalities. Interest in the nutritional status of patients with **renal failure** has increased with the understanding that poor nutrition predicts a poor outcome. This chapter on nutrition in chronic renal (kidney) failure (CRF) is from a comprehensive textbook that covers every clinical condition encountered in nephrology (the study of kidney disease). The author of this chapter discusses malnutrition, assessment of nutritional status, nutritional guidelines, monitoring and treatment, including the use of oral supplementation, tube feeding, supplementation of dialysate fluids, and appetite stimulants and growth factors. The author concludes that indices of malnutrition are powerful predictors of mortality in **end stage renal disease** (ESRD). The high prevalence of protein-energy malnutrition in this group is clearly related to multiple factors encountered both before and after renal replacement therapy (dialysis) has commenced. The chapter is clinically focused and extensively illustrated in full color. 8 figures. 4 tables. 28 references.

- **Bone and Mineral Metabolism in Chronic Renal Failure**

Source: in Johnson, R.J. and Feehally, J. Comprehensive Clinical Nephrology. 2nd ed. Orlando, FL: Mosby, Inc. 2003. p. 873-885.

Contact: Available from Mosby, Inc. Order Fulfillment Department, 6277 Sea Harbor Drive, Orlando FL 32887. (800) 321-5068. Fax (800)874-6418. E-mail: custserv.ehs@elsevier.com Website: www.elsevierhealth.com. PRICE: $199.00. ISBN: 723432589.

Summary: Disturbances of mineral metabolism are common during the course of chronic renal disease (CRF) and lead to serious and debilitating complications unless these abnormalities are addressed and treated. This chapter on bone and mineral metabolism in CRF is from a comprehensive textbook that covers every clinical condition encountered in nephrology (the study of kidney disease). The authors of this chapter discuss definitions, the epidemiology (incidence and prevalence) of these complications, pathogenesis, clinical manifestations of renal osteodystrophy, diagnosis and differential diagnosis, and treatment strategies. The chapter is clinically focused and extensively illustrated in full color. 14 figures. 2 tables. 28 references.

- **Nutrition in Patients with Chronic Renal Failure and Patients on Dialysis**

Source: in Nissenson, A.R., Fine, R.N., and Gentile, D.E. Clinical Dialysis. 3rd ed. Norwalk, CT: Appleton and Lange. 1995. p. 518-534.

Contact: Available from Appleton and Lange. 25 Van Zant Street, East Norwalk, CT 06855. PRICE: $215.00. ISBN: 0838513794.

Summary: For many years, dietary manipulation has been an important therapeutic intervention for patients with advanced renal disease.

Nutritional factors play a role in the morbidity and mortality of these patients, as well as in their quality of life and ultimate rehabilitative potential. This chapter, from a medical text on clinical dialysis, investigates the role of nutrition in patients with chronic **renal failure** (CRF) and patients on dialysis. The authors first outline the syndrome of malnutrition in patients with **renal failure.** Next, they discuss the causes of malnutrition in **renal failure,** including reduced nutritional intake, intercurrent illness, dialysis losses, and **uremia..** The authors stress the importance of accurately assessing the nutritional status of all patients with advanced renal disease in order to identify those patients who may need nutritional intervention and to monitor the effects of any therapeutic regimen. Assessment tools include history and physical examination, dietary history, anthropometry, serum proteins, and plasma amino acids. Protein restriction in patients with CRF can slow the progression of **renal failure** and delay the onset of uremic symptoms and associated metabolic disturbances once glomerular filtration rate (GFR) has fallen below 15 ml per minute. When the GFR falls below 5 ml per minute, dialysis therapy is usually required. Because dialysis therapy is associated with losses of protein and amino acids, the diet should be liberalized and protein intake increased. Additional topics include vitamin therapy and other supplements, nutrition in patients treated with peritoneal dialysis (PD), and intraperitoneal dialysis. 5 tables. 153 references. (AA-M).

- **Cardiovascular Disease in Chronic Renal Failure**

Source: in Johnson, R.J. and Feehally, J. Comprehensive Clinical Nephrology. 2nd ed. Orlando, FL: Mosby, Inc. 2003. p. 887-904.

Contact: Available from Mosby, Inc. Order Fulfillment Department, 6277 Sea Harbor Drive, Orlando FL 32887. (800) 321-5068. Fax (800)874-6418. E-mail: custserv.ehs@elsevier.com Website: www.elsevierhealth.com. PRICE: $199.00. ISBN: 723432589.

Summary: Life expectancy with **end stage renal disease** (ESRD) is poor despite modern renal replacement therapy (RRT, including dialysis and transplantation). Much of the premature death of these patients, particularly in the first few years of dialysis, is attributable to cardiovascular disease, including stroke, myocardial infarction, and heart failure. This chapter on cardiovascular disease in chronic renal (kidney) failure (CRF) is from a comprehensive textbook that covers every clinical condition encountered in nephrology (the study of kidney disease). The author of this chapter discusses epidemiology (incidence and prevalence), etiology and pathogenesis, clinical manifestations, management of common cardiovascular syndromes in **uremia,** the effects of hemodialysis and ultrafiltration on cardiovascular function, and the management of cardiovascular risk factors. The chapter is clinically focused and extensively illustrated in full color. 15 figures. 3 tables. 32 references.

- **Renal Dysfunction and Postoperative Renal Failure in Obstructive Jaundice**

Source: in Arroyo, V., et al, eds. Ascites and Renal Dysfunction in Liver Disease: Pathogenesis, Diagnosis, and Treatment. Malden, MA: Blackwell Science, Inc. 1999. p.79-98.

Contact: Available from Blackwell Science, Inc. 350 Main Street, Malden, MA 02148. (800) 215-1000 or (781)-388-8250. Fax (781) 388-8270. E-mail: csbooks@blacksci.com. Website: www.blackwellscience.com. PRICE: $125.00 plus shipping and handling. ISBN: 0632043423.

Summary: Patients with obstructive jaundice (OJ) have an increased risk for a wide array of postoperative complications, namely, bleeding, infections, poor wound healing, and kidney (renal) failure. The three major consequences of biliary obstruction: immunosuppression, malnutrition, and hemodynamic (blood flow) disturbances, are all implicated in the pathogenesis of these complications. This chapter on kidney dysfunction and postoperative **kidney failure** in OJ is from a textbook on ascites and renal dysfunction in liver disease. The author reviews evidence linking biliary obstruction with kidney dysfunction, emphasizing the pathogenesis (development) of this association according to the most recent experimental and clinical data. This knowledge will improve the perioperative care of patients with obstructive jaundice. The author notes that prevention of perioperative kidney dysfunction is best achieved by accurate monitoring of fluid replacement and diuresis, and avoidance of all potentially nephrotoxic drugs, particularly aminoglycoside antibiotics. Preoperative internal biliary drainage, coupled with appropriate rehydration and metabolic support, appears to be a promising adjunct for improving the condition of patients with OJ, particularly of those with severe hyperbilirubinemia, sepsis, or advanced malnutrition. 5 figures. 9 tables. 75 references.

- **Clinical Evaluation and Manifestations of Chronic Renal Failure**

Source: in Johnson, R.J. and Feehally, J. Comprehensive Clinical Nephrology. 2nd ed. Orlando, FL: Mosby, Inc. 2003. p. 857-872.

Contact: Available from Mosby, Inc. Order Fulfillment Department, 6277 Sea Harbor Drive, Orlando FL 32887. (800) 321-5068. Fax (800)874-6418. E-mail: custserv.ehs@elsevier.com Website: www.elsevierhealth.com. PRICE: $199.00. ISBN: 723432589.

Summary: The management of chronic **renal failure** (CRF) is now the dominant part of the work of a clinical nephrologist. This has come about because chronic kidney disease is easily uncovered by routine blood and urine tests and treatment for **end stage renal disease** (ESRD) is so successful and widely applied. Although supervision of patients receiving renal replacement therapy (RRT) is the undisputed domain of the nephrologist, care of patients with progressive renal insufficiency is as important, not least because it may be possible to delay progression or to halt a disease process. Many of the complications and long-term problems of **renal failure** start well before dialysis or renal transplantation are even being discussed, and there are a number of options for preventing or ameliorating these. This chapter on the clinical evaluation and manifestations of CRF is from a comprehensive textbook that covers every clinical condition encountered in nephrology (the study of kidney disease). The authors of this chapter discuss definition and incidence, the epidemiology (incidence and prevalence) of CRF, etiology and pathogenesis, clinical presentations (symptoms), the complications and consequences of CRF, the management of CRF, surgery in the patient with CRF, drug prescribing in CRF, and the management of terminal **uremia..** The chapter is clinically focused and extensively illustrated in full color. 4 figures. 7 tables. 26 references.

- **Gastrointestinal Disease in Patients With Chronic Renal Failure**

Source: in Nissenson, A.R., Fine, R.N., and Gentile, D.E., eds. Clinical Dialysis. 3rd ed. Norwalk, CT: Appleton and Lange. 1995. p. 607-617.

Contact: Available from Appleton and Lange. 25 Van Zant Street, P.O. Box 5630, Norwalk, CT 06856. (800) 423-1359 or (203) 838-4400. PRICE: $175.00. ISBN: 0838513794.

Summary: This chapter from a textbook on clinical dialysis covers gastrointestinal (GI) disease in patients with chronic **renal failure** (CRF). Topics include the types of upper GI symptoms common in patients with CRF; the pathogenesis of uremic GI lesions and upper GI tract bleeding; specific causes of GI tract bleeding in **renal failure,** including angiodysplasia, peptic ulcer disease, and Kaposi's sarcoma; chronic nausea and vomiting in the dialysis patient; GI medication in the dialysis patient, including the use of antiemetic therapy and prokinetic drugs and their use in gastroparesis; the causes of lower GI bleeding, including vascular telangectasia, colonic polyps, colitis, diverticular disease, and isolated idiopathic ulceration; abdominal emergencies in the patient on continuous ambulatory peritoneal dialysis (CAPD); and pancreatic disease in dialysis patients. 5 tables. 60 references.

- **End-Stage Renal Disease**

  Source: in Guiss, L.S., ed. Diabetes Surveillance 1997. Silver Spring, MD: Division of Diabetes Translation, Centers for Disease Control and Prevention (CDC). 1998. p. 193-212.

  Contact: Available from Division of Diabetes Translation, Centers for Disease Control and Prevention (CDC). P.O. Box 8728, Silver Spring, MD 20910. (877) 232-3422. Fax (301) 562-1050. E-mail: ccdinfo@cdc.gov. Website: www.cdc.gov/diabetes. PRICE: Single copy free.

  Summary: This chapter from the 1997 Diabetes Surveillance report offers statistics regarding diabetes and **end-stage renal disease** (ESRD), defined as **kidney failure** requiring dialysis or kidney transplant for survival. Diabetes accounts for more than a third of all new cases of ESRD in the United States, and persons with diabetes are the fastest growing group of recipients for kidney dialysis or transplantation. The number of new cases of ESRD attributable to diabetes increased from 7,017 in 1984 to 19,013 in 1993. This increase represents an underestimate because an unexplained undercount of ESRD incidence occurred in 1993. The age adjusted incidence of ESRD DM per 100,000 persons with diabetes was greater for blacks than for whites. The rate of increase in ESRD DM incidence per 100,000 persons with diabetes increased with age. The bulk of this chapter provides charts and graphs of these surveillance data. The introductory material (one page of text in the chapter) notes that these surveillance data do not answer whether this increase in ESRD DM among persons with diabetes is due to increased incidence of disease, increased use of treatment, increased recognition of the etiologic role of diabetes in ESRD, or a combination of these factors. 6 figures. 27 tables.

- **Options for Patients with End-Stage Renal Disease**

  Source: in Danovitch, G.M., ed. Handbook of Kidney Transplantation. 3rd ed. Philadelphia, PA: Lippincott Williams and Wilkins. 2000. p. 1-16.

  Contact: Available from Lippincott Williams and Wilkins. P.O. Box 1600, Hagerstown, MD 21741. (800) 638-3030 or (301) 223-2300. Fax (301) 223-2365. PRICE: $42.00 plus shipping and handling. ISBN: 0781720664.

  Summary: This chapter is from a handbook of kidney transplantation that provides practical information on therapy, patient monitoring, and patient care management. In this chapter, the authors outline options for patients with **end stage renal disease** (ESRD). Despite advances in knowledge and skill in treating chronic **renal failure** (CRF), patients with ESRD often remain unwell even when maintained by regular dialysis. Constitutional symptoms of fatigue and malaise persist despite the dramatic improvement that followed the introduction of erythropoietin for the management of the anemia of CRF. Progressive cardiovascular disease (CVD), peripheral and autonomic neuropathy, bone disease, and sexual dysfunction are common even in patients who receive adequate amounts of dialysis. For most patients with ESRD, kidney transplantation offers the greatest potential for restoring a healthy, productive life. However, practitioners of kidney transplantation must consider the clinical effects of ESRD on the overall health of renal transplantation candidates when this therapeutic option is first considered. The authors consider the demographics of the ESRD population, then outline each of the treatment options, including hemodialysis, peritoneal dialysis, and transplantation. The authors focus on issues of patient selection and when to initiate ESRD therapy. 5 figures. 2 tables. 13 references.

- **Calcium, Phosphorus, and Vitamin D Metabolism in Renal Disease and Chronic Renal Failure**

Source: in Kopple, J.D. and Massry, S.G. Nutritional Management of Renal Disease. Baltimore, MD: Williams and Wilkins. 1997. p. 341-369.

Contact: Available from Williams and Wilkins. 351 West Camden Street, Baltimore, MD 21201-2436. (800) 638-0672 or (410) 528-4223. Fax (800) 447-8438 or (410) 528-8550. PRICE: $99.00. ISBN: 068304740X.

Summary: This chapter is from a medical textbook on nutrition and metabolism of individuals with renal disease or **renal failure.** The authors discuss calcium, phosphorus, and vitamin D metabolism in renal disease and chronic **renal failure** (CRF). The authors begin with a brief review of normal physiologic control of calcium and phosphorus homeostasis and normal vitamin D and parathyroid hormone metabolism. Next, they discuss the effects of the failing kidney on mineral metabolism, secondary hyperparathyroidism, hyperphosphatemia, therapeutic interventions in predialysis patients, and control of phosphate retention and secondary hyperparathyroidism in dialysis patients. The authors conclude that dietary restriction of phosphorus intake and adequate dialysis therapy form the basis for management, but are usually insufficient to bring about adequate control. Calcium-based phosphate binders and hormonal vitamin D replacement are powerful adjuncts in regulating mineral pathophysiology. Despite these maneuvers, parathyroidectomy is still occasionally required. The authors provide an algorithm for the management of hyperphosphatemia and secondary hyperparathyroidism. Additional sections discuss the implications for bone disease (renal osteodystrophy), one of the more serious complications of disordered mineral metabolism in **renal failure;** implications for other complications; disturbances of mineral metabolism following renal transplantation; and disturbances of mineral and vitamin D metabolism in nephrotic syndrome. 5 figures. 124 references. (AA-M).

- **Anemia in Patients with Chronic Renal Failure and in Patients Undergoing Chronic Hemodialysis**

Source: in KT/DA (Kidney Transplant/Dialysis Association, Inc.). KT/DA Patient Handbook. 4th ed. Boston, MA: KT/DA (Kidney Transplant/Dialysis Association, Inc.). 2003. p. 131-134.

Contact: Available from KT/DA (Kidney Transplant/Dialysis Association, Inc.). P.O. Box 51362 GMF, Boston, MA 02205-1362. (781) 641-4000. Email: KTDA1@rcn.com. Website: www.ktda.org. PRICE: Full-text available online at no charge.

Summary: This chapter on anemia in patients with chronic renal (kidney) failure (CRF) and in patients undergoing chronic hemodialysis is from a book that was written to help kidney patients understand the forms of treatment available for their kidney disease and the impact of each form of treatment on the patient's quality of life. The authors define anemia as a reduction in the oxygen-carrying capacity of blood. The typical anemia in kidney disease is a result of a decreased production of red blood cells by the bone marrow. This defect in red blood cell production is largely explained by the inability of the failing kidneys to secrete the hormone erythropoietin. The authors describe the symptoms of anemia, the role of hemodialysis in this anemia, and treatment options, notably treatment with recombinant erythropoietin. The book is created and published by the Kidney Transplant/Dialysis Association, a non-profit, all-volunteer organization of dialysis and transplant patients, their families, and friends.

- **Carbohydrate Metabolism in Renal Failure**

Source: in Kopple, J.D. and Massry, S.G. Nutritional Management of Renal Disease. Baltimore, MD: Williams and Wilkins. 1997. p. 63-76.

Contact: Available from Williams and Wilkins. 351 West Camden Street, Baltimore, MD 21201-2436. (800) 638-0672 or (410) 528-4223. Fax (800) 447-8438 or (410) 528-8550. PRICE: $99.00. ISBN: 068304740X.

Summary: This chapter on carbohydrate metabolism is from a medical textbook on nutrition and metabolism of individuals with renal disease or **renal failure.** The authors note that many aspects of carbohydrate metabolism are impaired in patients with chronic **renal failure** (CRF). These derangements lead to glucose intolerance in these patients. The two major defects that underlie glucose intolerance in **uremia** are resistance to the peripheral action of insulin and impaired insulin secretion. When these two abnormalities are present in a particular patient, glucose intolerance ensues. Despite impaired insulin secretion, the increase in the blood levels of insulin in response to hyperglycemia may be decreased, normal, or increased. These variations are most likely due to differences in the degree of the impairment in insulin secretion or its metabolic clearance rate. The authors caution that these disturbances and the secondary hyperparathyroidism may all contribute to the increased risk for atherogenesis in patients with CRF. Postprandial (after meals) hyperglycemia in the glucose intolerant uremic patient may, by itself, be a risk factor for atherosclerotic cardiovascular disease. In addition, hyperinsulinemia and insulin resistant state may be associated with hypertension, which is an important risk factor for cardiac disease in **uremia**.. 2 figures. 1 table. 88 references. (AA-M).

- **Carnitine in Renal Failure**

Source: in Kopple, J.D. and Massry, S.G. Nutritional Management of Renal Disease. Baltimore, MD: Williams and Wilkins. 1997. p. 191-201.

Contact: Available from Williams and Wilkins. 351 West Camden Street, Baltimore, MD 21201-2436. (800) 638-0672 or (410) 528-4223. Fax (800) 447-8438 or (410) 528-8550. PRICE: $99.00. ISBN: 068304740X.

Summary: This chapter on carnitine in **renal failure** is from a medical textbook on nutrition and metabolism of individuals with renal disease or **renal failure**. Carnitine is found in mammalian cells and has a number of well-established roles in intermediary metabolism. In humans, carnitine is derived from dietary sources and from endogenous biosynthesis. Foods with high carnitine content include meat and dairy products, which is consistent with the high carnitine concentrations in muscle and milk. The author discusses the potential changes associated with **renal failure** that may impact carnitine metabolism and function. Glucose and fatty acid metabolism are clearly altered in **renal failure,** and carnitine metabolism is closely integrated with overall fuel homeostasis. Dietary recommendations for **renal failure** patients may inadvertently limit dietary carnitine intake. As the kidney may be an important site of carnitine biosynthesis, production rates may be altered in renal disease. Normal carnitine elimination occurs via urinary excretion, and this will be altered in **renal failure.** There are ample reports showing the beneficial effects of carnitine treatment in patients with **renal failure.** The effects of carnitine therapy to improve skeletal muscle function and decrease intradialytic symptoms are of particular clinical importance. The author concludes that decisions about the use of carnitine supplementation in **renal failure** patients must be individualized and must be considered as a therapeutic trial; the need for continued treatment should be reassessed at regular intervals based on objective measurements of efficacy. 3 figures. 3 tables. 42 references. (AA-M).

- **Drug Dosing and Toxicities in Renal Failure**

Source: in Mandal, A.K. and Nahman, N.S., Jr., eds. Kidney Disease in Primary Care. Baltimore, MD: Williams and Wilkins. 1998. p. 255-265.

Contact: Available from Williams and Wilkins. 351 West Camden Street, Baltimore, MD 21201-2436. (800) 638-0672 or (410) 528-4223. Fax (800) 447-8438 or (410) 528-8550. E-mail: custserv@wwilkins.com. PRICE: $39.95. ISBN: 0683300571.

Summary: This chapter on drug dosing and toxicities in **renal failure** is from a textbook that provides primary care physicians with practical approaches to common clinical problems of kidney diseases. Changes in drug absorption, distribution, metabolism, and excretion must be considered in the therapeutic management of patients with impaired renal function or **End Stage Renal Disease.**. The authors give general guidelines for the appropriate dosage adjustment of medications in patients with impaired renal function. Topics include the estimation of glomerular filtration rate (GFR), pharmacokinetics and pharmacodynamics (bioavailability, elimination coefficient and half-life, protein binding, volume of distribution), metabolism, and drug-induced nephrotoxicity (aminoglycosides, ACE inhibitors, amphotericin B, nonsteroidal anti-inflammatory agents, cisplatin, cyclosporine, radiographic contrast media, and nephrolithiasis or kidney stones). The authors note that gastrointestinal symptoms are common in renal patients and may prevent or delay oral absorption of drugs. Gastroparesis is especially common in renal patients with diabetes and may cause a delay in absorption of many drugs. 6 tables. 8 references.

- **Drug-Nutrient Interactions in Renal Failure**

Source: in Kopple, J.D. and Massry, S.G. Nutritional Management of Renal Disease. Baltimore, MD: Williams and Wilkins. 1997. p. 799-815.

Contact: Available from Williams and Wilkins. 351 West Camden Street, Baltimore, MD 21201-2436. (800) 638-0672 or (410) 528-4223. Fax (800) 447-8438 or (410) 528-8550. PRICE: $99.00. ISBN: 068304740X.

Summary: This chapter on drug-nutrient interactions is from a medical textbook on nutrition and metabolism of individuals with renal disease or **renal failure.** The author notes that, in patients with chronic **renal failure** (CRF) or **end-stage renal disease** (ESRD), drug-nutrient interactions may lead to overt nutritional deficiencies, particularly when the general nutritional status is poor or specific subclinical nutritional deficiencies already exist. The author reviews those drug-nutrient interactions that may result from medicines or food supplements that are commonly or occasionally used in patients with CRF or ESRD. Patients with advanced CRF and those on maintenance dialysis are often prescribed food supplements such as vitamins, iron preparations, or phosphate binders. Topics include the effect of food intake on drug absorption; the effects of nutrients on drug metabolism; the interactions of food supplements with drugs; drug-induced nutritional deficiencies, including vitamin, mineral, and trace-element deficiencies; interactions of cyclosporine A with nutrients; and enteral tube feeding and oral drug administration. 6 tables. 101 references. (AA-M).

- **Lipid Metabolism in Renal Disease and Renal Failure**

  Source: in Kopple, J.D. and Massry, S.G. Nutritional Management of Renal Disease. Baltimore, MD: Williams and Wilkins. 1997. p. 35-62.

  Contact: Available from Williams and Wilkins. 351 West Camden Street, Baltimore, MD 21201-2436. (800) 638-0672 or (410) 528-4223. Fax (800) 447-8438 or (410) 528-8550. PRICE: $99.00. ISBN: 068304740X.

  Summary: This chapter on lipid metabolism is from a medical textbook on nutrition and metabolism of individuals with renal disease or **renal failure.** In **uremia,** the distribution of lipid and apolipoproteins in the lipoprotein density classes is distorted. The disorder is complex and varies substantially within groups of patients treated with different renal replacement methods (e.g., hemodialysis, CAPD, transplantation). Abnormalities in lipid metabolism can be detected in the patient early as renal function begins to decline. The author summarizes the most characteristic patterns of serum lipids in patients with renal disease and **renal failure.** Guidelines for the detection, evaluation, and treatment of hypercholesterolemia in adults have been established in the U.S. and Europe. These guidelines recommend that total cholesterol levels be used for screening purposes. All persons in the so-called high category (cholesterol greater than 240 mg per dL) require measurements of low-density lipoprotein (LDL) cholesterol levels; the measurements are used as a guide to the selection of treatment. The chapter concludes with recommended treatment and patient care management strategies. 4 figures. 3 tables. 153 references. (AA-M).

- **Protein and Amino Acid Metabolism in Renal Disease and Renal Failure**

  Source: in Kopple, J.D. and Massry, S.G. Nutritional Management of Renal Disease. Baltimore, MD: Williams and Wilkins. 1997. p. 1-33.

Contact: Available from Williams and Wilkins. 351 West Camden Street, Baltimore, MD 21201-2436. (800) 638-0672 or (410) 528-4223. Fax (800) 447-8438 or (410) 528-8550. PRICE: $99.00. ISBN: 068304740X.

Summary: This chapter on protein and amino acid metabolism is from a medical textbook on nutrition and metabolism of individuals with renal disease or **renal failure.** The authors discuss alterations in protein and amino acid metabolism that are well recognized complications of acute and chronic **renal failure** and may contribute to wasting. As renal function declines, nitrogenous wastes accumulate, eventually resulting in symptomatic **uremia..** Changes in protein turnover and amino acid oxidation have also been described in the nephrotic syndrome when the glomerular filtration rate was normal, and in patients with early diabetic nephropathy. Finally, complications of **renal failure** (i.e., metabolic acidosis) may increase protein and amino acid catabolism and contribute to the loss of lean body mass. The authors note that recent advances in molecule and cellular biology have provided insight into the regulation of proteolysis and have indicated that accelerated protein catabolism in **renal failure** is due, at least in part, to activation of specific proteolytic pathways. Evidence that growth factors and inhibitors of proteolysis may block catabolism in experimental animals suggests a potential therapeutic role in patients with **renal failure.** 7 figures. 1 table. 141 references. (AA-M).

- **Rehabilitative Exercise Training in Chronic Renal Failure**

Source: in Kopple, J.D. and Massry, S.G. Nutritional Management of Renal Disease. Baltimore, MD: Williams and Wilkins. 1997. p. 817-841.

Contact: Available from Williams and Wilkins. 351 West Camden Street, Baltimore, MD 21201-2436. (800) 638-0672 or (410) 528-4223. Fax (800) 447-8438 or (410) 528-8550. PRICE: $99.00. ISBN: 068304740X.

Summary: This chapter on rehabilitative exercise training in chronic **renal failure** (CRF) is from a medical textbook on nutrition and metabolism of individuals with renal disease or **renal failure.** Exercise programs potentially have two distinct benefits for the patient with renal disease: psychologic and physiologic. The psychologic benefits of exercise are beginning to be understood; exercise programs generally have marked antidepressant effects. Exercise programs that focus on reaping these psychologic benefits can be quite successful in improving exercise tolerance and the overall quality of life. In contrast to programs designed to yield physiologic benefits, these programs can use exercise modalities and schedules at the convenience of the rehabilitation unit (i.e., more easily worked into the dialysis schedule). The author also summarizes exercise design features for physiologic gains for patients with CRF.

Topics include structural and biochemical changes induced by training in healthy persons; characteristics of an effective exercise training program; the causes of exercise intolerance in patients with **renal failure,** including anemia, myopathy, cardiovascular dysfunction, carnitine deficiency, and deconditioning; guidelines for exercise training programs in patients with CRF; and exercise prescription recommendations for chronic dialysis patients. 1 figure. 2 tables. 134 references. (AA-M).

- **Renal Failure**

Source: in Blandy, J. Lecture Notes on Urology. Malden, MA: Blackwell Science, Inc. 1998. p.112-120.

Contact: Available from Blackwell Science, Inc. 350 Main Street, Commerce Place, Malden, MA 02148. (800) 215-1000 or (617) 388-8250. Fax (617) 388-8270. E-mail: books@blacksci.com. Website: www.blackwell-science.com. PRICE: $39.95. ISBN: 0632042028.

Summary: This chapter on renal (kidney) failure is from an undergraduate medical textbook in the field of urology and urological surgery. The author discusses acute **renal failure** (ARF), chronic **renal failure** (CRF), dialysis, and renal transplantation. The causes of ARF fall into three main categories which often occur together: poor renal perfusion, renal tubular poisoning, and renal tubular blockage. Sometimes renal function deteriorates very slowly, and the patient may be kept well on a diet low in protein. But eventually, dialysis is called for, often because of intolerable symptoms. Much of the information is presented in diagrams or illustration format for ease of use. 9 figures. 13 references.

- **Renal Physiology and the Pathology of Renal Failure**

Source: in Gutch, C.F.; Stoner, M.H.; Corea, A.L. Review of Hemodialysis for Nurses and Dialysis Personnel. 6th ed. St. Louis, MO: Mosby. 1999. p. 25-34.

Contact: Available from Harcourt Publishers. Foots Cray High Street, Sidcup, Kent DA14 5HP UK. 02083085700. Fax 02083085702. E-mail: cservice@harcourt.com. Website: www.harcourt-international.com. PRICE: $37.95 plus shipping and handling. ISBN: 0815120990.

Summary: This chapter on renal physiology and the pathology of **renal failure** is from a nursing text that poses questions and then answers those questions with the aim of giving a good understanding of the basic principles, basic diseases, and basic problems in the treatment of kidney patients by dialysis. The author of the chapter reviews the two prime functions of the normal kidney: elimination of metabolic wastes and other toxic materials; and maintenance of a stable composition of the body's internal fluid environment. In addition, kidneys also have several endocrine functions including: production of renin, which affects sodium, fluid volume, and blood pressure; erythropoietin formation, which controls red cell production in the bone marrow; production of prostaglandins; and involvement in the kallikreinkinin system. Also, the normal kidney is a receptor site for several hormones: antidiuretic hormone (ADH), produced by the pituitary, which reduces the excretion of water; aldosterone, produced by the adrenal cortex, which promotes sodium retention and enhances secretion of potassium and hydrogen ion; and parathyroid hormone, which increases phosphorus and bicarbonate excretion and stimulates conversion of vitamin D to the active form. The author describes each of these functions in detail, and the related problems that occur during reduced kidney function or **kidney failure.** 3 figures. 1 table.

- **Causes, Manifestations, and Assessment of Malnutrition in Chronic Renal Failure**

Source: in Kopple, J.D. and Massry, S.G. Nutritional Management of Renal Disease. Baltimore, MD: Williams and Wilkins. 1997. p. 245-256.

Contact: Available from Williams and Wilkins. 351 West Camden Street, Baltimore, MD 21201-2436. (800) 638-0672 or (410) 528-4223. Fax (800) 447-8438 or (410) 528-8550. PRICE: $99.00. ISBN: 068304740X.

Summary: This chapter on the causes, manifestations, and assessment of malnutrition in chronic **renal failure** (CRF) is from a medical textbook on nutrition and metabolism of individuals with renal disease or **renal failure.** The author notes that patients with **chronic renal insufficiency** and those with **end-stage renal disease** (ESRD) often manifest signs of wasting and malnutrition. The initiation of dialysis therapy in the malnourished patient often fails to improve nutritional status. The author describes the causes of malnutrition in patients with **renal failure** and those treated with maintenance dialysis. Renal disease is associated with anorexia and alterations in taste; these symptoms may lead to decreased dietary intake and subsequent malnutrition. CAPD is also associated with abnormal patterns of dietary intake, due to the large amount of fluid in the peritoneal cavity and the effect of glucose absorption on appetite. Patients undergoing maintenance hemodialysis have reduced gastric emptying, and the frequent coexistence of diabetes mellitus may also be associated with gastroparesis, further suppressing intake. Frequent intercurrent illness may increase catabolism and further impair nutritional status. Inadequate dialysis is another possible cause of malnutrition in maintenance dialysis patients. The author also outlines the methods available to assess nutritional status in these patients. 1 figure. 2 tables. 52 references. (AA-M).

- **Epidemiology of Chronic Renal Failure and Guidelines for Initiation of Hemodialysis**

Source: in Wilson, S.E. Vascular Access: Principles and Practice. 4th ed. St. Louis, MO: Mosby, Inc. 2002. p. 76-81.

Contact: Available from Elsevier, Health Sciences Division, 11830 Westline Industrial Drive, St. Louis, MO 63146. (800) 325-4177. Website: www.us.elsevierhealth.com. PRICE: $99.00. ISBN: 0323011888.

Summary: This chapter on the epidemiology of chronic renal (kidney) failure (CRF) and guidelines for initiation of hemodialysis (HD) is from a text that reviews the principles and practice of vascular access, including that used for hemodialysis and for critical care, chemotherapy, and nutrition. Decisions concerning the timing of the initiation of dialysis are based on careful monitoring and evaluation of various clinical and biochemical features of **renal failure.** In this chapter, the authors provide a brief overview of the main clinical and biochemical manifestations of CRF. Topics include biochemical abnormalities, cardiovascular features, neurologic features, hematologic (blood) abnormalities, gastrointestinal abnormalities, immunologic abnormalities, endocrine abnormalities, and dermatologic (skin) abnormalities. The chapter concludes with brief sections offering guidelines for initiation of HD in CRF patients, and recommendations for vascular access. 1 table. 35 references.

- **Influences of Diet on the Progression of Chronic Renal Insufficiency**

Source: in Kopple, J.D. and Massry, S.G. Nutritional Management of Renal Disease. Baltimore, MD: Williams and Wilkins. 1997. p. 317-340.

Contact: Available from Williams and Wilkins. 351 West Camden Street, Baltimore, MD 21201-2436. (800) 638-0672 or (410) 528-4223. Fax (800) 447-8438 or (410) 528-8550. PRICE: $99.00. ISBN: 068304740X.

Summary: This chapter on the influences of diet on the progression of **chronic renal insufficiency** is from a medical textbook on nutrition and metabolism of individuals with renal disease or **renal failure.** The author notes that, in spite of intensive investigation, the mechanisms by which a low-protein diet could change the rate of loss of renal function have not been fully elucidated. In addition, the underlying mechanisms causing progressive loss of renal function have not been unequivocally identified, even in experimental animals. The author provides information designed to help readers make a rational decision about whether to implement nutritional therapy for a patient with progressive loss of renal function.

Topics covered include the nutritional adequacy of restricted diets; monitoring changes in renal function, including serum creatinine; low protein diets used to slow progress; assessment of dietary compliance; urea generation and protein nitrogen appearance; diabetic nephropathy and dietary protein restriction; supplemented low protein diets; and the Modification of Diet in Renal Disease (MDRD) Study. The author concludes that compliance with dietary protein restriction can be assessed reliably using available methods, and dietary regimens do not cause malnutrition if effort is made to ensure the nutritional adequacy of the diet actually ingested. Because there is evidence that dietary manipulation can slow progression in some patients, a low protein diet should be instituted in patients who have documented progressive renal insufficiency in spite of adequate treatment of hypertension. 4 figures. 1 table. 83 references. (AA-M).

- **Nutritional Management of Nondialyzed Patients with Chronic Renal Failure**

Source: in Kopple, J.D. and Massry, S.G. Nutritional Management of Renal Disease. Baltimore, MD: Williams and Wilkins. 1997. p. 479-531.

Contact: Available from Williams and Wilkins. 351 West Camden Street, Baltimore, MD 21201-2436. (800) 638-0672 or (410) 528-4223. Fax (800) 447-8438 or (410) 528-8550. PRICE: $99.00. ISBN: 068304740X.

Summary: This chapter on the nutritional management of nondialyzed patients with chronic **renal failure** (CRF) is from a medical textbook on nutrition and metabolism of individuals with renal disease or **renal failure.** The author stresses that the patient with CRF has alterations in both the dietary requirements and tolerance for most nutrients. Causes of these disorders include decreased (or occasionally increased) urinary, intestinal, and dermal excretion and intestinal absorption. Causes may also include altered metabolism of individual nutrients or their metabolites or products. The author also notes that the nutritional status of the patient undergoing maintenance hemodialysis or peritoneal dialysis is a strong predictor of morbidity and mortality. Other topics include training and monitoring the patient undergoing dietary therapy; dietary therapy for patients who are not yet receiving dialysis therapy, including recommended nutrient intakes; management of the patient with diabetic nephropathy; nutritional management during catabolic stress; and the use of growth factors. Detailed guidelines are provided for patient care management. 4 figures. 3 tables. 270 references. (AA-M).

- **Progression of Chronic Renal Failure**

  Source: in Johnson, R.J. and Feehally, J. Comprehensive Clinical Nephrology. 2nd ed. Orlando, FL: Mosby, Inc. 2003. p. 843-856.

  Contact: Available from Mosby, Inc. Order Fulfillment Department, 6277 Sea Harbor Drive, Orlando FL 32887. (800) 321-5068. Fax (800)874-6418. E-mail: custserv.ehs@elsevier.com Website: www.elsevierhealth.com. PRICE: $199.00. ISBN: 723432589.

  Summary: This chapter on the progression of chronic renal (kidney) failure (CRF) is from a comprehensive textbook that covers every clinical condition encountered in nephrology (the study of kidney disease). The authors of this chapter discuss definition and incidence, the epidemiology (incidence and prevalence) of CRF, natural history, factors affecting the progression of CRF, the mechanisms of progression of CRF, and clinical interventions in patients with CRF, including dietary interventions, and drug therapy. The authors conclude with a list of general recommendations for the management of patients with progressive CRF. The chapter is clinically focused and extensively illustrated in full color. 8 figures. 6 tables. 57 references.

- **Trace Element Metabolism in Renal Disease and Renal Failure**

  Source: in Kopple, J.D. and Massry, S.G. Nutritional Management of Renal Disease. Baltimore, MD: Williams and Wilkins. 1997. p. 395-414.

  Contact: Available from Williams and Wilkins. 351 West Camden Street, Baltimore, MD 21201-2436. (800) 638-0672 or (410) 528-4223. Fax (800) 447-8438 or (410) 528-8550. PRICE: $99.00. ISBN: 068304740X.

  Summary: This chapter on trace element metabolism is from a medical textbook on nutrition and metabolism of individuals with renal disease or **renal failure.** It is generally accepted that the term 'trace element' applies to elements that occur in the body at concentrations of less than 50 mg per kg under normal conditions. The definition of 'essential' trace elements is that the element should be present in healthy tissues; deficiency of the element consistently produces functional impairment; the abnormalities induced by the deficiency are always followed by specific biochemical changes; and addition of the element prevents or corrects these changes. Topics include methodology for the measurement of trace elements; trace element concentrations in **uremia;** the potential contribution of trace elements to the uremic syndrome, including impairment of renal function, susceptibility to cancer, cardiovascular disease, glucose intolerance, bone disease, anemia, enzyme dysfunction, encephalopathy and coma, and immune deficiency; factors affecting trace element concentration, including inadequate intake, decreased availability, impaired reabsorption, excessive excretion, and extracorporeal losses; specific examples relating to aluminum, lead, selenium and arsenic, zinc, vanadium, silicon, and chromium; and therapeutic considerations. The authors caution that the treatment of **uremia** by dialysis strategies may cause changes in trace element handling. Trace elements should be considered in the case of any unexplained toxic event in **uremia.**. 5 tables. 89 references. (AA-M).

- **Vitamin Metabolism and Requirements in Renal Disease and Renal Failure**

Source: in Kopple, J.D. and Massry, S.G. Nutritional Management of Renal Disease. Baltimore, MD: Williams and Wilkins. 1997. p. 415-477.

Contact: Available from Williams and Wilkins. 351 West Camden Street, Baltimore, MD 21201-2436. (800) 638-0672 or (410) 528-4223. Fax (800) 447-8438 or (410) 528-8550. PRICE: $99.00. ISBN: 068304740X.

Summary: This chapter on vitamin metabolism and requirements is from a medical textbook on nutrition and metabolism of individuals with renal disease or **renal failure.** The authors discuss several factors that may enhance the risk of abnormal vitamin levels in renal disease: decreased vitamin intake caused by anorexia, unpalatability of prescribed diets, or a dietary prescription that contains insufficient vitamins; increased degradation or endogenous clearance of vitamins from blood; elevated levels of vitamin binding proteins; losses of vitamins into dialysate; excretion of protein-bound vitamins by nephrotic patients; and interference of medicines with the absorption, excretion, and metabolism of vitamins. The authors review each of the common vitamins for its normal biochemistry and metabolism, the effect of renal disease and **renal failure** on these processes, and the clinical spectrum of vitamin disorders in these conditions. The authors propose guidelines concerning the needs for supplementation. Vitamins discussed are A, E, K, B1, B2, B6, B12, C, folates, niacin, biotin, and pantothenic acid. The authors conclude by calling for additional research to address vitamin supplementation in **renal failure** patients, particularly those on dialysis. 2 figures. 7 tables. 249 references. (AA-M).

- **Haemodialysis in Type 1 and Type 2 Diabetic Patients with End Stage Renal Failure**

Source: in Mogensen, C.E. Kidney and Hypertension in Diabetes Mellitus. 3rd ed. Norwell, MA: Kluwer Academic Publishers. 1997. p. 481-488.

Contact: Available from Kluwer Academic Publishers. 101 Philip Drive, Assinippi Park, Norwell, MA 02061. (617) 871-6600. Fax (617) 871-6528. PRICE: $130.00. ISBN: 0792343530.

Summary: This chapter, from a book on the kidney and hypertension in diabetes mellitus, addresses the use of hemodialysis in patients with **end-stage renal disease** (ESRD) and type 1 or type 2 diabetes. The authors consider epidemiology, survival and causes of death, predictors of survival, metabolic control while on renal replacement therapy (dialysis), managing diabetic complications while on renal replacement therapy, and kidney transplantation in the patient with diabetes. The authors note that the number of patients with diabetes entering renal replacement programs has increased in all Western countries. Hemodialysis is the preferred modality of treatment, hemofiltration and CAPD being used only in a minority of cases. The proportion of patients undergoing renal or combined renal and pancreatic transplantation is rising. Survival in patients with diabetes compared to nondiabetic patients is worse for all renal replacement modalities. This is mainly due to cardiovascular death. Cardiac death is poorly predicted by the level of blood pressure and blood pressure related target organ damage, while cholesterol and other lipid parameters are potent predictors. Common clinical problems in the dialysis patient with diabetes include metabolic control, visual disturbance, sequelae of autonomic polyneuropathy, amputation, and vascular access. 1 figure. 2 tables. 36 references. (AA-M).

- **Renal Failure and Secondary Hyperparathyroidism**

  Source: in Pellitteri, P.; McCaffrey, T.V. Endocrine Surgery of the Head and Neck. Florence, KY: Thomson Learning. 2003. p. 389-400.

  Contact: Available from Thomson Learning, Attn: Order Fulfillment. P.O. Box 6904 Florence, KY 41022 (800) 347-7707. Fax (800) 487-8488. E-mail: esales@thomsonlearning.com. Website: www.delmar.com. PRICE: $179.95 plus shipping and handling. ISBN: 076930091x.

  Summary: This chapter, from a textbook on endocrine surgery of the head and neck, covers renal (kidney) failure and secondary hyperparathyroidism (HPTH). The authors note that secondary HPTH is a complex process. Hyperplasia (overgrowth) of the parathyroid glands and increase in the serum PTH (parathyroid hormone) levels appear early in the development of renal disease. Medical treatment of HPTH is aimed at reducing serum phosphatase levels, increasing serum calcium levels, administering vitamin D analogs, and maintaining an appropriate metabolic equilibrium with adequate dialysis. The most common indications for surgical treatment of secondary HPTH are the development of renal osteodystrophy (bone disease), severe pruritus (itching) associated with HPTH, calciphylaxis, and tumoral calcinosis. Less clear indications for surgery are easy fatigability, proximal muscle weakness and anemia. Patients with secondary HPTH treated surgically can expect substantial improvements in bone and joint pain and pruritus in most cases. Amelioration of fatigue and generalized well being are often observed, albeit harder to quantify. Surgical techniques most commonly employed include subtotal parathyroidectomy and total parathyroidectomy with autotransplantation. There may be a role for minimally invasive approaches, such as endoscopic parathyroidectomy and percutaneous ethanol ablation, which are currently still investigational. 3 figures. 95 references.

- **Cholesterol Emboli: A Common Cause of Renal Failure**

Source: in Coggins, C.H., Hancock, E.W., and Levitt, L.J., eds. Annual Review of Medicine. Palo Alto, CA: Annual Reviews Inc. 1997. Volume 48: 375-385.

Contact: Available from Annual Reviews Inc. 4139 El Camino Way, P.O. Box 10139, Palo Alto, CA 94303-0139. (800) 523-8635. Fax (415) 424-0910. E-mail: service@annurev.org. PRICE: $60.00 for individuals; $120.00 for institutions. ISBN: 0824303555. ISSN: 00664219. Individual chapter reprints available from Annual Reviews Preprints and Reprints. (800) 347-8007 or (415) 259-5017. Base price $13.50 per article.

Summary: This chapter, from the Annual Review of Medicine, describes cholesterol emboli, a common cause of **renal failure.** Cholesterol embolization (CE), usually occurring in males in their sixth or seventh decade of life, can affect multiple organ systems, including the kidney. The author notes that interventive diagnostic procedures and aortic surgery greatly increase the risk of CE. Rapid or insidious progression of **renal failure** in association with surgical or diagnostic radiologic procedures should suggest this diagnosis. Progressive renal insufficiency in older patients with generalized arterial disease should suggest ischemic nephropathy secondary to bilateral renal artery stenosis, renal CE, or both. Recent worsening of hypertension is characteristic of either diagnosis. A number of clinical conditions can simulate renal CE, and final differentiation may be possible only by renal biopsy. The author stresses that aggressive, supportive management of renal CE is warranted because renal function may stabilize and, in a limited number of cases, may even improve. 2 figures. 2 tables. 44 references. (AA).

- **Bone Disease in Moderate Renal Failure: Cause, Nature, and Prevention**

  Source: in Coggins, C.H., Hancock, E.W., and Levitt, L.J., eds. Annual Review of Medicine. Palo Alto, CA: Annual Reviews Inc. 1997. Volume 48: 167-176.

  Contact: Available from Annual Reviews Inc. 4139 El Camino Way, P.O. Box 10139, Palo Alto, CA 94303-0139. (800) 523-8635. Fax (415) 424-0910. E-mail: service@annurev.org. PRICE: $60.00 for individuals; $120.00 for institutions. ISBN: 0824303555. ISSN: 00664219. Individual chapter reprints available from Annual Reviews Preprints and Reprints. (800) 347-8007 or (415) 259-5017. Base price $13.50 per article.

  Summary: This entry describes the cause, nature, and prevention of bone disease in moderate **renal failure.** Patients with **end-stage renal disease** (ESRD) present with two primary types of bone disorders: a high-turnover osteodystrophy characterized by osteitis fibrosa, and a low-turnover osteodystrophy characterized initially by osteomalacia and, more recently, by adynamic or aplastic bone disease. The author reviews the clinical presentation, pathogenesis, and laboratory findings of patients with these two disorders. The author discusses the important roles of phosphorus binding, vitamin D administration, and correction of acidosis in the prevention and treatment of bone disease in these patients. As renal function declines, dietary phosphorus intake should be restricted to prevent its accumulation. The author cautions that, although dialysis removes phosphate from the body, it is a rare dialysis patient who will not require phosphate binders in addition to dietary phosphorus restriction to control serum phosphate. Vitamin D sterols are effective in decreasing parathyroid hormone (PTH) secretion and bone turnover and in increasing serum calcium. Calcium carbonate is useful as a buffer against acidosis; it has been shown to increase the extracellular fluid bicarbonate concentration. Alkalosis should be avoided, as it promotes calcium phosphate deposit in soft tissues. 2 figures. 46 references. (AA-M).

- **Nutrition Support in Renal Failure**

  Source: in American Dietetic Association. Manual of Clinical Dietetics. Chicago, IL: American Dietetic Association. 1996. p. 327-342.

  Contact: Available from American Dietetic Association. 216 West Jackson Boulevard, Chicago, IL 60606. (800) 877-1600 or (312) 899-0040. Fax (312) 899-4899. PRICE: $59.95 for members, $70.00 for nonmembers. ISBN: 0880911530.

Summary: This section outlining guidelines for nutritional support in **renal failure** is from a manual that serves as a nutrition care guide for dietetics professionals, physicians, nurses, and other health professionals. The manual integrates current knowledge of nutrition, medical science, and food to set forth recommendations for healthy individuals and those for whom medical nutrition therapy (MNT) is indicated. The goal of nutrition support in **renal failure** is to achieve or maintain optimal nutritional status and preserve remaining kidney function through alterations in fluid, protein, and electrolyte intake. Nutrition support is used for patients with acute or chronic **renal failure** who are unable to meet nutrient requirements by oral intake. Impaired kidney function results in altered filtration, reabsorption, and excretion of metabolites and diminished urinary output. Hormonal function is also affected and may cause impaired vitamin D activation, impaired red blood cell synthesis, and glucose intolerance. The alterations differ with the cause of renal impairment; therefore, sodium, potassium, blood urea nitrogen (BUN), phosphate, urinary output, and the presence of acidosis must be monitored. The text notes the purpose, use, modifications, and adequacy of the diet. A separate section discusses enteral and parenteral nutrition, continuous arteriovenous hemofiltration, and the use of modified formulas (essential amino acids). 3 tables. 57 references. (AA-M).

- **Nutrition Management of Chronic Renal Insufficiency**

Source: in American Dietetic Association. Manual of Clinical Dietetics. Chicago, IL: American Dietetic Association. 1996. p. 521-534.

Contact: Available from American Dietetic Association. 216 West Jackson Boulevard, Chicago, IL 60606. (800) 877-1600 or (312) 899-0040. Fax (312) 899-4899. PRICE: $59.95 for members, $70.00 for nonmembers. ISBN: 0880911530.

Summary: This section providing guidelines for the nutritional management of **chronic renal insufficiency** (CRI) is from a manual that serves as a nutrition care guide for dietetics professionals, physicians, nurses, and other health professionals. The manual integrates current knowledge of nutrition, medical science, and food to set forth recommendations for healthy individuals and those for whom medical nutrition therapy (MNT) is indicated. CRI is characterized by a decrease in the kidney's ability to remove waste products as reflected by an increase in the serum creatinine level. The diet, often called the predialysis diet, is indicated for patients with CRI who do not yet require dialysis. The diet is restricted in two major areas: protein and phosphorus. The levels of sodium, potassium, fluid, and calories are based on individual needs. The text notes the purpose, use, modifications, and adequacy of the diet. The section also outlines the related physiology. Charts provide brief sample diets, food lists, and calculation figures for planning the CRI diet. 4 tables. 18 references. (AA-M).

- **Adequacy of Treatment for End-Stage Renal Disease in the United States**

Source: in Schrier, R.W., et al., eds. Advances in Internal Medicine. Vol 41. St. Louis, MO: Mosby-Year Book, Inc. 1996. p. 323-363.

Contact: Available from Mosby Year-Book, Inc. 11830 Westline Industrial Drive, St. Louis, MO 63146. (800) 426-4545. Fax (800) 535-9935. E-mail: customer.support@mosby.com. PRICE: $72.95. ISBN: 0815183143. ISSN: 00652822.

Summary: Whatever the cause of chronic or irreversible **renal failure,** when damage is complete, appearance of the more severe of the uremic symptoms permits the diagnosis of **end-stage renal disease** (ESRD). This chapter, from a yearbook of advances in internal medicine, considers the adequacy of treatment for ESRD in the United States. Topics include the origin of treatments for ESRD and the historical perspective of the development of different types of dialysis; expanding availability of treatments for ESRD, including the federally supported hemodialysis program; management of the ESRD program; selection and acceptance to therapy for ESRD; ESRD treatments, including transplantation, hemodialysis, and peritoneal dialysis; factors influencing the choice of modality; the prescription for dialysis adequacy; medical management, including access to blood or peritoneum, anemia, bone disease, and transplant care; mortality and morbidity considerations; and deficiencies in quality of ESRD care, including mortality in international comparisons, and contributory factors such as comparative treatment efficiency, patient selection, the effect of capped reimbursement rates, shortcuts to reuse, and medical management. In the final section, the authors present suggestions for improving the medical management of patients with ESRD. They discuss pre-ESRD care, increasing the dialysis dose, the role of the hemodialyzer membrane, improving access to transplantation, improving patient care, the role for the government, resolving patient-professional discord, and data collection and analysis. The authors conclude that the U.S. experiences with ESRD can be used as a model for American health care. 5 tables. 94 references.

## General Home References

In addition to references for kidney failure, you may want a general home medical guide that spans all aspects of home healthcare. The following list is a recent sample of such guides (sorted alphabetically by title; hyperlinks provide rankings, information, and reviews at Amazon.com):

- **Healthy Eating on a Renal Diet: A Cookbook for People With Kidney Disease** by The Renal Resource Center; Hardcover: 183 pages (December 1991); F A Davis Co; ASIN: 0803698879; http://www.amazon.com/exec/obidos/ASIN/0803698879/icongroupinter na

- **Kidney and Urinary Tract Diseases and Disorders Sourcebook: Basic Information About Kidney Stones, Urinary Incontinence, Bladder Disease, End Stage Renal Disease, Dialysis, and More, Along With Statistical and (Health Reference Series, Vol 21)** by Linda M. Ross (Editor), Peter Dresser (Editor); Hardcover: 602 pages (May 1997); Omnigraphics, Inc.; ISBN: 0780800796; http://www.amazon.com/exec/obidos/ASIN/0780800796/icongroupinter na

- **Urodynamics Made Easy** by Christopher R. Chapple, Scott A. MacDiarmid; Paperback -- 2nd edition (April 15, 2000), Churchill Livingstone; ISBN: 0443054630; http://www.amazon.com/exec/obidos/ASIN/0443054630/icongroupinter na

## Vocabulary Builder

The following vocabulary builder provides definitions of words used in this chapter that have not been defined in previous chapters:

**Ablation:** The removal of an organ by surgery. [NIH]

**Density:** The logarithm to the base 10 of the opacity of an exposed and processed film. [NIH]

**Dilution:** A diluted or attenuated medicine; in homeopathy, the diffusion of a given quantity of a medicinal agent in ten or one hundred times the same quantity of water. [NIH]

**Emboli:** Bit of foreign matter which enters the blood stream at one point and is carried until it is lodged or impacted in an artery and obstructs it. It may be a blood clot, an air bubble, fat or other tissue, or clumps of bacteria. [NIH]

**Fatigue:** The feeling of weariness of mind and body. [NIH]

**Hemodialyzer:** Apparatus for hemodialysis performing the functions of human kidneys in place of the damaged organs; highly specialized medical equipment used for treating kidney failure by passing the body's toxic substances through an external artificial kidney. [NIH]

**Pharmacodynamic:** Is concerned with the response of living tissues to chemical stimuli, that is, the action of drugs on the living organism in the absence of disease. [NIH]

**Rehabilitative:** Instruction of incapacitated individuals or of those affected with some mental disorder, so that some or all of their lost ability may be regained. [NIH]

**Sarcoma:** A malignant tumor of connective tissue or its derivatives. [NIH]

**Schematic:** Representative or schematic eye computed from the average of a large number of human eye measurements by Allvar Gullstrand. [NIH]

**Stimulants:** Any drug or agent which causes stimulation. [NIH]

**Translation:** The process whereby the genetic information present in the linear sequence of ribonucleotides in mRNA is converted into a corresponding sequence of amino acids in a protein. It occurs on the ribosome and is unidirectional. [NIH]

# CHAPTER 6. MULTIMEDIA ON KIDNEY FAILURE

## Overview

Information on kidney failure can come in a variety of formats. Among multimedia sources, video productions, slides, audiotapes, and computer databases are often available. In this chapter, we show you how to keep current on multimedia sources of information on kidney failure. We start with sources that have been summarized by federal agencies, and then show you how to find bibliographic information catalogued by the National Library of Medicine. If you see an interesting item, visit your local medical library to check on the availability of the title.

## Video Recordings

Most diseases do not have a video dedicated to them. If they do, they are often rather technical in nature. An excellent source of multimedia information on kidney failure is the Combined Health Information Database. You will need to limit your search to "video recording" and "kidney failure" using the "Detailed Search" option. Go directly to the following hyperlink: **http://chid.nih.gov/detail/detail.html**. To find video productions, use the drop boxes at the bottom of the search page where "You may refine your search by." Select the dates and language you prefer, and the format option "Videorecording (videotape, videocassette, etc.)." By making these selections and typing "kidney failure" (or synonyms) into the "For these words:" box, you will only receive results on video productions. The following is a typical result when searching for video recordings on kidney failure:

- **End-Stage Renal Disease: Preventing Dialysis Through Early Recognition and Intervention**

  Source: Secaucus, NJ: Network for Continuing Medical Education (NCME). 1992.

  Contact: Available from NCME. One Harmon Plaza, Secaucus, NJ 07094. (800) 223-0272 or, in New Jersey, (800) 624-2102, or (201) 867-3550. PRICE: $50 for 2-week rental or $75 for purchase. Available only to NCME subscribers; subscriber fees as of 1995 are $1,920 for VHS subscription, $2,120 for U-matic subscription.

  Summary: Although deaths in the United States from stroke and coronary artery disease are declining, the incidence of **renal failure,** another major consequence of hypertension, continues to grow. In this continuing education videotape program, viewers are taught early recognition of **end-stage renal disease** (ESRD) and appropriate intervention, in an attempt to eliminate or reduce the need for dialysis in hypertensive and diabetic patients. The program focuses on the identification of the very early signs of kidney impairment and the appropriate modes of therapy. (AA-M).

- **For the Nephrologist: Caring for People with Kidney Failure**

  Source: Madison, WI: Life Options Rehabilitation Program. 1998. (videocassette).

  Contact: Available from Life Options Rehabilitation Program. Medical Education Institute, Inc, 414 D'Onofrid Drive., Suite 200, Madison, WI 53719. (608) 833-8033. E-mail: lifeoptions@meiresearch.org. PRICE: Single copy free to health professionals only.

  Summary: This videocassette reminds nephrologists of the important role they play in improving the quality of life for each of their patients who are on chronic dialysis. The program emphasizes that the positive attitude of the physician is one of the most important factors in the successful rehabilitation of people on dialysis. The narrator briefly reviews topics such as good medical care and dialysis adequacy and then cover three areas where the nephrologist may have a great impact on the patient's life. The first area is to encourage hope, to support positive behaviors, and give honest advice, be it critical or positive. The second area focuses on the importance of providing information to patients so they can understand their treatments; this area includes referral to other care providers, such as dietitians and social workers. The third area encourages nephrologists to 'partner' with their patients, to reempower patients by giving them back the responsibility for their own care. The program emphasizes throughout the importance of really listening to patients and of taking time with them. The program features interviews with a variety of patients who have been on chronic dialysis. The program includes the toll free number of the Life Options Rehabilitation Center (800 468-7777) for viewers who would like additional information.

- **Chronic Renal Failure: Something You Can Live With**

  Source: Sharon, MA: BioMedical Video Incorporated. 1996. Videorecording.

  Contact: Available from BioMedical Video Incorporated. 619 Massapoag Avenue, Suite B, Sharon, MA, 02067. (617) 784-9700. (617) 784-5593.

  Summary: This videotape program helps parents of children diagnosed with chronic renal (kidney) failure (CRF) understand the care and management of the disease. The program reviews the history of advances in health care for infants with CRF, covers the anatomy and physiology of the kidney and its components, describes kidney function and monitoring tests (including BUN and creatinine), and discusses **end stage renal disease** (ESRD) and its management, including growth and nutrition, metabolism and metabolic problems, anemia, the use of home dialysis, recordkeeping, and the patient care team. The film includes interviews with health care providers and parents, as well as depictions of the every day care of the infant and young child with CRF.

- **Choices: Options for Living with Kidney Failure**

  Source: McGaw Park, IL: Baxter Healthcare Corporation. 1997 (videocassette).

  Contact: Available from community service section of Blockbuster video stores. PRICE: Free rental. Also available to health professionals from Baxter Healthcare Corporation. (888) 736-2543. 1620 Waukegan Road, McGaw Park, IL 60085.

  Summary: This videotape program helps viewers newly diagnosed with **kidney failure** to understand their treatment options and to make more informed choices for their own health care. The narrator reminds viewers that many members make up the health care team, but stresses that patients are the most important member of that team. The program reviews the functions of the kidneys, including clean the blood, make red blood cells, help maintain healthy bones and other bodily functions, balance body fluids and chemical levels, and retain valuable substances. Graphics demonstrate each of these functions. The narrator reviews the symptoms of **kidney failure,** and then real patients tell their own experiences of their movement into chronic **kidney failure.** The program outlines the common causes of chronic **kidney failure,** including diabetes, glomerulonephritis, hypertension (high blood pressure), polycystic kidney disease, and infections. The remainder of the program outlines each of the treatment options: hemodialysis, peritoneal dialysis, automated peritoneal dialysis (APD), and kidney transplantation. For each type, the program offers live footage of real patients using that treatment, drawings and graphics that demonstrate how the treatment works, and interviews with patients talking about how that treatment affects their lives. The program summarizes the reasons why each treatment option may be appropriate or inappropriate for a specific patient. The program concludes with a list of general guidelines that can help to reduce treatment side effects and with a list of associations to contact for more information.

- **Kidney Failure: Are You At Risk?**

  Source: Madison, WI: University of Wisconsin Hospitals and Clinics, Department of Outreach Education. 1998. (videocassette).

  Contact: Available from University of Wisconsin Hospital and Clinics. Picture of Health, 702 North Blackhawk Avenue, Suite 215, Madison, WI 53705-3357. (800) 757-4354 or (608) 263-6510. Fax (608) 262-7172. PRICE: $19.95 plus shipping and handling; bulk copies available. Order number 051498B.

  Summary: This videotape program, moderated by Mary Lee, discusses **end stage renal disease** and the prevention or delay of **kidney failure.** The program features Dr. Bryan Becker, a nephrologist (kidney specialist). Dr. Becker explores the epidemiology of the recent trend of increasing levels of **kidney failure,** discussing the aging population, better diagnostics, and better rates of survival. Dr. Becker then reviews the physiology of the kidneys, noting that kidneys control fluids and electrolytes (sodium, potassium, chloride) in the body, regulate the acid base balance, help metabolize proteins and carbohydrates, and remove creatinine (a muscle breakdown product). Different kidney diseases have a varying impact on kidney function. More than 50 percent of **kidney failure** is caused by two diseases: diabetes mellitus and hypertension; other causes include heredity, illnesses, inflammation, toxicity, kidney cancer, and trauma to the kidney (e.g., automobile accidents). The symptoms of kidney disease (which can be largely silent) can include protein in the urine, hypertension, elevated creatinine levels, decrease in urine output, swelling in the feet (edema, or fluid accumulation), and an increase in nocturia (urinating at night). **End stage renal disease** (ESRD) is defined as loss of 90 percent or more of kidney function. Dr. Becker discusses screening and identifying patients who may be at risk of kidney disease, then debunks various myths about kidney disease, on the topics of one kidney versus two kidneys, dialysis, and transplantation. Dr. Becker emphasizes that kidney disease, while treatable, has a great impact on lifestyle, diet, caretaking, finances, family and support systems, and heart disease. Prevention strategies include identifying high risk patients, avoiding nephrotoxic medications (including ibuprofen), monitoring the diet, controlling blood pressure, controlling blood glucose levels (for people with diabetes), and educating oneself about kidney disease. The program concludes by referring viewers to the National Kidney and Urologic Diseases Information Clearinghouse (**www.niddk.nih.gov**).

## Audio Recordings

The Combined Health Information Database contains abstracts on audio productions. To search CHID, go directly to the following hyperlink: **http://chid.nih.gov/detail/detail.html**. To find audio productions, use the drop boxes at the bottom of the search page where "You may refine your search by." Select the dates and language you prefer, and the format option "Sound Recordings." By making these selections and typing "kidney failure" (or synonyms) into the "For these words:" box, you will only receive results on sound recordings (again, most diseases do not have results, so do not expect to find many). The following is a typical result when searching for sound recordings on kidney failure:

- **Diet and the Retardation of the Progression of Chronic Renal Failure**

  Source: Bethlehem, PA: St. Luke's Hospital. 1991.

  Contact: Available from St. Luke's Hospital. Nutrition Services-Renal, 801 Ostrum Street, Bethlehem, PA 18015. (215) 954-4000. ATTN: Emilia Johns. PRICE: Contact directly for details.

  Summary: This audiocassette presents a program from a one-day symposium, held in October 1991, that focuses on the nutritional assessment and nutritional intervention in the treatment of patients with chronic **renal failure** (CRF). The speaker, Joel D. Kopple, a professor of medicine and public health, discusses diet and the retardation of the progression of CRF. Special attention is directed at the nutritional aspects of the treatment of the patient in the earlier stages of CRF. The symposium was designed for dietitians and for students studying to become dietitians.

# CHAPTER 7. PERIODICALS AND NEWS ON KIDNEY FAILURE

## Overview

Keeping up on the news relating to kidney failure can be challenging. Subscribing to targeted periodicals can be an effective way to stay abreast of recent developments on kidney failure. Periodicals include newsletters, magazines, and academic journals.

In this chapter, we suggest a number of news sources and present various periodicals that cover kidney failure beyond and including those which are published by patient associations mentioned earlier. We will first focus on news services, and then on periodicals. News services, press releases, and newsletters generally use more accessible language, so if you do chose to subscribe to one of the more technical periodicals, make sure that it uses language you can easily follow.

## News Services and Press Releases

Well before articles show up in newsletters or the popular press, they may appear in the form of a press release or a public relations announcement. One of the simplest ways of tracking press releases on kidney failure is to search the news wires. News wires are used by professional journalists, and have existed since the invention of the telegraph. Today, there are several major "wires" that are used by companies, universities, and other organizations to announce new medical breakthroughs. In the following sample of sources, we will briefly describe how to access each service. These services only post recent news intended for public viewing.

### PR Newswire

Perhaps the broadest of the wires is PR Newswire Association, Inc. To access this archive, simply go to **http://www.prnewswire.com**. Below the search box, select the option "The last 30 days." In the search box, type "kidney failure" or synonyms. The search results are shown by order of relevance. When reading these press releases, do not forget that the sponsor of the release may be a company or organization that is trying to sell a particular product or therapy. Their views, therefore, may be biased.

### Reuters Health

The Reuters' Medical News and Health eLine databases can be very useful in exploring news archives relating to kidney failure. While some of the listed articles are free to view, others can be purchased for a nominal fee. To access this archive, go to **http://www.reutershealth.com/en/index.html** and search by "kidney failure" (or synonyms). The following was recently listed in this archive for kidney failure:

- **Drugs cut kidney failure risk in lupus patients**
  Source: Reuters Health eLine
  Date: March 04, 2004

- **Susceptibility genes may explain high rate of diabetic kidney failure in blacks**
  Source: Reuters Medical News
  Date: November 14, 2003

- **Reasons for the unabated rise in kidney failure in the US remain unresolved**
  Source: Reuters Medical News
  Date: May 29, 2003

- **Daily dialysis for kidney failure lengthens life**
  Source: Reuters Health eLine
  Date: January 30, 2002

### The NIH

Within MEDLINEplus, the NIH has made an agreement with the New York Times Syndicate, the AP News Service, and Reuters to deliver news that can be browsed by the public. Search news releases at **http://www.nlm.nih.gov/medlineplus/alphanews_a.html.** MEDLINEplus allows you to browse across an alphabetical index. Or you can search by date at **http://www.nlm.nih.gov/medlineplus/newsbydate.html**. Often, news items are indexed by MEDLINEplus within their search engine.

### Business Wire

Business Wire is similar to PR Newswire. To access this archive, simply go to **http://www.businesswire.com**. You can scan the news by industry category or company name.

### Market Wire

Market Wire is more focused on technology than the other wires. To browse the latest press releases by topic, such as alternative medicine, biotechnology, fitness, healthcare, legal, nutrition, and pharmaceuticals, log on to Market Wire's Medical/Health channel at the following hyperlink **http://www.marketwire.com/mw/release_index?channel=MedicalHealth**. Market Wire's home page is **http://www.marketwire.com/mw/home**. From here, type "kidney failure" (or synonyms) into the search box, and click on "Search News." As this service is technology oriented, you may wish to use it when searching for press releases covering diagnostic procedures or tests.

### Search Engines

Free-to-view news can also be found in the news section of your favorite search engines (see the health news page at Yahoo: **http://dir.yahoo.com/Health/News_and_Media/,** or use this Web site's general news search page **http://news.yahoo.com/.** Type in "kidney failure" (or synonyms). If you know the name of a company that is relevant to kidney failure, you can go to any stock trading Web site (such as **www.etrade.com**) and search for the company name there. News items across various news sources are reported on indicated hyperlinks.

### BBC

Covering news from a more European perspective, the British Broadcasting Corporation (BBC) allows the public free access to their news archive located at **http://www.bbc.co.uk/**. Search by "kidney failure" (or synonyms).

## Newsletters on Kidney Failure

Given their focus on current and relevant developments, newsletters are often more useful to patients than academic articles. You can find newsletters using the Combined Health Information Database (CHID). You will need to use the "Detailed Search" option. To access CHID, go directly to the following hyperlink: **http://chid.nih.gov/detail/detail.html**. Your investigation must limit the search to "Newsletter" and "kidney failure." Go to the bottom of the search page where "You may refine your search by." Select the dates and language that you prefer. For the format option, select "Newsletter." By making these selections and typing in "kidney failure" or synonyms into the "For these words:" box, you will only receive results on newsletters. The following list was generated using the options described above:

- **Kidney Failure in Sarcoidosis**

  Source: Sarcoidosis Networking. 8(3): 3. 2000.

  Contact: Available from Sarcoid Network Association. Sarcoidosis Networking, 13925 80th Street East, Puyallup, WA 98372-3614. Email: sarcoidosis_network@prodigy.net.

  Summary: Sarcoidosis is a chronic, progressive systemic granulomatous (causing lesions) disease of unknown cause (etiology), involving almost any organ or tissue, including the skin, lungs, lymph nodes, liver, spleen, eyes, and small bones of the hands or feet. This brief article, from a newsletter for patients with sarcoidosis, reviews the complications of **kidney failure** in sarcoidosis. Granulomatous infiltration of the kidney may be present in as many as 40 percent of patients with sarcoidosis, but it is rarely extensive enough to cause renal (kidney) dysfunction. The lesions are usually responsive to steroid therapy. **Kidney failure** has also been diagnosed in patients with sarcoidosis without the presence of lesions, possibly due to hypercalcemia (too much calcium in the blood), involvement of the glomerular filter system, and renal arteritis (inflammation of the arteries of the kidney), which may be associated with severe high blood pressure. It is recommended that all people with active sarcoidosis be screened for hypercalciuria (high levels of calcium in the urine). This may precede development of hypercalcemia, which should be treated. Glucocorticoids are the main choice of therapy and do seem to reduce levels of urinary calcium to normal within a few days. People with sarcoidosis may also have severe pain; the frequent use of pain medication can be another cause of **kidney failure.** People who take pain medication should ask their physicians to evaluate their kidneys on a regular basis. 9 references.

## Newsletter Articles

If you choose not to subscribe to a newsletter, you can nevertheless find references to newsletter articles. We recommend that you use the Combined Health Information Database, while limiting your search criteria to "newsletter articles." Again, you will need to use the "Detailed Search" option at **http://chid.nih.gov/detail/detail.html**. Go to the bottom of the search page where "You may refine your search by." Select the dates and language that you prefer. For the format option, select "Newsletter Article."

By making these selections, and typing in "kidney failure" (or synonyms) into the "For these words:" box, you will only receive results on newsletter articles. You should check back periodically with this database as it is updated every 3 months. The following is a typical result when searching for newsletter articles on kidney failure:

- **Overcoming the Changes of Kidney Failure and Dialysis**

  Source: Renal Rehabilitation Report. 9(2): 1, 6-8. Summer 2001.

  Contact: Available from Life Options Rehabilitation Program. Medical Education Institute, Inc, 414 D'Onofrid Drive., Suite 200, Madison, WI 53719. (608) 833-8033. E-mail: lifeoptions@meiresearch.org.

  Summary: From the moment individuals become aware they are beginning to lose kidney function, their lives change. Schedules that may have been relatively free of day to day health care concerns must soon be adapted to include a changing diet, new medications, multiple medical appointments, and eventually a complex regimen of life saving dialysis treatments. This article reviews the changes that a patient undergoes when coming to terms with a chronic illness such as **kidney failure.** The author emphasizes that, to enjoy a long and full life, people with kidney disease must not only receive good clinical care, they must also commit to rehabilitation. Because there is no cure, complete recovery is not a realistic goal, but rehabilitation can be. To return to a near normal life, people with a chronic illness must be willing to take responsibility for their own care. A recent study identified four changed circumstances that people on dialysis commonly face on their way to rehabilitation: an uncertain future and the risk of death; constraints on such usual activities as eating, drinking, traveling, and exercising; dialysis treatment itself; and repeated setbacks in health. One sidebar offers tips to help patients come to terms: recognize oneself as a changed person, acknowledge that circumstances have changed, see the value in one's changed self and changed life, learn to adjust, and take control of one's own health and life. Health care providers are encouraged to help patients face **kidney failure** with optimism and self determination, recognizing that these may not be easy tasks to achieve. 10 references.

- **Calcitriol Replacement in Renal Failure**

Source: OsteoDynamics. 3(1): 1-2. Spring 1995.

Contact: Available from Abbott Renal Care. Abbott Laboratories, Abbott Park, IL 60064-3537. (800) 457-9472.

Summary: In this newsletter article, the author familiarizes readers with the benefits of calcitriol replacement in patients on dialysis. Topics covered include the discovery and biosynthesis of calcitriol; its mechanism of action; how **end-stage renal disease** (ESRD) affects calcitriol; synthetic calcitriol (Calcijex); and present calcitriol uses. The author notes that almost every patient who is referred to a dialysis unit for treatment of ESRD is already affected by low levels of calcitriol. Although symptoms may be minimal, or even absent, the consequences of long term calcitriol deprivation will worsen without treatment.

- **Kidney Failure: Early Detection Is Key**

Source: Mayo Clinic Health Letter. 18(10): 1-3. October 2000.

Contact: Available from Mayo Clinic Health Letter. Subscription Services, P.O. Box 53889, Boulder, CO 80322-3889. (800) 333-9037 or (303) 604-1465.

Summary: This health information newsletter article describes the role of early detection in the adequate treatment of **kidney failure.** The author notes that **kidney failure** (the term for a decline in kidney function) is becoming more common because people are living longer with chronic illnesses that can harm their kidneys. To preserve kidney function, it is important to manage conditions that can affect the kidneys, as well as to recognize and treat **kidney failure** as early as possible. The article briefly reviews the anatomy and function of the kidneys, which not only filter out waste products but also regulate certain chemicals in the body, produce several important hormones (for manufacturing red blood cells), regulate blood pressure, and maintain bone calcium. The majority of people who need dialysis because of **kidney failure** have diabetes mellitus, hypertension (high blood pressure), or both. The symptoms of **kidney failure** may go unrecognized until substantial damage has occurred and kidney function is at just a small fraction of the normal level. The destruction of the filtering nephrons in the kidney can result in symptoms including a prolonged flulike illness, headaches, fatigue, itchiness over the entire body, a need to urinate less or more often, loss of appetite, and nausea and vomiting. When fewer nephrons are functioning, wastes and fluids accumulate in the blood. However, simple blood tests and urinalysis done during a routine exam may detect **kidney failure** even before symptoms show up. The article concludes by reminding readers of the importance of controlling high blood pressure in order to prevent or delay **kidney failure,** the need to control blood glucose (sugar) levels for people with diabetes, and the concept of maintaining adequate and healthy nutrition and fluid levels (including avoiding toxic drugs or herbal supplements). One sidebar reviews the most common tests of kidney function which check for creatinine, blood urea nitrogen (BUN), and proteinuria (protein in the urine). 2 figures.

## Academic Periodicals covering Kidney Failure

Academic periodicals can be a highly technical yet valuable source of information on kidney failure. We have compiled the following list of periodicals known to publish articles relating to kidney failure and which are currently indexed within the National Library of Medicine's PubMed database (follow hyperlinks to view more information, summaries, etc., for each). In addition to these sources, to keep current on articles written on kidney failure published by any of the periodicals listed below, you can follow the hyperlink indicated or go to **www.ncbi.nlm.nih.gov/pubmed**. Type the periodical's name into the search box to find the latest studies published.

If you want complete details about the historical contents of a periodical, you can also visit **http://www.ncbi.nlm.nih.gov/entrez/jrbrowser.cgi**. Here, type in the name of the journal or its abbreviation, and you will receive an index of published articles. At **http://locatorplus.gov/** you can retrieve more indexing information on medical periodicals (e.g. the name of the publisher). Select the button "Search LOCATORplus." Then type in the name of the journal and select the advanced search option "Journal Title Search." The following is a sample of periodicals which publish articles on kidney failure:

- **American Heart Journal. (Am Heart J)**
  http://www.ncbi.nlm.nih.gov/entrez/jrbrowser.cgi?field=0&regexp=American+Heart+Journal&dispmax=20&dispstart=0

- **American Journal of Hypertension: Journal of the American Society of Hypertension. (Am J Hypertens)**
  http://www.ncbi.nlm.nih.gov/entrez/jrbrowser.cgi?field=0&regexp=American+Journal+of+Hypertension+:+Journal+of+the+American+Society+of+Hypertension&dispmax=20&dispstart=0

- **American Journal of Kidney Diseases: the Official Journal of the National Kidney Foundation. (Am J Kidney Dis)**
  http://www.ncbi.nlm.nih.gov/entrez/jrbrowser.cgi?field=0&regexp=American+Journal+of+Kidney+Diseases+:+the+Official+Journal+of+the+National+Kidney+Foundation&dispmax=20&dispstart=0

- **American Journal of Nephrology. (Am J Nephrol)**
  http://www.ncbi.nlm.nih.gov/entrez/jrbrowser.cgi?field=0&regexp=American+Journal+of+Nephrology&dispmax=20&dispstart=0

- **Annals of Emergency Medicine. (Ann Emerg Med)**
  http://www.ncbi.nlm.nih.gov/entrez/jrbrowser.cgi?field=0&regexp=Annals+of+Emergency+Medicine&dispmax=20&dispstart=0

- **Archives of Neurology. (Arch Neurol)**
  http://www.ncbi.nlm.nih.gov/entrez/jrbrowser.cgi?field=0&regexp=Archives+of+Neurology&dispmax=20&dispstart=0

- **Archives of Pediatrics & Adolescent Medicine. (Arch Pediatr Adolesc Med)**
  http://www.ncbi.nlm.nih.gov/entrez/jrbrowser.cgi?field=0&regexp=Archives+of+Pediatrics+&+Adolescent+Medicine&dispmax=20&dispstart=0

- **Artificial Organs. (Artif Organs)**
  http://www.ncbi.nlm.nih.gov/entrez/jrbrowser.cgi?field=0&regexp=Artificial+Organs&dispmax=20&dispstart=0

- **British Journal of Urology. (Br J Urol)**
  http://www.ncbi.nlm.nih.gov/entrez/jrbrowser.cgi?field=0&regexp=British+Journal+of+Urology&dispmax=20&dispstart=0

- **British Medical Journal (Clinical Research Ed.. (Br Med J (Clin Res Ed))**
  http://www.ncbi.nlm.nih.gov/entrez/jrbrowser.cgi?field=0&regexp=British+Medical+Journal+(Clinical+Research+Ed.+&dispmax=20&dispstart=0

- **British Medical Journal. (Br Med J)**
  http://www.ncbi.nlm.nih.gov/entrez/jrbrowser.cgi?field=0&regexp=British+Medical+Journal&dispmax=20&dispstart=0

- **Clinical Pediatrics. (Clin Pediatr (Phila))**
  http://www.ncbi.nlm.nih.gov/entrez/jrbrowser.cgi?field=0&regexp=Clinical+Pediatrics&dispmax=20&dispstart=0

- **Clinical Pharmacology and Therapeutics. (Clin Pharmacol Ther)**
  http://www.ncbi.nlm.nih.gov/entrez/jrbrowser.cgi?field=0&regexp=Clinical+Pharmacology+and+Therapeutics&dispmax=20&dispstart=0

- **European Journal of Clinical Pharmacology. (Eur J Clin Pharmacol)**
  http://www.ncbi.nlm.nih.gov/entrez/jrbrowser.cgi?field=0&regexp=European+Journal+of+Clinical+Pharmacology&dispmax=20&dispstart=0

- **European Journal of Nuclear Medicine and Molecular Imaging. (Eur J Nucl Med Mol Imaging)**
  http://www.ncbi.nlm.nih.gov/entrez/jrbrowser.cgi?field=0&regexp=European+Journal+of+Nuclear+Medicine+and+Molecular+Imaging&dispmax=20&dispstart=0

- **Expert Opinion on Pharmacotherapy. (Expert Opin Pharmacother)**
  http://www.ncbi.nlm.nih.gov/entrez/jrbrowser.cgi?field=0&regexp=Expert+Opinion+on+Pharmacotherapy&dispmax=20&dispstart=0

- **Hepatology (Baltimore, Md. (Hepatology))**
  http://www.ncbi.nlm.nih.gov/entrez/jrbrowser.cgi?field=0&regexp=Hepatology+(Baltimore,+Md.+&dispmax=20&dispstart=0

- **International Journal of Dermatology. (Int J Dermatol)**
  http://www.ncbi.nlm.nih.gov/entrez/jrbrowser.cgi?field=0&regexp=International+Journal+of+Dermatology&dispmax=20&dispstart=0

- **International Urology and Nephrology. (Int Urol Nephrol)**
  http://www.ncbi.nlm.nih.gov/entrez/jrbrowser.cgi?field=0&regexp=International+Urology+and+Nephrology&dispmax=20&dispstart=0

- **Jama: the Journal of the American Medical Association. (JAMA)**
  http://www.ncbi.nlm.nih.gov/entrez/jrbrowser.cgi?field=0&regexp=Jama+:+the+Journal+of+the+American+Medical+Association&dispmax=20&dispstart=0

- **Journal of Clinical Epidemiology. (J Clin Epidemiol)**
  http://www.ncbi.nlm.nih.gov/entrez/jrbrowser.cgi?field=0&regexp=Journal+of+Clinical+Epidemiology&dispmax=20&dispstart=0

- **Journal of Clinical Microbiology. (J Clin Microbiol)**
  http://www.ncbi.nlm.nih.gov/entrez/jrbrowser.cgi?field=0&regexp=Journal+of+Clinical+Microbiology&dispmax=20&dispstart=0

- **Journal of Medical Engineering & Technology. (J Med Eng Technol)**
  http://www.ncbi.nlm.nih.gov/entrez/jrbrowser.cgi?field=0&regexp=Journal+of+Medical+Engineering+&+Technology&dispmax=20&dispstart=0

- **Journal of Pediatric Health Care: Official Publication of National Association of Pediatric Nurse Associates & Practitioners. (J Pediatr Health Care)**
  http://www.ncbi.nlm.nih.gov/entrez/jrbrowser.cgi?field=0&regexp=Journal+of+Pediatric+Health+Care+:+Official+Publication+of+National+Association+of+Pediatric+Nurse+Associates+&+Practitioners&dispmax=20&dispstart=0

- **Journal of Renal Nutrition: the Official Journal of the Council on Renal Nutrition of the National Kidney Foundation. (J Ren Nutr)**
  http://www.ncbi.nlm.nih.gov/entrez/jrbrowser.cgi?field=0&regexp=Journal+of+Renal+Nutrition+:+the+Official+Journal+of+the+Council+on+Renal+Nutrition+of+the+National+Kidney+Foundation&dispmax=20&dispstart=0

- **Journal of the American Academy of Dermatology. (J Am Acad Dermatol)**
  http://www.ncbi.nlm.nih.gov/entrez/jrbrowser.cgi?field=0&regexp=Journal+of+the+American+Academy+of+Dermatology&dispmax=20&dispstart=0

- **Journal of the American Dietetic Association. (J Am Diet Assoc)**
  http://www.ncbi.nlm.nih.gov/entrez/jrbrowser.cgi?field=0&regexp=Journal+of+the+American+Dietetic+Association&dispmax=20&dispstart=0

- **Kidney International. Supplement. (Kidney Int Suppl)**
  http://www.ncbi.nlm.nih.gov/entrez/jrbrowser.cgi?field=0&regexp=Kidney+International.+Supplement&dispmax=20&dispstart=0

- **Medical Decision Making: an International Journal of the Society for Medical Decision Making. (Med Decis Making)**
http://www.ncbi.nlm.nih.gov/entrez/jrbrowser.cgi?field=0&regexp=Medical+Decision+Making+:+an+International+Journal+of+the+Society+for+Medical+Decision+Making&dispmax=20&dispstart=0

- **Medical Hypotheses. (Med Hypotheses)**
http://www.ncbi.nlm.nih.gov/entrez/jrbrowser.cgi?field=0&regexp=Medical+Hypotheses&dispmax=20&dispstart=0

- **Nature Genetics. (Nat Genet)**
http://www.ncbi.nlm.nih.gov/entrez/jrbrowser.cgi?field=0&regexp=Nature+Genetics&dispmax=20&dispstart=0

- **Nephrology, Dialysis, Transplantation: Official Publication of the European Dialysis and Transplant Association - European Renal Association. (Nephrol Dial Transplant)**
http://www.ncbi.nlm.nih.gov/entrez/jrbrowser.cgi?field=0&regexp=Nephrology,+Dialysis,+Transplantation+:+Official+Publication+of+the+European+Dialysis+and+Transplant+Association+-+European+Renal+Association&dispmax=20&dispstart=0

- **Nutrition Reviews. (Nutr Rev)**
http://www.ncbi.nlm.nih.gov/entrez/jrbrowser.cgi?field=0&regexp=Nutrition+Reviews&dispmax=20&dispstart=0

- **Pediatrics in Review / American Academy of Pediatrics. (Pediatr Rev)**
http://www.ncbi.nlm.nih.gov/entrez/jrbrowser.cgi?field=0&regexp=Pediatrics+in+Review+/+American+Academy+of+Pediatrics&dispmax=20&dispstart=0

- **Redox Report: Communications in Free Radical Research. (Redox Rep)**
http://www.ncbi.nlm.nih.gov/entrez/jrbrowser.cgi?field=0&regexp=Redox+Report+:+Communications+in+Free+Radical+Research&dispmax=20&dispstart=0

- **Scandinavian Journal of Clinical and Laboratory Investigation. (Scand J Clin Lab Invest)**
http://www.ncbi.nlm.nih.gov/entrez/jrbrowser.cgi?field=0&regexp=Scandinavian+Journal+of+Clinical+and+Laboratory+Investigation&dispma

x=20&dispstart=0

- **Social Science & Medicine (1982). (Soc Sci Med)**
  http://www.ncbi.nlm.nih.gov/entrez/jrbrowser.cgi?field=0&regexp=So
  cial+Science+&+Medicine+(1982)&dispmax=20&dispstart=0

- **Swiss Medical Weekly: Official Journal of the Swiss Society of Infectious Diseases, the Swiss Society of Internal Medicine, the Swiss Society of Pneumology. (Swiss Med Wkly)**
  http://www.ncbi.nlm.nih.gov/entrez/jrbrowser.cgi?field=0&regexp=Sw
  iss+Medical+Weekly+:+Official+Journal+of+the+Swiss+Society+of+Infec
  tious+Diseases,+the+Swiss+Society+of+Internal+Medicine,+the+Swiss+S
  ociety+of+Pneumology&dispmax=20&dispstart=0

- **The American Journal of Clinical Nutrition. (Am J Clin Nutr)**
  http://www.ncbi.nlm.nih.gov/entrez/jrbrowser.cgi?field=0&regexp=Th
  e+American+Journal+of+Clinical+Nutrition&dispmax=20&dispstart=0

- **The American Journal of the Medical Sciences. (Am J Med Sci)**
  http://www.ncbi.nlm.nih.gov/entrez/jrbrowser.cgi?field=0&regexp=Th
  e+American+Journal+of+the+Medical+Sciences&dispmax=20&dispstart
  =0

- **The Annals of Pharmacotherapy. (Ann Pharmacother)**
  http://www.ncbi.nlm.nih.gov/entrez/jrbrowser.cgi?field=0&regexp=Th
  e+Annals+of+Pharmacotherapy&dispmax=20&dispstart=0

- **The Journal of Clinical Endocrinology and Metabolism. (J Clin Endocrinol Metab)**
  http://www.ncbi.nlm.nih.gov/entrez/jrbrowser.cgi?field=0&regexp=Th
  e+Journal+of+Clinical+Endocrinology+and+Metabolism&dispmax=20&
  dispstart=0

- **The Journal of Heart and Lung Transplantation: the Official Publication of the International Society for Heart Transplantation. (J Heart Lung Transplant)**
  http://www.ncbi.nlm.nih.gov/entrez/jrbrowser.cgi?field=0&regexp=Th
  e+Journal+of+Heart+and+Lung+Transplantation+:+the+Official+Publica
  tion+of+the+International+Society+for+Heart+Transplantation&dispmax
  =20&dispstart=0

- **The Journal of Laboratory and Clinical Medicine. (J Lab Clin Med)**
  http://www.ncbi.nlm.nih.gov/entrez/jrbrowser.cgi?field=0&regexp=The+Journal+of+Laboratory+and+Clinical+Medicine&dispmax=20&dispstart=0

- **The Journal of Pediatrics. (J Pediatr)**
  http://www.ncbi.nlm.nih.gov/entrez/jrbrowser.cgi?field=0&regexp=The+Journal+of+Pediatrics&dispmax=20&dispstart=0

- **The New England Journal of Medicine. (N Engl J Med)**
  http://www.ncbi.nlm.nih.gov/entrez/jrbrowser.cgi?field=0&regexp=The+New+England+Journal+of+Medicine&dispmax=20&dispstart=0

- **Transplantation Proceedings. (Transplant Proc)**
  http://www.ncbi.nlm.nih.gov/entrez/jrbrowser.cgi?field=0&regexp=Transplantation+Proceedings&dispmax=20&dispstart=0

# CHAPTER 8. PHYSICIAN GUIDELINES AND DATABASES

## Overview

Doctors and medical researchers rely on a number of information sources to help patients with their conditions. Many will subscribe to journals or newsletters published by their professional associations or refer to specialized textbooks or clinical guides published for the medical profession. In this chapter, we focus on databases and Internet-based guidelines created or written for this professional audience.

## NIH Guidelines

For the more common diseases, The National Institutes of Health publish guidelines that are frequently consulted by physicians. Publications are typically written by one or more of the various NIH Institutes. For physician guidelines, commonly referred to as "clinical" or "professional" guidelines, you can visit the following Institutes:

- Office of the Director (OD); guidelines consolidated across agencies available at **http://www.nih.gov/health/consumer/conkey.htm**

- National Institute of General Medical Sciences (NIGMS); fact sheets available at **http://www.nigms.nih.gov/news/facts/**

- National Library of Medicine (NLM); extensive encyclopedia (A.D.A.M., Inc.) with guidelines:
  **http://www.nlm.nih.gov/medlineplus/healthtopics.html**

- National Institute of Diabetes and Digestive and Kidney Diseases (NIDDK); guidelines available at
  **http://www.niddk.nih.gov/health/health.htm**

## NIH Databases

In addition to the various Institutes of Health that publish professional guidelines, the NIH has designed a number of databases for professionals.[22] Physician-oriented resources provide a wide variety of information related to the biomedical and health sciences, both past and present. The format of these resources varies. Searchable databases, bibliographic citations, full text articles (when available), archival collections, and images are all available. The following are referenced by the National Library of Medicine:[23]

- **Bioethics:** Access to published literature on the ethical, legal and public policy issues surrounding healthcare and biomedical research. This information is provided in conjunction with the Kennedy Institute of Ethics located at Georgetown University, Washington, D.C.: **http://www.nlm.nih.gov/databases/databases_bioethics.html**

- **HIV/AIDS Resources:** Describes various links and databases dedicated to HIV/ AIDS research: **http://www.nlm.nih.gov/pubs/factsheets/aidsinfs.html**

- **NLM Online Exhibitions:** Describes "Exhibitions in the History of Medicine": **http://www.nlm.nih.gov/exhibition/exhibition.html**. Additional resources for historical scholarship in medicine: **http://www.nlm.nih.gov/hmd/hmd.html**

- **Biotechnology Information:** Access to public databases. The National Center for Biotechnology Information conducts research in computational biology, develops software tools for analyzing genome data, and disseminates biomedical information for the better understanding of molecular processes affecting human health and disease: **http://www.ncbi.nlm.nih.gov/**

- **Population Information:** The National Library of Medicine provides access to worldwide coverage of population, family planning, and related health issues, including family planning technology and programs, fertility, and population law and policy: **http://www.nlm.nih.gov/databases/databases_population.html**

- **Cancer Information:** Access to caner-oriented databases: **http://www.nlm.nih.gov/databases/databases_cancer.html**

---

[22] Remember, for the general public, the National Library of Medicine recommends the databases referenced in MEDLINE*plus* (**http://medlineplus.gov/** or **http://www.nlm.nih.gov/medlineplus/databases.html**).
[23] See **http://www.nlm.nih.gov/databases/databases.html**.

- **Profiles in Science:** Offering the archival collections of prominent twentieth-century biomedical scientists to the public through modern digital technology: **http://www.profiles.nlm.nih.gov/**

- **Chemical Information:** Provides links to various chemical databases and references: **http://sis.nlm.nih.gov/Chem/ChemMain.html**

- **Clinical Alerts:** Reports the release of findings from the NIH-funded clinical trials where such release could significantly affect morbidity and mortality: **http://www.nlm.nih.gov/databases/alerts/clinical_alerts.html**

- **Space Life Sciences:** Provides links and information to space-based research (including NASA): **http://www.nlm.nih.gov/databases/databases_space.html**

- **MEDLINE:** Bibliographic database covering the fields of medicine, nursing, dentistry, veterinary medicine, the healthcare system, and the pre-clinical sciences: **http://www.nlm.nih.gov/databases/databases_medline.html**

- **Toxicology and Environmental Health Information (TOXNET):** Databases covering toxicology and environmental health: **http://sis.nlm.nih.gov/Tox/ToxMain.html**

- **Visible Human Interface:** Anatomically detailed, three-dimensional representations of normal male and female human bodies: **http://www.nlm.nih.gov/research/visible/visible_human.html**

While all of the above references may be of interest to physicians who study and treat kidney failure, the following are particularly noteworthy.

### The NLM Gateway[24]

The NLM (National Library of Medicine) Gateway is a Web-based system that lets users search simultaneously in multiple retrieval systems at the U.S. National Library of Medicine (NLM). It allows users of NLM services to initiate searches from one Web interface, providing "one-stop searching" for many of NLM's information resources or databases.[25] One target audience for the Gateway is the Internet user who is new to NLM's online resources and does not know what information is available or how best to search for it. This audience may include physicians and other healthcare providers,

---

[24] Adapted from NLM: **http://gateway.nlm.nih.gov/gw/Cmd?Overview.x**.

[25] The NLM Gateway is currently being developed by the Lister Hill National Center for Biomedical Communications (LHNCBC) at the National Library of Medicine (NLM) of the National Institutes of Health (NIH).

researchers, librarians, students, and, increasingly, patients, their families, and the public.[26] To use the NLM Gateway, simply go to the search site at **http://gateway.nlm.nih.gov/gw/Cmd**. Type "kidney failure" (or synonyms) into the search box and click "Search." The results will be presented in a tabular form, indicating the number of references in each database category.

**Results Summary**

| Category | Items Found |
|---|---|
| Journal Articles | 75199 |
| Books / Periodicals / Audio Visual | 680 |
| Consumer Health | 916 |
| Meeting Abstracts | 69 |
| Other Collections | 371 |
| Total | 77235 |

**HSTAT**[27]

HSTAT is a free, Web-based resource that provides access to full-text documents used in healthcare decision-making.[28] HSTAT's audience includes healthcare providers, health service researchers, policy makers, insurance companies, consumers, and the information professionals who serve these groups. HSTAT provides access to a wide variety of publications, including clinical practice guidelines, quick-reference guides for clinicians, consumer health brochures, evidence reports and technology assessments from the Agency for Healthcare Research and Quality (AHRQ), as well as AHRQ's Put Prevention Into Practice.[29] Simply search by "kidney failure" (or synonyms) at the following Web site: **http://text.nlm.nih.gov**.

---

[26] Other users may find the Gateway useful for an overall search of NLM's information resources. Some searchers may locate what they need immediately, while others will utilize the Gateway as an adjunct tool to other NLM search services such as PubMed® and MEDLINEplus®. The Gateway connects users with multiple NLM retrieval systems while also providing a search interface for its own collections. These collections include various types of information that do not logically belong in PubMed, LOCATORplus, or other established NLM retrieval systems (e.g., meeting announcements and pre-1966 journal citations). The Gateway will provide access to the information found in an increasing number of NLM retrieval systems in several phases.

[27] Adapted from HSTAT: **http://www.nlm.nih.gov/pubs/factsheets/hstat.html**.

[28] The HSTAT URL is **http://hstat.nlm.nih.gov/**.

[29] Other important documents in HSTAT include: the National Institutes of Health (NIH) Consensus Conference Reports and Technology Assessment Reports; the HIV/AIDS Treatment Information Service (ATIS) resource documents; the Substance Abuse and Mental Health Services Administration's Center for Substance Abuse Treatment (SAMHSA/CSAT) Treatment Improvement Protocols (TIP) and Center for Substance Abuse Prevention

## Coffee Break: Tutorials for Biologists[30]

Some patients may wish to have access to a general healthcare site that takes a scientific view of the news and covers recent breakthroughs in biology that may one day assist physicians in developing treatments. To this end, we recommend "Coffee Break," a collection of short reports on recent biological discoveries. Each report incorporates interactive tutorials that demonstrate how bioinformatics tools are used as a part of the research process. Currently, all Coffee Breaks are written by NCBI staff.[31] Each report is about 400 words and is usually based on a discovery reported in one or more articles from recently published, peer-reviewed literature.[32] This site has new articles every few weeks, so it can be considered an online magazine of sorts, and intended for general background information. You can access Coffee Break at **http://www.ncbi.nlm.nih.gov/Coffeebreak/**.

---

(SAMHSA/CSAP) Prevention Enhancement Protocols System (PEPS); the Public Health Service (PHS) Preventive Services Task Force's *Guide to Clinical Preventive Services*; the independent, nonfederal Task Force on Community Services *Guide to Community Preventive Services*; and the Health Technology Advisory Committee (HTAC) of the Minnesota Health Care Commission (MHCC) health technology evaluations.

[30] Adapted from **http://www.ncbi.nlm.nih.gov/Coffeebreak/Archive/FAQ.html**.

[31] The figure that accompanies each article is frequently supplied by an expert external to NCBI, in which case the source of the figure is cited. The result is an interactive tutorial that tells a biological story.

[32] After a brief introduction that sets the work described into a broader context, the report focuses on how a molecular understanding can provide explanations of observed biology and lead to therapies for diseases. Each vignette is accompanied by a figure and hypertext links that lead to a series of pages that interactively show how NCBI tools and resources are used in the research process.

## Other Commercial Databases

In addition to resources maintained by official agencies, other databases exist that are commercial ventures addressing medical professionals. Here are some examples that may interest you:

- **CliniWeb International:** Index and table of contents to selected clinical information on the Internet; see **http://www.ohsu.edu/cliniweb/**.

- **Medical World Search:** Searches full text from thousands of selected medical sites on the Internet; see **http://www.mwsearch.com/**.

# CHAPTER 9. DISSERTATIONS ON KIDNEY FAILURE

## Overview

University researchers are active in studying almost all known diseases. The result of research is often published in the form of Doctoral or Master's dissertations. You should understand, therefore, that applied diagnostic procedures and/or therapies can take many years to develop after the thesis that proposed the new technique or approach was written.

In this chapter, we will give you a bibliography on recent dissertations relating to kidney failure. You can read about these in more detail using the Internet or your local medical library. We will also provide you with information on how to use the Internet to stay current on dissertations.

## Dissertations on Kidney Failure

*ProQuest Digital Dissertations* is the largest archive of academic dissertations available. From this archive, we have compiled the following list covering dissertations devoted to kidney failure. You will see that the information provided includes the dissertation's title, its author, and the author's institution. To read more about the following, simply use the Internet address indicated. The following covers recent dissertations dealing with kidney failure:

- **Economic analysis of end-stage renal disease treatments (cost-effectiveness, Logit; Maryland)** by Garner, Thesia Isedora, PhD from University of Maryland College Park, 1984, 351 pages
  http://wwwlib.umi.com/dissertations/fullcit/8506527

- **Evaluation of the cost effectiveness of Medicare's End Stage Renal Disease program** by Shih, Ya-Chen Tina, PhD from Stanford University, 1996, 87 pages
  http://wwwlib.umi.com/dissertations/fullcit/9723418

## Keeping Current

As previously mentioned, an effective way to stay current on dissertations dedicated to kidney failure is to use the database called *ProQuest Digital Dissertations* via the Internet, located at the following Web address: **http://wwwlib.umi.com/dissertations.** The site allows you to freely access the last two years of citations and abstracts. Ask your medical librarian if the library has full and unlimited access to this database. From the library, you should be able to do more complete searches than with the limited 2-year access available to the general public.

# PART III. APPENDICES

## ABOUT PART III

Part III is a collection of appendices on general medical topics which may be of interest to patients with kidney failure and related conditions.

# APPENDIX A. RESEARCHING YOUR MEDICATIONS

## Overview

There are a number of sources available on new or existing medications which could be prescribed to patients with kidney failure. While a number of hard copy or CD-Rom resources are available to patients and physicians for research purposes, a more flexible method is to use Internet-based databases. In this chapter, we will begin with a general overview of medications. We will then proceed to outline official recommendations on how you should view your medications. You may also want to research medications that you are currently taking for other conditions as they may interact with medications for kidney failure. Research can give you information on the side effects, interactions, and limitations of prescription drugs used in the treatment of kidney failure. Broadly speaking, there are two sources of information on approved medications: public sources and private sources. We will emphasize free-to-use public sources.

## Your Medications: The Basics[33]

The Agency for Health Care Research and Quality has published extremely useful guidelines on how you can best participate in the medication aspects of kidney failure. Taking medicines is not always as simple as swallowing a pill. It can involve many steps and decisions each day. The AHCRQ recommends that patients with kidney failure take part in treatment decisions. Do not be afraid to ask questions and talk about your concerns. By taking a moment to ask questions early, you may avoid problems later. Here are some points to cover each time a new medicine is prescribed:

---

[33] This section is adapted from AHCRQ: **http://www.ahcpr.gov/consumer/ncpiebro.htm**.

- Ask about all parts of your treatment, including diet changes, exercise, and medicines.

- Ask about the risks and benefits of each medicine or other treatment you might receive.

- Ask how often you or your doctor will check for side effects from a given medication.

Do not hesitate to ask what is important to you about your medicines. You may want a medicine with the fewest side effects, or the fewest doses to take each day. You may care most about cost, or how the medicine might affect how you live or work. Or, you may want the medicine your doctor believes will work the best. Telling your doctor will help him or her select the best treatment for you.

Do not be afraid to "bother" your doctor with your concerns and questions about medications for kidney failure. You can also talk to a nurse or a pharmacist. They can help you better understand your treatment plan. Feel free to bring a friend or family member with you when you visit your doctor. Talking over your options with someone you trust can help you make better choices, especially if you are not feeling well. Specifically, ask your doctor the following:

- The name of the medicine and what it is supposed to do.

- How and when to take the medicine, how much to take, and for how long.

- What food, drinks, other medicines, or activities you should avoid while taking the medicine.

- What side effects the medicine may have, and what to do if they occur.

- If you can get a refill, and how often.

- About any terms or directions you do not understand.

- What to do if you miss a dose.

- If there is written information you can take home (most pharmacies have information sheets on your prescription medicines; some even offer large-print or Spanish versions).

Do not forget to tell your doctor about all the medicines you are currently taking (not just those for kidney failure). This includes prescription medicines and the medicines that you buy over the counter. Then your doctor can avoid giving you a new medicine that may not work well with the medications you take now. When talking to your doctor, you may wish to prepare a list of medicines you currently take, the reason you take them, and how you take them. Be sure to include the following information for each:

- Name of medicine

- Reason taken

- Dosage

- Time(s) of day

Also include any over-the-counter medicines, such as:

- Laxatives

- Diet pills

- Vitamins

- Cold medicine

- Aspirin or other pain, headache, or fever medicine

- Cough medicine

- Allergy relief medicine

- Antacids

- Sleeping pills

- Others (include names)

## Learning More about Your Medications

Because of historical investments by various organizations and the emergence of the Internet, it has become rather simple to learn about the medications your doctor has recommended for kidney failure. One such source is the United States Pharmacopeia. In 1820, eleven physicians met in Washington, D.C. to establish the first compendium of standard drugs for the United States. They called this compendium the "U.S. Pharmacopeia (USP)." Today, the USP is a non-profit organization consisting of 800 volunteer scientists, eleven elected officials, and 400 representatives of state associations and colleges of medicine and pharmacy. The USP is located in Rockville, Maryland, and its home page is located at **www.usp.org**. The USP currently provides standards for over 3,700 medications. The resulting USP DI® Advice for the Patient® can be accessed through the National Library of Medicine of the National Institutes of Health. The database is partially derived from lists of federally approved medications in the Food and Drug Administration's (FDA) Drug Approvals database.[34]

While the FDA database is rather large and difficult to navigate, the Phamacopeia is both user-friendly and free to use. It covers more than 9,000 prescription and over-the-counter medications. To access this database, simply type the following hyperlink into your Web browser: **http://www.nlm.nih.gov/medlineplus/druginformation.html**. To view examples of a given medication (brand names, category, description, preparation, proper use, precautions, side effects, etc.), simply follow the hyperlinks indicated within the United States Pharmacopeia (USP).

Of course, we as editors cannot be certain as to what medications you are taking. Therefore, we have compiled a list of medications associated with the treatment of kidney failure. Once again, due to space limitations, we only list a sample of medications and provide hyperlinks to ample documentation (e.g. typical dosage, side effects, drug-interaction risks, etc.). The following drugs have been mentioned in the Pharmacopeia and other sources as being potentially applicable to kidney failure:

### Amlodipine

- **Systemic - U.S. Brands:** Norvasc
  http://www.nlm.nih.gov/medlineplus/druginfo/uspdi/202670.html

### Amlodipine and Benazepril

- **Systemic - U.S. Brands:** Lotrel
  http://www.nlm.nih.gov/medlineplus/druginfo/uspdi/203634.html

### Angiotensin-converting Enzyme (ACE) Inhibitors

- **ACE - U.S. Brands:** Accupril; Aceon; Altace; Capoten; Lotensin; Mavik; Monopril; Prinivil; Univasc; Vasotec; Zestril
  http://www.nlm.nih.gov/medlineplus/druginfo/uspdi/202044.html

### Angiotensin-converting Enzyme (ACE) Inhibitors and Hydrochlorothiazide

- **ACE - U.S. Brands:** Accuretic; Capozide; Lotensin HCT; Prinzide; Uniretic; Vaseretic; Zestoretic

---

[34] Though cumbersome, the FDA database can be freely browsed at the following site: **www.fda.gov/cder/da/da.htm**.

http://www.nlm.nih.gov/medlineplus/druginfo/uspdi/202045.ht
ml

## Beta-adrenergic Blocking Agents and Thiazide Diuretics

- **Systemic - U.S. Brands:** Corzide 40/5; Corzide 80/5; Inderide;
  Inderide LA; Lopressor HCT; Tenoretic 100; Tenoretic 50; Timolide
  10-25; Ziac
  http://www.nlm.nih.gov/medlineplus/druginfo/uspdi/202088.ht
  ml

## Calcium Channel Blocking Agents

- **Systemic - U.S. Brands:** Adalat; Adalat CC; Calan; Calan SR;
  Cardene; Cardizem; Cardizem CD; Cardizem SR; Dilacor-XR;
  DynaCirc; Isoptin; Isoptin SR; Nimotop; Norvasc; Plendil;
  Procardia; Procardia XL; Vascor; Verelan
  http://www.nlm.nih.gov/medlineplus/druginfo/uspdi/202107.ht
  ml

## Candesartan

- **Systemic - U.S. Brands:** Atacand
  http://www.nlm.nih.gov/medlineplus/druginfo/uspdi/203598.ht
  ml

## Carvedilol

- **Systemic - U.S. Brands:** Coreg
  http://www.nlm.nih.gov/medlineplus/druginfo/uspdi/203636.ht
  ml

## Clonidine

- **Systemic - U.S. Brands:** Catapres; Catapres-TTS-1; Catapres-TTS-2;
  Catapres-TTS-3
  http://www.nlm.nih.gov/medlineplus/druginfo/uspdi/202152.ht
  ml

## Clonidine and Chlorthalidone

- **Systemic - U.S. Brands:** Combipres
  http://www.nlm.nih.gov/medlineplus/druginfo/uspdi/202153.ht
  ml

### Darbepoetin alfa

- **Systemic - U.S. Brands:** Aranesp
  http://www.nlm.nih.gov/medlineplus/druginfo/uspdi/500331.ht
  ml

### Diuretics, Loop

- **Systemic - U.S. Brands:** Bumex; Edecrin; Lasix; Myrosemide
  http://www.nlm.nih.gov/medlineplus/druginfo/uspdi/202205.ht
  ml

### Diuretics, Potassium-sparing

- **Systemic - U.S. Brands:** Aldactone; Dyrenium; Midamor
  http://www.nlm.nih.gov/medlineplus/druginfo/uspdi/202206.ht
  ml

### Diuretics, Potassium-sparing, and Hydrochlorothiazide

- **Systemic - U.S. Brands:** Aldactazide; Dyazide; Maxzide;
  Moduretic; Spirozide
  http://www.nlm.nih.gov/medlineplus/druginfo/uspdi/202207.ht
  ml

### Diuretics, Thiazide

- **Systemic - U.S. Brands:** Aquatensen; Diucardin; Diulo; Diuril;
  Enduron; Esidrix; Hydro-chlor; Hydro-D; HydroDIURIL;
  Hydromox; Hygroton; Metahydrin; Microzide; Mykrox; Naqua;
  Naturetin; Oretic; Renese; Saluron; Thalitone; Trichlorex; Zaroxolyn
  http://www.nlm.nih.gov/medlineplus/druginfo/uspdi/202208.ht
  ml

### Doxazosin

- **Systemic - U.S. Brands:** Cardura
  http://www.nlm.nih.gov/medlineplus/druginfo/uspdi/202629.ht
  ml

### Enalapril and Felodipine

- **Systemic - U.S. Brands:** Lexxel
  http://www.nlm.nih.gov/medlineplus/druginfo/uspdi/203638.ht
  ml

### Eplerenone

- **Systemic - U.S. Brands:** Inspra
  http://www.nlm.nih.gov/medlineplus/druginfo/uspdi/500431.ht
  ml

### Eprosartan

- **Systemic - U.S. Brands:** Teveten
  http://www.nlm.nih.gov/medlineplus/druginfo/uspdi/500044.ht
  ml

### Guanabenz

- **Systemic - U.S. Brands:** Wytensin
  http://www.nlm.nih.gov/medlineplus/druginfo/uspdi/202271.ht
  ml

### Guanadrel

- **Systemic - U.S. Brands:** Hylorel
  http://www.nlm.nih.gov/medlineplus/druginfo/uspdi/202272.ht
  ml

### Guanethidine

- **Systemic - U.S. Brands:** Ismelin
  http://www.nlm.nih.gov/medlineplus/druginfo/uspdi/202273.ht
  ml

### Guanfacine

- **Systemic - U.S. Brands:** Tenex
  http://www.nlm.nih.gov/medlineplus/druginfo/uspdi/202275.ht
  ml

### Hydralazine and Hydrochlorothiazide

- **Systemic - U.S. Brands:** Apresazide
  http://www.nlm.nih.gov/medlineplus/druginfo/uspdi/202286.ht
  ml

### Indapamide

- **Systemic - U.S. Brands:** Lozol
  http://www.nlm.nih.gov/medlineplus/druginfo/uspdi/202296.ht
  ml

### Irbesartan

- **Systemic - U.S. Brands:** Avapro
  http://www.nlm.nih.gov/medlineplus/druginfo/uspdi/203379.html

### Losartan

- **Systemic - U.S. Brands:** Cozaar
  http://www.nlm.nih.gov/medlineplus/druginfo/uspdi/202767.html

### Losartan and Hydrochlorothiazide

- **Systemic - U.S. Brands:** Hyzaar
  http://www.nlm.nih.gov/medlineplus/druginfo/uspdi/203639.html

### Mecamylamine

- **Systemic - U.S. Brands:** Inversine
  http://www.nlm.nih.gov/medlineplus/druginfo/uspdi/202340.html

### Methyldopa

- **Systemic - U.S. Brands:** Aldomet
  http://www.nlm.nih.gov/medlineplus/druginfo/uspdi/202359.html

### Methyldopa and Thiazide Diuretics

- **Systemic - U.S. Brands:** Aldoclor; Aldoril
  http://www.nlm.nih.gov/medlineplus/druginfo/uspdi/202360.html

### Minoxidil

- **Systemic - U.S. Brands:** Loniten
  http://www.nlm.nih.gov/medlineplus/druginfo/uspdi/202373.html

### Nisoldipine

- **Systemic - U.S. Brands:** Sular
  http://www.nlm.nih.gov/medlineplus/druginfo/uspdi/203431.html

## Olmesartan

- **Systemic - U.S. Brands:** Benicar
  http://www.nlm.nih.gov/medlineplus/druginfo/uspdi/500393.ht
  ml

## Prazosin

- **Systemic - U.S. Brands:** Minipress
  http://www.nlm.nih.gov/medlineplus/druginfo/uspdi/202475.ht
  ml

## Prazosin and Polythiazide

- **Systemic - U.S. Brands:** Minizide
  http://www.nlm.nih.gov/medlineplus/druginfo/uspdi/202476.ht
  ml

## Rauwolfia Alkaloids

- **Systemic - U.S. Brands:** Harmonyl; Raudixin; Rauval; Rauverid;
  Serpalan; Wolfina
  http://www.nlm.nih.gov/medlineplus/druginfo/uspdi/202503.ht
  ml

## Rauwolfia Alkaloids and Thiazide Diuretics

- **Systemic - U.S. Brands:** Demi-Regroton; Diupres; Diurigen with
  Reserpine; Diutensen-R; Enduronyl; Enduronyl Forte; Oreticyl;
  Oreticyl Forte; Rauzide; Regroton
  http://www.nlm.nih.gov/medlineplus/druginfo/uspdi/202504.ht
  ml

## Reserpine, Hydralazine, and Hydrochlorothiazide

- **Systemic - U.S. Brands:** Cam-Ap-Es; Cherapas; Ser-A-Gen;
  Seralazide; Ser-Ap-Es; Serpazide; Tri-Hydroserpine; Unipres
  http://www.nlm.nih.gov/medlineplus/druginfo/uspdi/202506.ht
  ml

## Telmisartan

- **Systemic - U.S. Brands:** Micardis
  http://www.nlm.nih.gov/medlineplus/druginfo/uspdi/203710.ht
  ml

### Telmisartan and Hydrochlorothiazide

- **Systemic - U.S. Brands:** Micardis HCT
  http://www.nlm.nih.gov/medlineplus/druginfo/uspdi/500333.ht
  ml

### Terazosin

- **Systemic - U.S. Brands:** Hytrin
  http://www.nlm.nih.gov/medlineplus/druginfo/uspdi/202546.ht
  ml

### Torsemide

- **Systemic - U.S. Brands:** Demadex
  http://www.nlm.nih.gov/medlineplus/druginfo/uspdi/202740.ht
  ml

### Trandolapril and Verapamil

- **Systemic - U.S. Brands:** Tarka
  http://www.nlm.nih.gov/medlineplus/druginfo/uspdi/203641.ht
  ml

### Valsartan

- **Systemic - U.S. Brands:** Diovan
  http://www.nlm.nih.gov/medlineplus/druginfo/uspdi/203478.ht
  ml

### Valsartan and Hydrochlorothiazide

- **Systemic - U.S. Brands:** Diovan HCT
  http://www.nlm.nih.gov/medlineplus/druginfo/uspdi/203577.ht
  ml

### Vitamin D and Related Compounds

- **Systemic - U.S. Brands:** Calciferol; Calciferol Drops; Calcijex;
  Calderol; DHT; DHT Intensol; Drisdol; Drisdol Drops; Hectorol;
  Hytakerol; Rocaltrol; Zemplar
  http://www.nlm.nih.gov/medlineplus/druginfo/uspdi/202597.ht
  ml

# Commercial Databases

In addition to the medications listed in the USP above, a number of commercial sites are available by subscription to physicians and their institutions. You may be able to access these sources from your local medical library or your doctor's office.

### Reuters Health Drug Database

The Reuters Health Drug Database can be searched by keyword at the hyperlink: **http://www.reutershealth.com/frame2/drug.html**.

### Mosby's GenRx

Mosby's GenRx database (also available on CD-Rom and book format) covers 45,000 drug products including generics and international brands. It provides prescribing information, drug interactions, and patient information. Information can be obtained at the following hyperlink: **http://www.genrx.com/Mosby/PhyGenRx/group.html**.

### PDR*health*

The PDR*health* database is a free-to-use, drug information search engine that has been written for the public in layman's terms. It contains FDA-approved drug information adapted from the Physicians' Desk Reference (PDR) database. PDR*health* can be searched by brand name, generic name, or indication. It features multiple drug interactions reports. Search PDR*health* at **http://www.pdrhealth.com/drug_info/index.html**.

### Other Web Sites

A number of additional Web sites discuss drug information. As an example, you may like to look at **www.drugs.com** which reproduces the information in the Pharmacopeia as well as commercial information. You may also want to consider the Web site of the Medical Letter, Inc. which allows users to download articles on various drugs and therapeutics for a nominal fee: **http://www.medletter.com/**.

## Researching Orphan Drugs

Orphan drugs are a special class of pharmaceuticals used by patients who are unaffected by existing treatments or with illnesses for which no known drug is effective. Orphan drugs are most commonly prescribed or developed for "rare" diseases or conditions.[35] According to the FDA, an orphan drug (or biological) may already be approved, or it may still be experimental. A drug becomes an "orphan" when it receives orphan designation from the Office of Orphan Products Development at the FDA.[36] Orphan designation qualifies the sponsor to receive certain benefits from the U.S. Government in exchange for developing the drug. The drug must then undergo the new drug approval process as any other drug would. To date, over 1000 orphan products have been designated, and over 200 have been approved for marketing. Historically, the approval time for orphan products as a group has been considerably shorter than the approval time for other drugs. This is due to the fact that many orphan products receive expedited review because they are developed for serious or life-threatening diseases.

The cost of orphan products is determined by the sponsor of the drug and can vary greatly. Reimbursement rates for drug expenses are set by each insurance company and outlined in your policy. Insurance companies will generally reimburse for orphan products that have been approved for marketing, but may not reimburse for products that are considered experimental. Consult your insurance company about specific reimbursement policies. If an orphan product has been approved for marketing, it will be available through the normal pharmaceutical supply channels. If the product has not been approved, the sponsor may make the product available on a compassionate-use basis.[37]

Although the list of orphan drugs is revised on a daily basis, you can quickly research orphan drugs that might be applicable to kidney failure using the

---

[35] The U.S. Food and Drug Administration defines a rare disease or condition as "any disease or condition which affects less than 200,000 persons in the United States, or affects more than 200,000 in the United States and for which there is no reasonable expectation that the cost of developing and making available in the United States a drug for such disease or condition will be recovered from sales in the United States of such drug." Adapted from the U.S. Food and Drug Administration: **http://www.fda.gov/opacom/laws/orphandg.htm**.

[36] The following is adapted from the U.S. Food and Drug Administration: **http://www.fda.gov/orphan/faq/index.htm**.

[37] For contact information on sponsors of orphan products, contact the Office of Orphan Products Development (**http://www.fda.gov/orphan/**). General inquiries may be routed to the main office: Office of Orphan Products Development (HF-35), Food and Drug Administration, 5600 Fishers Lane, Rockville, MD 20857; Voice: (301) 827-3666 or (800) 300-7469; FAX: (301) 443-4915.

database managed by the National Organization for Rare Disorders, Inc. (NORD), located at **www.raredisease.org**. Simply go to their general search page and select "Orphan Drug Designation Database." On this page (**http://www.rarediseases.org/search/noddsearch.html**), type "kidney failure" or a synonym into the search box and click "Submit Query." When you see a list of drugs, understand that not all of the drugs may be relevant. Some may have been withdrawn from orphan status. Write down or print out the name of each drug and the relevant contact information. Visit the Pharmacopeia Web site and type the name of each orphan drug into the search box on **http://www.nlm.nih.gov/medlineplus/druginformation.html**. Read about each drug in detail and consult your doctor to find out if you might benefit from these medications. You or your physician may need to contact the sponsor or NORD.

NORD conducts "early access programs for investigational new drugs (IND) under the Food and Drug Administration's (FDA's) approval 'Treatment INDs' programs which allow for a limited number of individuals to receive investigational drugs before FDA marketing approval." If the orphan product about which you are seeking information is approved for marketing, information on side effects can be found on the product's label. If the product is not approved, you or your physician should consult the sponsor.

The following is a list of orphan drugs currently listed in the NORD Orphan Drug Designation Database for kidney failure or related conditions:

- **Somatropin for Injection (trade name: Nutropin)**
  http://www.rarediseases.org/nord/search/nodd_full?code=100

- **Levocarnitine (trade name: Carnitor)**
  http://www.rarediseases.org/nord/search/nodd_full?code=235

- **Epoetin alfa (trade name: Epogen)**
  http://www.rarediseases.org/nord/search/nodd_full?code=364

- **Epoetin Alpha (trade name: Procrit)**
  http://www.rarediseases.org/nord/search/nodd_full?code=381

- **Epoetin beta (trade name: Marogen)**
  http://www.rarediseases.org/nord/search/nodd_full?code=400

- **Erythropoietin (recombinant human)**
  http://www.rarediseases.org/nord/search/nodd_full?code=447

- **Anaritide acetate (trade name: Auriculin)**
  http://www.rarediseases.org/nord/search/nodd_full?code=558

- **Calcium acetate (trade name: Phos-Lo)**
  http://www.rarediseases.org/nord/search/nodd_full?code=606

- **Calcium acetate**
  http://www.rarediseases.org/nord/search/nodd_full?code=609

- **Calcium carbonate (trade name: R&D calcium /600)**
  http://www.rarediseases.org/nord/search/nodd_full?code=611

- **Icodextrin 7.5% with Electrolytes Peritoneal Dialy (trade name: Extraneal (with 7.5% Icodextrin) Peritoneal Dialys)**
  http://www.rarediseases.org/nord/search/nodd_full?code=841

- **Alpha-melanocye stimulating hormone**
  http://www.rarediseases.org/nord/search/nodd_full?code=842

- **Alpha-melanocyte stimulating hormone**
  http://www.rarediseases.org/nord/search/nodd_full?code=875

## Contraindications and Interactions (Hidden Dangers)

Some of the medications mentioned in the previous discussions can be problematic for patients with kidney failure--not because they are used in the treatment process, but because of contraindications, or side effects. Medications with contraindications are those that could react with drugs used to treat kidney failure or potentially create deleterious side effects in patients with kidney failure. You should ask your physician about any contraindications, especially as these might apply to other medications that you may be taking for common ailments.

Drug-drug interactions occur when two or more drugs react with each other. This drug-drug interaction may cause you to experience an unexpected side effect. Drug interactions may make your medications less effective, cause unexpected side effects, or increase the action of a particular drug. Some drug interactions can even be harmful to you.

Be sure to read the label every time you use a nonprescription or prescription drug, and take the time to learn about drug interactions. These precautions may be critical to your health. You can reduce the risk of potentially harmful drug interactions and side effects with a little bit of knowledge and common sense.

Drug labels contain important information about ingredients, uses, warnings, and directions which you should take the time to read and understand. Labels also include warnings about possible drug interactions. Further, drug labels may change as new information becomes available. This is why it's especially important to read the label every time you use a medication. When your doctor prescribes a new drug, discuss all over-the-counter and prescription medications, dietary supplements, vitamins, botanicals, minerals and herbals you take as well as the foods you eat. Ask your pharmacist for the package insert for each prescription drug you take. The package insert provides more information about potential drug interactions.

## A Final Warning

At some point, you may hear of alternative medications from friends, relatives, or in the news media. Advertisements may suggest that certain alternative drugs can produce positive results for patients with kidney failure. Exercise caution--some of these drugs may have fraudulent claims, and others may actually hurt you. The Food and Drug Administration (FDA) is the official U.S. agency charged with discovering which medications are likely to improve the health of patients with kidney failure. The FDA warns patients to watch out for[38]:

- Secret formulas (real scientists share what they know)

- Amazing breakthroughs or miracle cures (real breakthroughs don't happen very often; when they do, real scientists do not call them amazing or miracles)

- Quick, painless, or guaranteed cures

- If it sounds too good to be true, it probably isn't true.

If you have any questions about any kind of medical treatment, the FDA may have an office near you. Look for their number in the blue pages of the phone book. You can also contact the FDA through its toll-free number, 1-888-INFO-FDA (1-888-463-6332), or on the World Wide Web at **www.fda.gov**.

## General References

In addition to the resources provided earlier in this chapter, the following general references describe medications (sorted alphabetically by title; hyperlinks provide rankings, information and reviews at Amazon.com):

- **Complete Guide to Prescription and Nonprescription Drugs 2001 (Complete Guide to Prescription and Nonprescription Drugs, 2001)** by H. Winter Griffith, Paperback 16th edition (2001), Medical Surveillance;

---

[38] This section has been adapted from **http://www.fda.gov/opacom/lowlit/medfraud.html**.

ISBN: 0942447417;
http://www.amazon.com/exec/obidos/ASIN/039952634X/icongroupinterna

- **The Essential Guide to Prescription Drugs, 2001** by James J. Rybacki, James W. Long; Paperback - 1274 pages (2001), Harper Resource; ISBN: 0060958162;
http://www.amazon.com/exec/obidos/ASIN/0060958162/icongroupinterna

- **Handbook of Commonly Prescribed Drugs** by G. John Digregorio, Edward J. Barbieri; Paperback 16th edition (2001), Medical Surveillance; ISBN: 0942447417;
http://www.amazon.com/exec/obidos/ASIN/0942447417/icongroupinterna

- **Johns Hopkins Complete Home Encyclopedia of Drugs 2nd ed.** by Simeon Margolis (Ed.), Johns Hopkins; Hardcover - 835 pages (2000), Rebus; ISBN: 0929661583;
http://www.amazon.com/exec/obidos/ASIN/0929661583/icongroupinterna

- **Medical Pocket Reference: Drugs 2002** by Springhouse Paperback 1st edition (2001), Lippincott Williams & Wilkins Publishers; ISBN: 1582550964;
http://www.amazon.com/exec/obidos/ASIN/1582550964/icongroupinterna

- **PDR** by Medical Economics Staff, Medical Economics Staff Hardcover - 3506 pages 55th edition (2000), Medical Economics Company; ISBN: 1563633752;
http://www.amazon.com/exec/obidos/ASIN/1563633752/icongroupinterna

- **Pharmacy Simplified: A Glossary of Terms** by James Grogan; Paperback - 432 pages, 1st edition (2001), Delmar Publishers; ISBN: 0766828581;
http://www.amazon.com/exec/obidos/ASIN/0766828581/icongroupinterna

- **Physician Federal Desk Reference** by Christine B. Fraizer; Paperback 2nd edition (2001), Medicode Inc; ISBN: 1563373971;
http://www.amazon.com/exec/obidos/ASIN/1563373971/icongroupinterna

- **Physician's Desk Reference Supplements** Paperback - 300 pages, 53 edition (1999), ISBN: 1563632950;
http://www.amazon.com/exec/obidos/ASIN/1563632950/icongroupinterna

## Vocabulary Builder

The following vocabulary builder provides definitions of words used in this chapter that have not been defined in previous chapters:

**Compassionate:** A process for providing experimental drugs to very sick patients who have no treatment options. [NIH]

**Zestril:** A heart drug. [NIH]

# APPENDIX B. RESEARCHING ALTERNATIVE MEDICINE

## Overview

Complementary and alternative medicine (CAM) is one of the most contentious aspects of modern medical practice. You may have heard of these treatments on the radio or on television. Maybe you have seen articles written about these treatments in magazines, newspapers, or books. Perhaps your friends or doctor have mentioned alternatives.

In this chapter, we will begin by giving you a broad perspective on complementary and alternative therapies. Next, we will introduce you to official information sources on CAM relating to kidney failure. Finally, at the conclusion of this chapter, we will provide a list of readings on kidney failure from various authors. We will begin, however, with the National Center for Complementary and Alternative Medicine's (NCCAM) overview of complementary and alternative medicine.

## What Is CAM?[39]

Complementary and alternative medicine (CAM) covers a broad range of healing philosophies, approaches, and therapies. Generally, it is defined as those treatments and healthcare practices which are not taught in medical schools, used in hospitals, or reimbursed by medical insurance companies. Many CAM therapies are termed "holistic," which generally means that the healthcare practitioner considers the whole person, including physical, mental, emotional, and spiritual health. Some of these therapies are also known as "preventive," which means that the practitioner educates and

---

[39] Adapted from the NCCAM: **http://nccam.nih.gov/health/whatiscam/#4**.

treats the person to prevent health problems from arising, rather than treating symptoms after problems have occurred.

People use CAM treatments and therapies in a variety of ways. Therapies are used alone (often referred to as alternative), in combination with other alternative therapies, or in addition to conventional treatment (sometimes referred to as complementary). Complementary and alternative medicine, or "integrative medicine," includes a broad range of healing philosophies, approaches, and therapies. Some approaches are consistent with physiological principles of Western medicine, while others constitute healing systems with non-Western origins. While some therapies are far outside the realm of accepted Western medical theory and practice, others are becoming established in mainstream medicine.

Complementary and alternative therapies are used in an effort to prevent illness, reduce stress, prevent or reduce side effects and symptoms, or control or cure disease. Some commonly used methods of complementary or alternative therapy include mind/body control interventions such as visualization and relaxation, manual healing including acupressure and massage, homeopathy, vitamins or herbal products, and acupuncture.

## What Are the Domains of Alternative Medicine?[40]

The list of CAM practices changes continually. The reason being is that these new practices and therapies are often proved to be safe and effective, and therefore become generally accepted as "mainstream" healthcare practices. Today, CAM practices may be grouped within five major domains: (1) alternative medical systems, (2) mind-body interventions, (3) biologically-based treatments, (4) manipulative and body-based methods, and (5) energy therapies. The individual systems and treatments comprising these categories are too numerous to list in this sourcebook. Thus, only limited examples are provided within each.

### Alternative Medical Systems

Alternative medical systems involve complete systems of theory and practice that have evolved independent of, and often prior to, conventional biomedical approaches. Many are traditional systems of medicine that are

---

[40] Adapted from the NCCAM: **http://nccam.nih.gov/health/whatiscam/#4.**

practiced by individual cultures throughout the world, including a number of venerable Asian approaches.

Traditional oriental medicine emphasizes the balance or disturbances of qi (pronounced chi) or vital energy in health and disease, respectively. Traditional oriental medicine consists of a group of techniques and methods including acupuncture, herbal medicine, oriental massage, and qi gong (a form of energy therapy). Acupuncture involves stimulating specific anatomic points in the body for therapeutic purposes, usually by puncturing the skin with a thin needle.

Ayurveda is India's traditional system of medicine. Ayurvedic medicine (meaning "science of life") is a comprehensive system of medicine that places equal emphasis on body, mind, and spirit. Ayurveda strives to restore the innate harmony of the individual. Some of the primary Ayurvedic treatments include diet, exercise, meditation, herbs, massage, exposure to sunlight, and controlled breathing.

Other traditional healing systems have been developed by the world's indigenous populations. These populations include Native American, Aboriginal, African, Middle Eastern, Tibetan, and Central and South American cultures. Homeopathy and naturopathy are also examples of complete alternative medicine systems.

Homeopathic medicine is an unconventional Western system that is based on the principle that "like cures like," i.e., that the same substance that in large doses produces the symptoms of an illness, in very minute doses cures it. Homeopathic health practitioners believe that the more dilute the remedy, the greater its potency. Therefore, they use small doses of specially prepared plant extracts and minerals to stimulate the body's defense mechanisms and healing processes in order to treat illness.

Naturopathic medicine is based on the theory that disease is a manifestation of alterations in the processes by which the body naturally heals itself and emphasizes health restoration rather than disease treatment. Naturopathic physicians employ an array of healing practices, including the following: diet and clinical nutrition, homeopathy, acupuncture, herbal medicine, hydrotherapy (the use of water in a range of temperatures and methods of applications), spinal and soft-tissue manipulation, physical therapies (such as those involving electrical currents, ultrasound, and light), therapeutic counseling, and pharmacology.

### Mind-Body Interventions

Mind-body interventions employ a variety of techniques designed to facilitate the mind's capacity to affect bodily function and symptoms. Only a select group of mind-body interventions having well-documented theoretical foundations are considered CAM. For example, patient education and cognitive-behavioral approaches are now considered "mainstream." On the other hand, complementary and alternative medicine includes meditation, certain uses of hypnosis, dance, music, and art therapy, as well as prayer and mental healing.

### Biological-Based Therapies

This category of CAM includes natural and biological-based practices, interventions, and products, many of which overlap with conventional medicine's use of dietary supplements. This category includes herbal, special dietary, orthomolecular, and individual biological therapies.

Herbal therapy employs an individual herb or a mixture of herbs for healing purposes. An herb is a plant or plant part that produces and contains chemical substances that act upon the body. Special diet therapies, such as those proposed by Drs. Atkins, Ornish, Pritikin, and Weil, are believed to prevent and/or control illness as well as promote health. Orthomolecular therapies aim to treat disease with varying concentrations of chemicals such as magnesium, melatonin, and mega-doses of vitamins. Biological therapies include, for example, the use of laetrile and shark cartilage to treat cancer and the use of bee pollen to treat autoimmune and inflammatory diseases.

### Manipulative and Body-Based Methods

This category includes methods that are based on manipulation and/or movement of the body. For example, chiropractors focus on the relationship between structure and function, primarily pertaining to the spine, and how that relationship affects the preservation and restoration of health. Chiropractors use manipulative therapy as an integral treatment tool.

In contrast, osteopaths place particular emphasis on the musculoskeletal system and practice osteopathic manipulation. Osteopaths believe that all of the body's systems work together and that disturbances in one system may have an impact upon function elsewhere in the body. Massage therapists manipulate the soft tissues of the body to normalize those tissues.

### Energy Therapies

Energy therapies focus on energy fields originating within the body (biofields) or those from other sources (electromagnetic fields). Biofield therapies are intended to affect energy fields (the existence of which is not yet experimentally proven) that surround and penetrate the human body. Some forms of energy therapy manipulate biofields by applying pressure and/or manipulating the body by placing the hands in or through these fields. Examples include Qi gong, Reiki and Therapeutic Touch.

Qi gong is a component of traditional oriental medicine that combines movement, meditation, and regulation of breathing to enhance the flow of vital energy (qi) in the body, improve blood circulation, and enhance immune function. Reiki, the Japanese word representing Universal Life Energy, is based on the belief that, by channeling spiritual energy through the practitioner, the spirit is healed and, in turn, heals the physical body. Therapeutic Touch is derived from the ancient technique of "laying-on of hands." It is based on the premises that the therapist's healing force affects the patient's recovery and that healing is promoted when the body's energies are in balance. By passing their hands over the patient, these healers identify energy imbalances.

Bioelectromagnetic-based therapies involve the unconventional use of electromagnetic fields to treat illnesses or manage pain. These therapies are often used to treat asthma, cancer, and migraine headaches. Types of electromagnetic fields which are manipulated in these therapies include pulsed fields, magnetic fields, and alternating current or direct current fields.

## Can Alternatives Affect My Treatment?

A critical issue in pursuing complementary alternatives mentioned thus far is the risk that these might have undesirable interactions with your medical treatment. It becomes all the more important to speak with your doctor who can offer advice on the use of alternatives. Official sources confirm this view. Though written for women, we find that the National Women's Health Information Center's advice on pursuing alternative medicine is appropriate for patients of both genders and all ages.[41]

---

[41] Adapted from **http://www.4woman.gov/faq/alternative.htm**.

### Is It Okay to Want Both Traditional and Alternative or Complementary Medicine?

Should you wish to explore non-traditional types of treatment, be sure to discuss all issues concerning treatments and therapies with your healthcare provider, whether a physician or practitioner of complementary and alternative medicine. Competent healthcare management requires knowledge of both conventional and alternative therapies you are taking for the practitioner to have a complete picture of your treatment plan.

The decision to use complementary and alternative treatments is an important one. Consider before selecting an alternative therapy, the safety and effectiveness of the therapy or treatment, the expertise and qualifications of the healthcare practitioner, and the quality of delivery. These topics should be considered when selecting any practitioner or therapy.

### National Center for Complementary and Alternative Medicine

The National Center for Complementary and Alternative Medicine (NCCAM) of the National Institutes of Health (**http://nccam.nih.gov**) has created a link to the National Library of Medicine's databases to allow patients to search for articles that specifically relate to kidney failure and complementary medicine. To search the database, go to **www.nlm.nih.gov/nccam/camonpubmed.html**. Select "CAM on PubMed." Enter "kidney failure" (or synonyms) into the search box. Click "Go." The following references provide information on particular aspects of complementary and alternative medicine (CAM) that are related to kidney failure:

- **A controlled trial of the effect of folate supplements on homocysteine, lipids and hemorheology in end-stage renal disease.**
  Author(s): McGregor D, Shand B, Lynn K.
  Source: Nephron. 2000 July; 85(3): 215-20.
  http://www.ncbi.nlm.nih.gov/entrez/query.fcgi?cmd=Retrieve&db=pubmed&dopt=Abstract&list_uids=10867536

- **Accelerated atherosclerosis, dyslipidemia, and oxidative stress in end-stage renal disease.**
  Author(s): Mathur S, Devaraj S, Jialal I.

Source: Current Opinion in Nephrology and Hypertension. 2002 March; 11(2): 141-7. Review.

http://www.ncbi.nlm.nih.gov/entrez/query.fcgi?cmd=Retrieve&db=pubmed&dopt=Abstract&list_uids=11856905

- **Activity of (-)-epigallocatechin 3-O-gallate against oxidative stress in rats with adenine-induced renal failure.**
  Author(s): Nakagawa T, Yokozawa T, Sano M, Takeuchi S, Kim M, Minamoto S.
  Source: Journal of Agricultural and Food Chemistry. 2004 April 7; 52(7): 2103-7.
  http://www.ncbi.nlm.nih.gov/entrez/query.fcgi?cmd=Retrieve&db=pubmed&dopt=Abstract&list_uids=15053559

- **Acupoints massage in improving the quality of sleep and quality of life in patients with end-stage renal disease.**
  Author(s): Tsay SL, Rong JR, Lin PF.
  Source: Journal of Advanced Nursing. 2003 April; 42(2): 134-42.
  http://www.ncbi.nlm.nih.gov/entrez/query.fcgi?cmd=Retrieve&db=pubmed&dopt=Abstract&list_uids=12670382

- **Acupressure and fatigue in patients with end-stage renal disease-a randomized controlled trial.**
  Author(s): Tsay SL.
  Source: International Journal of Nursing Studies. 2004 January; 41(1): 99-106.
  http://www.ncbi.nlm.nih.gov/entrez/query.fcgi?cmd=Retrieve&db=pubmed&dopt=Abstract&list_uids=14670399

- **Acupressure and quality of sleep in patients with end-stage renal disease--a randomized controlled trial.**
  Author(s): Tsay SL, Chen ML.
  Source: International Journal of Nursing Studies. 2003 January; 40(1): 1-7.
  http://www.ncbi.nlm.nih.gov/entrez/query.fcgi?cmd=Retrieve&db=pubmed&dopt=Abstract&list_uids=12550145

- **Acute renal failure due to the herbal remedy CKLS.**
  Author(s): Adesunloye BA.
  Source: The American Journal of Medicine. 2003 October 15; 115(6): 506-7.
  http://www.ncbi.nlm.nih.gov/entrez/query.fcgi?cmd=Retrieve&db=pubmed&dopt=Abstract&list_uids=14563511

- **Anorexia in end-stage renal disease: pathophysiology and treatment.**
  Author(s): Aguilera A, Selgas R, Diez JJ, Bajo MA, Codoceo R, Alvarez V.
  Source: Expert Opinion on Pharmacotherapy. 2001 November; 2(11): 1825-38. Review.
  http://www.ncbi.nlm.nih.gov/entrez/query.fcgi?cmd=Retrieve&db=pubmed&dopt=Abstract&list_uids=11825320

- **Cholesterol metabolism in patients with chronic renal failure on hemodialysis.**
  Author(s): Igel-Korcagova A, Raab P, Brensing KA, Poge U, Klehr HU, Igel M, von Bergmann K, Sudhop T.
  Source: Journal of Nephrology. 2003 November-December; 16(6): 850-4.
  http://www.ncbi.nlm.nih.gov/entrez/query.fcgi?cmd=Retrieve&db=pubmed&dopt=Abstract&list_uids=14736012

- **Dietary CLA decreased weight loss and extended survival following the onset of kidney failure in NZB/W F1 mice.**
  Author(s): Yang M, Cook ME.
  Source: Lipids. 2003 January; 38(1): 21-4.
  http://www.ncbi.nlm.nih.gov/entrez/query.fcgi?cmd=Retrieve&db=pubmed&dopt=Abstract&list_uids=12669815

- **Effect of a keto acid-amino acid supplement on the metabolism and renal elimination of branched-chain amino acids in patients with chronic renal insufficiency on a low protein diet.**
  Author(s): Teplan V, Schuck O, Horackova M, Skibova J, Holecek M.
  Source: Wiener Klinische Wochenschrift. 2000 October 27; 112(20): 876-81.
  http://www.ncbi.nlm.nih.gov/entrez/query.fcgi?cmd=Retrieve&db=pubmed&dopt=Abstract&list_uids=11244613

- **Effect of Aerva lanata on cisplatin and gentamicin models of acute renal failure.**
  Author(s): Shirwaikar A, Issac D, Malini S.
  Source: Journal of Ethnopharmacology. 2004 January; 90(1): 81-6.
  http://www.ncbi.nlm.nih.gov/entrez/query.fcgi?cmd=Retrieve&db=pubmed&dopt=Abstract&list_uids=14698513

- **Effects of carnitine supplementation on muscle metabolism by the use of magnetic resonance spectroscopy and near-infrared spectroscopy in end-stage renal disease.**
  Author(s): Vaux EC, Taylor DJ, Altmann P, Rajagopalan B, Graham K, Cooper R, Bonomo Y, Styles P.

Source: Nephron. Clinical Practice [electronic Resource]. 2004; 97(2): C41-8.
http://www.ncbi.nlm.nih.gov/entrez/query.fcgi?cmd=Retrieve&db=pubmed&dopt=Abstract&list_uids=15218329

- **Effects of dietary fat and polyunsaturated fatty acids in dogs with naturally developing chronic renal failure.**
  Author(s): Bauer JE, Markwell PJ, Rawlings JM, Senior DE.
  Source: J Am Vet Med Assoc. 1999 December 1; 215(11): 1588-91. Review. No Abstract Available.
  http://www.ncbi.nlm.nih.gov/entrez/query.fcgi?cmd=Retrieve&db=pubmed&dopt=Abstract&list_uids=14567419

- **Estimation of glomerular filtration rate in older patients with chronic renal insufficiency: is the modification of diet in renal disease formula an improvement?**
  Author(s): Lamb EJ, Webb MC, Simpson DE, Coakley AJ, Newman DJ, O'Riordan SE.
  Source: Journal of the American Geriatrics Society. 2003 July; 51(7): 1012-7.
  http://www.ncbi.nlm.nih.gov/entrez/query.fcgi?cmd=Retrieve&db=pubmed&dopt=Abstract&list_uids=12834524

- **Glycyrrhizin ameliorates renal function defects in the early-phase of ischemia-induced acute renal failure.**
  Author(s): Kang DG, Sohn EJ, Mun YJ, Woo WH, Lee HS.
  Source: Phytotherapy Research: Ptr. 2003 September; 17(8): 947-51.
  http://www.ncbi.nlm.nih.gov/entrez/query.fcgi?cmd=Retrieve&db=pubmed&dopt=Abstract&list_uids=13680831

- **High prevalence of fenfluramine-related aortic regurgitation in women with end-stage renal disease secondary to Chinese herb nephropathy.**
  Author(s): Unger P, Nortier J, Muniz Martinez MC, Plein D, Vandenbossche JL, Vereerstraeten P, Vanherweghem JL.
  Source: Nephrology, Dialysis, Transplantation: Official Publication of the European Dialysis and Transplant Association - European Renal Association. 2003 May; 18(5): 906-10.
  http://www.ncbi.nlm.nih.gov/entrez/query.fcgi?cmd=Retrieve&db=pubmed&dopt=Abstract&list_uids=12686663

- **Homocysteine lowering effect of different multivitamin preparations in patients with end-stage renal disease.**

Author(s): Dierkes J, Domrose U, Bosselmann KP, Neumann KH, Luley C.

Source: Journal of Renal Nutrition: the Official Journal of the Council on Renal Nutrition of the National Kidney Foundation. 2001 April; 11(2): 67-72.

http://www.ncbi.nlm.nih.gov/entrez/query.fcgi?cmd=Retrieve&db=pubmed&dopt=Abstract&list_uids=11295026

- **Hypertension as cause of end-stage renal disease: lessons from international registries.**
  Author(s): Valderrabano F, Gomez-Campdera F, Jones EH.
  Source: Kidney International. Supplement. 1998 December; 68: S60-6. Review.
  http://www.ncbi.nlm.nih.gov/entrez/query.fcgi?cmd=Retrieve&db=pubmed&dopt=Abstract&list_uids=9839286

- **Incidence of side-effects associated with high-dose ferric gluconate in patients with severe chronic renal failure.**
  Author(s): Bastani B, Jain A, Pandurangan G.
  Source: Nephrology (Carlton). 2003 February; 8(1): 8-10.
  http://www.ncbi.nlm.nih.gov/entrez/query.fcgi?cmd=Retrieve&db=pubmed&dopt=Abstract&list_uids=15012743

- **Increased body lead burden--cause or consequence of chronic renal insufficiency?**
  Author(s): Marsden PA.
  Source: The New England Journal of Medicine. 2003 January 23; 348(4): 345-7.
  http://www.ncbi.nlm.nih.gov/entrez/query.fcgi?cmd=Retrieve&db=pubmed&dopt=Abstract&list_uids=12540649

- **Intravenous iron supplementation in end-stage renal disease patients.**
  Author(s): Matzke GR.
  Source: American Journal of Kidney Diseases: the Official Journal of the National Kidney Foundation. 1999 March; 33(3): 595-7.
  http://www.ncbi.nlm.nih.gov/entrez/query.fcgi?cmd=Retrieve&db=pubmed&dopt=Abstract&list_uids=10070926

- **Over-the-counter remedies in chronic renal insufficiency: risks versus benefits.**
  Author(s): Dykeman-Sharpe J.

Source: Cannt J. 2003 April-June; 13(2): 17-28; Quiz 28-30. Review.
http://www.ncbi.nlm.nih.gov/entrez/query.fcgi?cmd=Retrieve&db=pu
bmed&dopt=Abstract&list_uids=14535226

- **Pamidronate in a girl with chronic renal insufficiency dependent on parenteral nutrition.**
  Author(s): Duke JL, Jones DP, Frizzell NK, Chesney RW, Hak EB.
  Source: Pediatric Nephrology (Berlin, Germany). 2003 July; 18(7): 714-7. Epub 2003 May 15.
  http://www.ncbi.nlm.nih.gov/entrez/query.fcgi?cmd=Retrieve&db=pu
  bmed&dopt=Abstract&list_uids=12750976

- **Parenteral iron supplementation in patients with end stage renal disease.**
  Author(s): Vogel SC.
  Source: Anna J. 1998 December; 25(6): 625-30. Review.
  http://www.ncbi.nlm.nih.gov/entrez/query.fcgi?cmd=Retrieve&db=pu
  bmed&dopt=Abstract&list_uids=10188399

- **Parenteral iron use in the management of anemia in end-stage renal disease patients.**
  Author(s): Bailie GR, Johnson CA, Mason NA.
  Source: American Journal of Kidney Diseases: the Official Journal of the National Kidney Foundation. 2000 January; 35(1): 1-12. Review.
  http://www.ncbi.nlm.nih.gov/entrez/query.fcgi?cmd=Retrieve&db=pu
  bmed&dopt=Abstract&list_uids=10620537

- **Plasma thrombopoietin levels in liver cirrhosis and kidney failure.**
  Author(s): Stockelberg D, Andersson P, Bjornsson E, Bjork S, Wadenvik H.
  Source: Journal of Internal Medicine. 1999 November; 246(5): 471-5.
  http://www.ncbi.nlm.nih.gov/entrez/query.fcgi?cmd=Retrieve&db=pu
  bmed&dopt=Abstract&list_uids=10583716

- **Protective effects of glycyrrhizin on gentamicin-induced acute renal failure in rats.**
  Author(s): Sohn EJ, Kang DG, Lee HS.
  Source: Pharmacology & Toxicology. 2003 September; 93(3): 116-22.
  http://www.ncbi.nlm.nih.gov/entrez/query.fcgi?cmd=Retrieve&db=pu
  bmed&dopt=Abstract&list_uids=12969435

- **Proteinuria patterns and their association with subsequent end-stage renal disease in IgA nephropathy.**
  Author(s): Donadio JV, Bergstralh EJ, Grande JP, Rademcher DM.
  Source: Nephrology, Dialysis, Transplantation: Official Publication of the European Dialysis and Transplant Association - European Renal Association. 2002 July; 17(7): 1197-203.
  http://www.ncbi.nlm.nih.gov/entrez/query.fcgi?cmd=Retrieve&db=pubmed&dopt=Abstract&list_uids=12105241

- **Remnant-like particle-cholesterol concentrations in patients with type 2 diabetes mellitus and end-stage renal disease.**
  Author(s): Hirany S, O'Byrne D, Devaraj S, Jialal I.
  Source: Clinical Chemistry. 2000 May; 46(5): 667-72.
  http://www.ncbi.nlm.nih.gov/entrez/query.fcgi?cmd=Retrieve&db=pubmed&dopt=Abstract&list_uids=10794749

- **Response of hyperhomocysteinemia to folic acid supplementation in patients with end-stage renal disease.**
  Author(s): Dierkes J, Domrose U, Ambrosch A, Bosselmann HP, Neumann KH, Luley C.
  Source: Clinical Nephrology. 1999 February; 51(2): 108-15.
  http://www.ncbi.nlm.nih.gov/entrez/query.fcgi?cmd=Retrieve&db=pubmed&dopt=Abstract&list_uids=10069646

- **Safety of new phosphate binders for chronic renal failure.**
  Author(s): Loghman-Adham M.
  Source: Drug Safety: an International Journal of Medical Toxicology and Drug Experience. 2003; 26(15): 1093-115. Review.
  http://www.ncbi.nlm.nih.gov/entrez/query.fcgi?cmd=Retrieve&db=pubmed&dopt=Abstract&list_uids=14640773

- **Safety profile of a high dose ferric gluconate in patients with severe chronic renal insufficiency.**
  Author(s): Jain AK, Bastani B.
  Source: Journal of Nephrology. 2002 November-December; 15(6): 681-3.
  http://www.ncbi.nlm.nih.gov/entrez/query.fcgi?cmd=Retrieve&db=pubmed&dopt=Abstract&list_uids=12495284

- **Serum isoflavones and soya food intake in Japanese, Thai and American end-stage renal disease patients on chronic haemodialysis.**
  Author(s): Fanti P, Stephenson TJ, Kaariainen IM, Rezkalla B, Tsukamoto Y, Morishita T, Nomura M, Kitiyakara C, Custer LJ, Franke AA.

Source: Nephrology, Dialysis, Transplantation: Official Publication of the European Dialysis and Transplant Association - European Renal Association. 2003 September; 18(9): 1862-8.

http://www.ncbi.nlm.nih.gov/entrez/query.fcgi?cmd=Retrieve&db=pubmed&dopt=Abstract&list_uids=12937236

- **Sevelamer hydrochloride, a phosphate binder, protects against deterioration of renal function in rats with progressive chronic renal insufficiency.**
  Author(s): Nagano N, Miyata S, Obana S, Kobayashi N, Fukushima N, Burke SK, Wada M.
  Source: Nephrology, Dialysis, Transplantation: Official Publication of the European Dialysis and Transplant Association - European Renal Association. 2003 October; 18(10): 2014-23.
  http://www.ncbi.nlm.nih.gov/entrez/query.fcgi?cmd=Retrieve&db=pubmed&dopt=Abstract&list_uids=13679475

- **Supplementation with vitamin B12 decreases homocysteine and methylmalonic acid but also serum folate in patients with end-stage renal disease.**
  Author(s): Dierkes J, Domrose U, Ambrosch A, Schneede J, Guttormsen AB, Neumann KH, Luley C.
  Source: Metabolism: Clinical and Experimental. 1999 May; 48(5): 631-5.
  http://www.ncbi.nlm.nih.gov/entrez/query.fcgi?cmd=Retrieve&db=pubmed&dopt=Abstract&list_uids=10337865

- **The effect of acupressure with massage on fatigue and depression in patients with end-stage renal disease.**
  Author(s): Cho YC, Tsay SL.
  Source: The Journal of Nursing Research: Jnr. 2004 March; 12(1): 51-9.
  http://www.ncbi.nlm.nih.gov/entrez/query.fcgi?cmd=Retrieve&db=pubmed&dopt=Abstract&list_uids=15136963

- **Trends in the incidence of renal replacement therapy for end-stage renal disease in Europe, 1990-1999.**
  Author(s): Stengel B, Billon S, Van Dijk PC, Jager KJ, Dekker FW, Simpson K, Briggs JD.

Source: Nephrology, Dialysis, Transplantation: Official Publication of the European Dialysis and Transplant Association - European Renal Association. 2003 September; 18(9): 1824-33.
http://www.ncbi.nlm.nih.gov/entrez/query.fcgi?cmd=Retrieve&db=pubmed&dopt=Abstract&list_uids=12937231

- **Update on dialytic management of acute renal failure.**
  Author(s): Teehan GS, Liangos O, Jaber BL.
  Source: Journal of Intensive Care Medicine. 2003 May-June; 18(3): 130-8. Review.
  http://www.ncbi.nlm.nih.gov/entrez/query.fcgi?cmd=Retrieve&db=pubmed&dopt=Abstract&list_uids=14984631

- **Use of electrotherapy to reverse expanding cutaneous gangrene in end-stage renal disease.**
  Author(s): Goldman RJ, Brewley BI, Cohen R, Rudnick M.
  Source: Advances in Skin & Wound Care. 2003 December; 16(7): 363-6.
  http://www.ncbi.nlm.nih.gov/entrez/query.fcgi?cmd=Retrieve&db=pubmed&dopt=Abstract&list_uids=14688644

- **Vitamin E supplementation increases circulating vitamin E metabolites tenfold in end-stage renal disease patients.**
  Author(s): Smith KS, Lee CL, Ridlington JW, Leonard SW, Devaraj S, Traber MG.
  Source: Lipids. 2003 August; 38(8): 813-9.
  http://www.ncbi.nlm.nih.gov/entrez/query.fcgi?cmd=Retrieve&db=pubmed&dopt=Abstract&list_uids=14577659

## Additional Web Resources

A number of additional Web sites offer encyclopedic information covering CAM and related topics. The following is a representative sample:

- Alternative Medicine Foundation, Inc.: **http://www.herbmed.org/**

- AOL: **http://search.aol.com/cat.adp?id=169&layer=&from=subcats**

- Chinese Medicine: **http://www.newcenturynutrition.com/**

- Family Village: **http://www.familyvillage.wisc.edu/med_altn.htm**

- Google: **http://directory.google.com/Top/Health/Alternative/**

- Open Directory Project: **http://dmoz.org/Health/Alternative/**

- TPN.com: **http://www.tnp.com/**

- Yahoo.com: **http://dir.yahoo.com/Health/Alternative_Medicine/**

- WebMD®Health: **http://my.webmd.com/drugs_and_herbs**

- WholeHealthMD.com:
  **http://www.wholehealthmd.com/reflib/0,1529,,00.html**

The following is a specific Web list relating to kidney failure; please note that any particular subject below may indicate either a therapeutic use, or a contraindication (potential danger), and does not reflect an official recommendation:

- **General Overview**

  **Abdominal Wall Inflammation**
  Source: Integrative Medicine Communications; www.drkoop.com

  **Amenorrhea**
  Source: Integrative Medicine Communications; www.drkoop.com

  **Amyloidosis**
  Source: Integrative Medicine Communications; www.drkoop.com

  **Atherosclerosis**
  Source: Healthnotes, Inc.; www.healthnotes.com

  **Bone Loss**
  Source: Integrative Medicine Communications; www.drkoop.com

  **Capillary Fragility**
  Source: Healthnotes, Inc.; www.healthnotes.com

  **Cataracts (prevention)**
  Source: Prima Communications, Inc.www.personalhealthzone.com

  **Congestive Heart Failure**
  Source: Integrative Medicine Communications; www.drkoop.com

  **Diabetes**
  Source: Prima Communications, Inc.www.personalhealthzone.com

**Food Poisoning**
Source: Integrative Medicine Communications; www.drkoop.com

**Heat Exhaustion**
Source: Integrative Medicine Communications; www.drkoop.com

**High Cholesterol**
Source: Integrative Medicine Communications; www.drkoop.com

**High Homocysteine**
Source: Healthnotes, Inc.; www.healthnotes.com

**Hypercholesterolemia**
Source: Integrative Medicine Communications; www.drkoop.com

**Hyperparathyroidism**
Source: Integrative Medicine Communications; www.drkoop.com

**Hypothermia**
Source: Integrative Medicine Communications; www.drkoop.com

**Leukemia**
Source: Integrative Medicine Communications; www.drkoop.com

**Osteoporosis**
Source: Integrative Medicine Communications; www.drkoop.com

**Osteoporosis**
Source: Prima Communications, Inc.www.personalhealthzone.com

**Peritonitis**
Source: Integrative Medicine Communications; www.drkoop.com

**Prostate Cancer**
Source: Integrative Medicine Communications; www.drkoop.com

**Scleroderma**
Source: Integrative Medicine Communications; www.drkoop.com

**Tuberculosis**
Source: Integrative Medicine Communications; www.drkoop.com

- **Herbs and Supplements**

   **Aesculus**
   Alternative names: Horse Chestnut; Aesculus hippocastanum L.
   Source: Alternative Medicine Foundation, Inc.;
   www.amfoundation.org

   **Aluminum Hydroxide**
   Source: Healthnotes, Inc.; www.healthnotes.com

   **Amino Acids Overview**
   Source: Healthnotes, Inc.; www.healthnotes.com

   **Aristolochia**
   Alternative names: Snakeroot, Guaco; Aristolochia sp
   Source: Alternative Medicine Foundation, Inc.;
   www.amfoundation.org

   **Astragalus**
   Alternative names: Astragalus membranaceus
   Source: Healthnotes, Inc.; www.healthnotes.com

   **Astragalus Mem**
   Alternative names: Huang-Qi; Astragalus membranaceus
   Source: Alternative Medicine Foundation, Inc.;
   www.amfoundation.org

   **Astragalus Sp**
   Alternative names: Vetch, Rattlepod, Locoweed; Astragalus sp.
   Source: Alternative Medicine Foundation, Inc.;
   www.amfoundation.org

   **Branched-Chain Amino Acids**
   Source: Healthnotes, Inc.; www.healthnotes.com

   **Chitosan**
   Source: Healthnotes, Inc.; www.healthnotes.com

   **Deferoxamine**
   Source: Healthnotes, Inc.; www.healthnotes.com

   **DHEA (Dehydroepiandrosterone)**
   Source: Prima Communications, Inc.www.personalhealthzone.com

**Dong Quai**
Alternative names: Angelica sinensis
Source: Healthnotes, Inc.; www.healthnotes.com

**EDTA**
Source: Integrative Medicine Communications; www.drkoop.com

**Ethylenediaminetetraacetic Acid (EDTA)**
Source: Integrative Medicine Communications; www.drkoop.com

**Etodolac**
Source: Healthnotes, Inc.; www.healthnotes.com

**Fumaric Acid**
Source: Healthnotes, Inc.; www.healthnotes.com

**Glycyrrhiza**
Alternative names: Licorice; Glycyrrhiza glabra L.
Source: Alternative Medicine Foundation, Inc.;
www.amfoundation.org

**Ibuprofen**
Source: Healthnotes, Inc.; www.healthnotes.com

**Inositol**
Source: Healthnotes, Inc.; www.healthnotes.com

**Ipriflavone**
Source: Healthnotes, Inc.; www.healthnotes.com

**Juniper**
Alternative names: Juniperus communis
Source: Healthnotes, Inc.; www.healthnotes.com

**Ketorolac**
Source: Healthnotes, Inc.; www.healthnotes.com

**Loop Diuretics**
Source: Integrative Medicine Communications; www.drkoop.com

**L-tyrosine**
Source: Healthnotes, Inc.; www.healthnotes.com

**Nabumetone**
Source: Healthnotes, Inc.; www.healthnotes.com

**Oxaprozin**
Source: Healthnotes, Inc.; www.healthnotes.com

**Panax**
Alternative names: Ginseng; Panax ginseng
Source: Alternative Medicine Foundation, Inc.;
www.amfoundation.org

**Pennyroyal**
Alternative names: Hedeoma pulegoides, Mentha pulegium
Source: Healthnotes, Inc.; www.healthnotes.com

**Peppermint**
Source: Prima Communications, Inc.www.personalhealthzone.com

**Phosphatidylserine (PS)**
Source: WholeHealthMD.com, LLC.; www.wholehealthmd.com
Hyperlink:
http://www.wholehealthmd.com/refshelf/substances_view/0,1525,
813,00.html

**Plantago Psyllium**
Alternative names: Psyllium, Ispaghula; Plantago psyllium/ovata
Source: Alternative Medicine Foundation, Inc.;
www.amfoundation.org

**Uncaria Catclaw**
Alternative names: Cat's Claw, Uno de Gato; Uncaria tomentosa
(Willd.) D.C.
Source: Alternative Medicine Foundation, Inc.;
www.amfoundation.org

## General References

A good place to find general background information on CAM is the
National Library of Medicine. It has prepared within the MEDLINEplus
system an information topic page dedicated to complementary and
alternative medicine. To access this page, go to the MEDLINEplus site at:

**www.nlm.nih.gov/medlineplus/alternativemedicine.html.** This Web site provides a general overview of various topics and can lead to a number of general sources. The following additional references describe, in broad terms, alternative and complementary medicine (sorted alphabetically by title; hyperlinks provide rankings, information, and reviews at Amazon.com):

- **Alternative Medicine for Dummies** by James Dillard (Author); Audio Cassette, Abridged edition (1998), Harper Audio; ISBN: 0694520659; **http://www.amazon.com/exec/obidos/ASIN/0694520659/icongroupinterna**

- **Complementary and Alternative Medicine Secrets** by W. Kohatsu (Editor); Hardcover (2001), Hanley & Belfus; ISBN: 1560534400; **http://www.amazon.com/exec/obidos/ASIN/1560534400/icongroupinterna**

- **Dictionary of Alternative Medicine** by J. C. Segen; Paperback-2nd edition (2001), Appleton & Lange; ISBN: 0838516211; **http://www.amazon.com/exec/obidos/ASIN/0838516211/icongroupinterna**

- **Eat, Drink, and Be Healthy: The Harvard Medical School Guide to Healthy Eating** by Walter C. Willett, MD, et al; Hardcover - 352 pages (2001), Simon & Schuster; ISBN: 0684863375; **http://www.amazon.com/exec/obidos/ASIN/0684863375/icongroupinterna**

- **Encyclopedia of Natural Medicine, Revised 2nd Edition** by Michael T. Murray, Joseph E. Pizzorno; Paperback - 960 pages, 2nd Rev edition (1997), Prima Publishing; ISBN: 0761511571; **http://www.amazon.com/exec/obidos/ASIN/0761511571/icongroupinterna**

- **Integrative Medicine: An Introduction to the Art & Science of Healing** by Andrew Weil (Author); Audio Cassette, Unabridged edition (2001), Sounds True; ISBN: 1564558541; **http://www.amazon.com/exec/obidos/ASIN/1564558541/icongroupinterna**

- **New Encyclopedia of Herbs & Their Uses** by Deni Bown; Hardcover - 448 pages, Revised edition (2001), DK Publishing; ISBN: 078948031X; **http://www.amazon.com/exec/obidos/ASIN/078948031X/icongroupinterna**

- **Textbook of Complementary and Alternative Medicine** by Wayne B. Jonas; Hardcover (2003), Lippincott, Williams & Wilkins; ISBN:

0683044370;
**http://www.amazon.com/exec/obidos/ASIN/0683044370/icongroupinter na**

For additional information on complementary and alternative medicine, ask your doctor or write to:

**National Center for Complementary and Alternative Medicine Clearinghouse**
National Institutes of Health
P. O. Box 8218
Silver Spring, MD 20907-8218

## Vocabulary Builder

The following vocabulary builder provides definitions of words used in this chapter that have not been defined in previous chapters:

**Communis:** Common tendon of the rectus group of muscles that surrounds the optic foramen and a portion of the superior orbital fissure, to the anterior margin of which it is attached at the spina recti lateralis. [NIH]

**Exhaustion:** The feeling of weariness of mind and body. [NIH]

**Gallate:** Antioxidant present in tea. [NIH]

# APPENDIX C. RESEARCHING NUTRITION

## Overview

Since the time of Hippocrates, doctors have understood the importance of diet and nutrition to patients' health and well-being. Since then, they have accumulated an impressive archive of studies and knowledge dedicated to this subject. Based on their experience, doctors and healthcare providers may recommend particular dietary supplements to patients with kidney failure. Any dietary recommendation is based on a patient's age, body mass, gender, lifestyle, eating habits, food preferences, and health condition. It is therefore likely that different patients with kidney failure may be given different recommendations. Some recommendations may be directly related to kidney failure, while others may be more related to the patient's general health. These recommendations, themselves, may differ from what official sources recommend for the average person.

In this chapter we will begin by briefly reviewing the essentials of diet and nutrition that will broadly frame more detailed discussions of kidney failure. We will then show you how to find studies dedicated specifically to nutrition and kidney failure.

## Food and Nutrition: General Principles

### What Are Essential Foods?

Food is generally viewed by official sources as consisting of six basic elements: (1) fluids, (2) carbohydrates, (3) protein, (4) fats, (5) vitamins, and (6) minerals. Consuming a combination of these elements is considered to be a healthy diet:

- **Fluids** are essential to human life as 80-percent of the body is composed of water. Water is lost via urination, sweating, diarrhea, vomiting, diuretics (drugs that increase urination), caffeine, and physical exertion.

- **Carbohydrates** are the main source for human energy (thermoregulation) and the bulk of typical diets. They are mostly classified as being either simple or complex. Simple carbohydrates include sugars which are often consumed in the form of cookies, candies, or cakes. Complex carbohydrates consist of starches and dietary fibers. Starches are consumed in the form of pastas, breads, potatoes, rice, and other foods. Soluble fibers can be eaten in the form of certain vegetables, fruits, oats, and legumes. Insoluble fibers include brown rice, whole grains, certain fruits, wheat bran and legumes.

- **Proteins** are eaten to build and repair human tissues. Some foods that are high in protein are also high in fat and calories. Food sources for protein include nuts, meat, fish, cheese, and other dairy products.

- **Fats** are consumed for both energy and the absorption of certain vitamins. There are many types of fats, with many general publications recommending the intake of unsaturated fats or those low in cholesterol.

Vitamins and minerals are fundamental to human health, growth, and, in some cases, disease prevention. Most are consumed in your diet (exceptions being vitamins K and D which are produced by intestinal bacteria and sunlight on the skin, respectively). Each vitamin and mineral plays a different role in health. The following outlines essential vitamins:

- **Vitamin A** is important to the health of your eyes, hair, bones, and skin; sources of vitamin A include foods such as eggs, carrots, and cantaloupe.

- **Vitamin B$^1$**, also known as thiamine, is important for your nervous system and energy production; food sources for thiamine include meat, peas, fortified cereals, bread, and whole grains.

- **Vitamin B$^2$**, also known as riboflavin, is important for your nervous system and muscles, but is also involved in the release of proteins from nutrients; food sources for riboflavin include dairy products, leafy vegetables, meat, and eggs.

- **Vitamin B$^3$**, also known as niacin, is important for healthy skin and helps the body use energy; food sources for niacin include peas, peanuts, fish, and whole grains

- **Vitamin B$^6$**, also known as pyridoxine, is important for the regulation of cells in the nervous system and is vital for blood formation; food sources for pyridoxine include bananas, whole grains, meat, and fish.

- **Vitamin B¹² is vital for a healthy nervous system and for the growth of red blood cells in bone marrow; food sources for vitamin B¹² include yeast, milk, fish, eggs, and meat.**

- **Vitamin C** allows the body's immune system to fight various diseases, strengthens body tissue, and improves the body's use of iron; food sources for vitamin C include a wide variety of fruits and vegetables.

- **Vitamin D** helps the body absorb calcium which strengthens bones and teeth; food sources for vitamin D include oily fish and dairy products.

- **Vitamin E** can help protect certain organs and tissues from various degenerative diseases; food sources for vitamin E include margarine, vegetables, eggs, and fish.

- **Vitamin K** is essential for bone formation and blood clotting; common food sources for vitamin K include leafy green vegetables.

- **Folic Acid** maintains healthy cells and blood and, when taken by a pregnant woman, can prevent her fetus from developing neural tube defects; food sources for folic acid include nuts, fortified breads, leafy green vegetables, and whole grains.

It should be noted that it is possible to overdose on certain vitamins which become toxic if consumed in excess (e.g. vitamin A, D, E and K).

Like vitamins, minerals are chemicals that are required by the body to remain in good health. Because the human body does not manufacture these chemicals internally, we obtain them from food and other dietary sources. The more important minerals include:

- **Calcium** is needed for healthy bones, teeth, and muscles, but also helps the nervous system function; food sources for calcium include dry beans, peas, eggs, and dairy products.

- **Chromium** is helpful in regulating sugar levels in blood; food sources for chromium include egg yolks, raw sugar, cheese, nuts, beets, whole grains, and meat.

- **Fluoride** is used by the body to help prevent tooth decay and to reinforce bone strength; sources of fluoride include drinking water and certain brands of toothpaste.

- **Iodine** helps regulate the body's use of energy by synthesizing into the hormone thyroxine; food sources include leafy green vegetables, nuts, egg yolks, and red meat.

- **Iron** helps maintain muscles and the formation of red blood cells and certain proteins; food sources for iron include meat, dairy products, eggs, and leafy green vegetables.

- **Magnesium** is important for the production of DNA, as well as for healthy teeth, bones, muscles, and nerves; food sources for magnesium include dried fruit, dark green vegetables, nuts, and seafood.

- **Phosphorous** is used by the body to work with calcium to form bones and teeth; food sources for phosphorous include eggs, meat, cereals, and dairy products.

- **Selenium** primarily helps maintain normal heart and liver functions; food sources for selenium include wholegrain cereals, fish, meat, and dairy products.

- **Zinc** helps wounds heal, the formation of sperm, and encourage rapid growth and energy; food sources include dried beans, shellfish, eggs, and nuts.

The United States government periodically publishes recommended diets and consumption levels of the various elements of food. Again, your doctor may encourage deviations from the average official recommendation based on your specific condition. To learn more about basic dietary guidelines, visit the Web site: **http://www.health.gov/dietaryguidelines/**. Based on these guidelines, many foods are required to list the nutrition levels on the food's packaging. Labeling Requirements are listed at the following site maintained by the Food and Drug Administration: **http://www.cfsan.fda.gov/~dms/lab-cons.html**. When interpreting these requirements, the government recommends that consumers become familiar with the following abbreviations before reading FDA literature:[42]

- **DVs (Daily Values):** A new dietary reference term that will appear on the food label. It is made up of two sets of references, DRVs and RDIs.

- **DRVs (Daily Reference Values):** A set of dietary references that applies to fat, saturated fat, cholesterol, carbohydrate, protein, fiber, sodium, and potassium.

- **RDIs (Reference Daily Intakes):** A set of dietary references based on the Recommended Dietary Allowances for essential vitamins and minerals and, in selected groups, protein. The name "RDI" replaces the term "U.S. RDA."

---

[42] Adapted from the FDA: **http://www.fda.gov/fdac/special/foodlabel/dvs.html**.

- **RDAs (Recommended Dietary Allowances):** A set of estimated nutrient allowances established by the National Academy of Sciences. It is updated periodically to reflect current scientific knowledge.

## What Are Dietary Supplements?[43]

Dietary supplements are widely available through many commercial sources, including health food stores, grocery stores, pharmacies, and by mail. Dietary supplements are provided in many forms including tablets, capsules, powders, gel-tabs, extracts, and liquids. Historically in the United States, the most prevalent type of dietary supplement was a multivitamin/mineral tablet or capsule that was available in pharmacies, either by prescription or "over the counter." Supplements containing strictly herbal preparations were less widely available. Currently in the United States, a wide array of supplement products are available, including vitamin, mineral, other nutrients, and botanical supplements as well as ingredients and extracts of animal and plant origin.

The Office of Dietary Supplements (ODS) of the National Institutes of Health is the official agency of the United States which has the expressed goal of acquiring "new knowledge to help prevent, detect, diagnose, and treat disease and disability, from the rarest genetic disorder to the common cold."[44] According to the ODS, dietary supplements can have an important impact on the prevention and management of disease and on the maintenance of health.[45] The ODS notes that considerable research on the effects of dietary supplements has been conducted in Asia and Europe where the use of plant products, in particular, has a long tradition. However, the overwhelming majority of supplements have not been studied scientifically. To explore the role of dietary supplements in the improvement of health care, the ODS plans, organizes, and supports conferences, workshops, and

---

[43] This discussion has been adapted from the NIH:
**http://ods.od.nih.gov/showpage.aspx?pageid=46.**
[44] Contact: The Office of Dietary Supplements, National Institutes of Health, Building 31, Room 1B29, 31 Center Drive, MSC 2086, Bethesda, Maryland 20892-2086, Tel: (301) 435-2920, Fax: (301) 480-1845, E-mail: ods@nih.gov.
[45] Adapted from **http://ods.od.nih.gov/showpage.aspx?pageid=2.** The Dietary Supplement Health and Education Act defines dietary supplements as "a product (other than tobacco) intended to supplement the diet that bears or contains one or more of the following dietary ingredients: a vitamin, mineral, amino acid, herb or other botanical; or a dietary substance for use to supplement the diet by increasing the total dietary intake; or a concentrate, metabolite, constituent, extract, or combination of any ingredient described above; and intended for ingestion in the form of a capsule, powder, softgel, or gelcap, and not represented as a conventional food or as a sole item of a meal or the diet."

symposia on scientific topics related to dietary supplements. The ODS often works in conjunction with other NIH Institutes and Centers, other government agencies, professional organizations, and public advocacy groups.

To learn more about official information on dietary supplements, visit the ODS site at **http://dietary-supplements.info.nih.gov/**. Or contact:

> **The Office of Dietary Supplements**
> National Institutes of Health
> Building 31, Room 1B29
> 31 Center Drive, MSC 2086
> Bethesda, Maryland 20892-2086
> Tel: (301) 435-2920
> Fax: (301) 480-1845
> E-mail: ods@nih.gov

## Finding Studies on Kidney Failure

The NIH maintains an office dedicated to patient nutrition and diet. The National Institutes of Health's Office of Dietary Supplements (ODS) offers a searchable bibliographic database called the IBIDS (International Bibliographic Information on Dietary Supplements). The IBIDS contains over 460,000 scientific citations and summaries about dietary supplements and nutrition as well as references to published international, scientific literature on dietary supplements such as vitamins, minerals, and botanicals.[46] IBIDS is available to the public free of charge through the ODS Internet page: **http://ods.od.nih.gov/databases/ibids.html**.

After entering the search area, you have three choices: (1) IBIDS Consumer Database, (2) Full IBIDS Database, or (3) Peer Reviewed Citations Only. We recommend that you start with the Consumer Database. While you may not find references for the topics that are of most interest to you, check back periodically as this database is frequently updated. More studies can be found by searching the Full IBIDS Database. Healthcare professionals and researchers generally use the third option, which lists peer-reviewed citations. In all cases, we suggest that you take advantage of the "Advanced

---

[46] Adapted from **http://ods.od.nih.gov**. IBIDS is produced by the Office of Dietary Supplements (ODS) at the National Institutes of Health to assist the public, healthcare providers, educators, and researchers in locating credible, scientific information on dietary supplements. IBIDS was developed and will be maintained through an interagency partnership with the Food and Nutrition Information Center of the National Agricultural Library, U.S. Department of Agriculture.

Search" option that allows you to retrieve up to 100 fully explained references in a comprehensive format. Type "kidney failure" (or synonyms) into the search box. To narrow the search, you can also select the "Title" field. The following is a typical result when searching for recently indexed consumer information on kidney failure:

- **Nutritional strategies for the treatment of chronic renal failure in children.**
  Source: Georgalas, A. Goffi, J. Dwyer, J. Nutrition-today (USA). (August 1993). volume 28(4) page 24-28.

Additional consumer oriented references include:

- **Effect of intensive treatment of diabetes of the risk of death or renal failure in NIDDM and IDDM.**
  Author(s): Heart of America Diabetes Research Foundation, North Kansas City, MO 64116, USA.
  Source: Hellman, R Regan, J Rosen, H Diabetes-Care. 1997 March; 20(3): 258-64 0149-5992

The following information is typical of that found when using the "Full IBIDS Database" when searching using "kidney failure" (or a synonym):

- **Acute renal failure during dextran-40 antithrombotic prophylaxis: report of two microsurgical cases.**
  Author(s): Department of Plastic and Reconstructive Surgery at Antoni van Leeuwenhoek Hospital, Amsterdam, The Netherlands.
  Source: Vos, Sanne C B Hage, J Joris Woerdeman, Leonie A E Noordanus, Robert P Ann-Plast-Surg. 2002 February; 48(2): 193-6 0148-7043

- **Continuous haemofiltration in acute renal failure with prostacyclin as the sole anti-haemostatic agent.**
  Author(s): Dipartimento di Clinica Medica, Nefrologia & Scienze della Prevenzione, Universita degli Studi di Parma, Via Gramsci 14, 43100 Parma, Italy. enrico.fiaccadori@unipr.it
  Source: Fiaccadori, E Maggiore, U Rotelli, C Minari, M Melfa, L Cappe, G Cabassi, A Intensive-Care-Med. 2002 May; 28(5): 586-93 0342-4642

- **Effects of the anti-ulcer agents ecabet sodium, cimetidine and sucralfate on acetylsalicylic acid-induced gastric mucosal damage deteriorated by renal failure in rats.**
  Source:

- **Experimental renal failure and iron overload: a histomorphometric study in the alveolar bone of rats.**
  Author(s): Department of Histology, School of Dentistry, University of Buenos Aires, Argentina. patricia@histo.odon.uba.ar
  Source: Mandalunis, P Gibaja, F Ubios, A M Exp-Toxicol-Pathol. 2002 August; 54(2): 85-90 0940-2993

- **Immobilization-related hypercalcemia after renal failure in burn injury.**
  Author(s): Division of Endocrinology and Metabolism, Loyola University Medical Center, Maywood, Illinois 60153, USA.
  Source: Peralta, M C Gordon, D L Endocr-Pract. 2002 May-June; 8(3): 213-6 1530-891X

- **Information and counselling for patients approaching end-stage renal failure in selected centres across Europe.**
  Author(s): Renal Unit, Lister Hospital, Stevenage, UK.
  Source: Da Silva Gane, Maria Goovaerts, Tony Elseviers, Monique M Lindley, Elizabeth J EDTNA-ERCA-J. 2002 Jan-Mar; 28(1): 49-55 1019-083X

- **Isoniazid-induced seizures with secondary rhabdomyolysis and associated acute renal failure in a dog.**
  Author(s): Ocean Avenue Veterinary Hospital, San Francisco, CA 94112, USA.
  Source: Haburjak, J J Spangler, W L J-Small-Anim-Pract. 2002 April; 43(4): 182-6 0022-4510

- **Severe chronic renal failure in association with oxycodone addiction: a new form of fibrillary glomerulopathy.**
  Author(s): Department of Anatomical Pathology, St. Vincent's Hospital, Fitzroy, Victoria, Australia.
  Source: Hill, P Dwyer, K Kay, T Murphy, B Hum-Pathol. 2002 August; 33(8): 783-7 0046-8177

- **Time-course of iodine elimination by hemodialysis in patients with renal failure after angiography.**
  Author(s): Department of Medicine, Division of Nephrology and Dialysis, Social Insurance Chuo General Hospital, Tokyo, Japan. shinodatmd@par.odn.ne.jp
  Source: Shinoda, T Hata, T Nakajima, K Yoshimoto, H Niwa, A Ther-Apher. 2002 December; 6(6): 437-42 1091-6660

## Federal Resources on Nutrition

In addition to the IBIDS, the United States Department of Health and Human Services (HHS) and the United States Department of Agriculture (USDA) provide many sources of information on general nutrition and health. Recommended resources include:

- healthfinder®, HHS's gateway to health information, including diet and nutrition: **http://www.healthfinder.gov/scripts/SearchContext.asp?topic=238&page=0**

- The United States Department of Agriculture's Web site dedicated to nutrition information: **www.nutrition.gov**

- The Food and Drug Administration's Web site for federal food safety information: **www.foodsafety.gov**

- The National Action Plan on Overweight and Obesity sponsored by the United States Surgeon General: **http://www.surgeongeneral.gov/topics/obesity/**

- The Center for Food Safety and Applied Nutrition has an Internet site sponsored by the Food and Drug Administration and the Department of Health and Human Services: **http://vm.cfsan.fda.gov/**

- Center for Nutrition Policy and Promotion sponsored by the United States Department of Agriculture: **http://www.usda.gov/cnpp/**

- Food and Nutrition Information Center, National Agricultural Library sponsored by the United States Department of Agriculture: **http://www.nal.usda.gov/fnic/**

- Food and Nutrition Service sponsored by the United States Department of Agriculture: **http://www.fns.usda.gov/fns/**

## Additional Web Resources

A number of additional Web sites offer encyclopedic information covering food and nutrition. The following is a representative sample:

- AOL: **http://search.aol.com/cat.adp?id=174&layer=&from=subcats**

- Family Village: **http://www.familyvillage.wisc.edu/med_nutrition.html**

- Google: **http://directory.google.com/Top/Health/Nutrition/**

- Open Directory Project: **http://dmoz.org/Health/Nutrition/**

- Yahoo.com: **http://dir.yahoo.com/Health/Nutrition/**

- WebMD®Health: **http://my.webmd.com/nutrition**

- WholeHealthMD.com:
  **http://www.wholehealthmd.com/reflib/0,1529,,00.html**

The following is a specific Web list relating to kidney failure; please note that any particular subject below may indicate either a therapeutic use, or a contraindication (potential danger), and does not reflect an official recommendation:

- **Vitamins**

  **Folic Acid**
  Source: Healthnotes, Inc.; www.healthnotes.com

  **Niacin**
  Source: WholeHealthMD.com, LLC.; www.wholehealthmd.com
  Hyperlink:
  http://www.wholehealthmd.com/refshelf/substances_view/0,1525, 892,00.html

  **Pyridoxine**
  Source: Integrative Medicine Communications; www.drkoop.com

  **Vitamin B6**
  Source: Healthnotes, Inc.; www.healthnotes.com

  **Vitamin B6 (Pyridoxine)**
  Source: Integrative Medicine Communications; www.drkoop.com

  **Vitamin C**
  Source: Healthnotes, Inc.; www.healthnotes.com

  **Vitamin C**
  Source: Prima Communications, Inc.www.personalhealthzone.com

- **Minerals**

  **Biotin**
  Source: Integrative Medicine Communications; www.drkoop.com

**Calcium**
Source: Integrative Medicine Communications; www.drkoop.com

**Calcium**
Source: WholeHealthMD.com, LLC.; www.wholehealthmd.com
Hyperlink:
http://www.wholehealthmd.com/refshelf/substances_view/0,1525,
884,00.html

**Calcium Acetate**
Source: Healthnotes, Inc.; www.healthnotes.com

**Chromium**
Source: Healthnotes, Inc.; www.healthnotes.com

**Chromium**
Source: Prima Communications, Inc.www.personalhealthzone.com

**Chromium**
Source: WholeHealthMD.com, LLC.; www.wholehealthmd.com
Hyperlink:
http://www.wholehealthmd.com/refshelf/substances_view/0,1525,
10018,00.html

**Naproxen/Naproxen Sodium**
Source: Healthnotes, Inc.; www.healthnotes.com

**Potassium**
Source: Healthnotes, Inc.; www.healthnotes.com

**Potassium**
Source: Integrative Medicine Communications; www.drkoop.com

**Potassium Chloride**
Source: Healthnotes, Inc.; www.healthnotes.com

**Vitamin H (Biotin)**
Source: Integrative Medicine Communications; www.drkoop.com

- **Food and Diet**

  ### Diabetes
  Source: Healthnotes, Inc.; www.healthnotes.com

  ### The Zone Diet
  Source: Healthnotes, Inc.; www.healthnotes.com

# APPENDIX D. FINDING MEDICAL LIBRARIES

## Overview

At a medical library you can find medical texts and reference books, consumer health publications, specialty newspapers and magazines, as well as medical journals. In this Appendix, we show you how to quickly find a medical library in your area.

## Preparation

Before going to the library, highlight the references mentioned in this sourcebook that you find interesting. Focus on those items that are not available via the Internet, and ask the reference librarian for help with your search. He or she may know of additional resources that could be helpful to you. Most importantly, your local public library and medical libraries have Interlibrary Loan programs with the National Library of Medicine (NLM), one of the largest medical collections in the world. According to the NLM, most of the literature in the general and historical collections of the National Library of Medicine is available on interlibrary loan to any library. NLM's interlibrary loan services are only available to libraries. If you would like to access NLM medical literature, then visit a library in your area that can request the publications for you.[47]

---

[47] Adapted from the NLM: **http://www.nlm.nih.gov/psd/cas/interlibrary.html**.

## Finding a Local Medical Library

The quickest method to locate medical libraries is to use the Internet-based directory published by the National Network of Libraries of Medicine (NN/LM). This network includes 4626 members and affiliates that provide many services to librarians, health professionals, and the public. To find a library in your area, simply visit **http://nnlm.gov/members/adv.html** or call 1-800-338-7657.

## Medical Libraries in the U.S. and Canada

In addition to the NN/LM, the National Library of Medicine (NLM) lists a number of libraries with reference facilities that are open to the public. The following is the NLM's list and includes hyperlinks to each library's Web site. These Web pages can provide information on hours of operation and other restrictions. The list below is a small sample of libraries recommended by the National Library of Medicine (sorted alphabetically by name of the U.S. state or Canadian province where the library is located)[48]:

- **Alabama:** Health InfoNet of Jefferson County (Jefferson County Library Cooperative, Lister Hill Library of the Health Sciences), **http://www.uab.edu/infonet/**

- **Alabama:** Richard M. Scrushy Library (American Sports Medicine Institute)

- **Arizona:** Samaritan Regional Medical Center: The Learning Center (Samaritan Health System, Phoenix, Arizona), **http://www.samaritan.edu/library/bannerlibs.htm**

- **California:** Kris Kelly Health Information Center (St. Joseph Health System, Humboldt), **http://www.humboldt1.com/~kkhic/index.html**

- **California:** Community Health Library of Los Gatos, **http://www.healthlib.org/orgresources.html**

- **California:** Consumer Health Program and Services (CHIPS) (County of Los Angeles Public Library, Los Angeles County Harbor-UCLA Medical Center Library) - Carson, CA, **http://www.colapublib.org/services/chips.html**

- **California:** Gateway Health Library (Sutter Gould Medical Foundation)

- **California:** Health Library (Stanford University Medical Center), **http://www-med.stanford.edu/healthlibrary/**

---

[48] Abstracted from **http://www.nlm.nih.gov/medlineplus/libraries.html**.

- **California:** Patient Education Resource Center - Health Information and Resources (University of California, San Francisco), **http://sfghdean.ucsf.edu/barnett/PERC/default.asp**

- **California:** Redwood Health Library (Petaluma Health Care District), **http://www.phcd.org/rdwdlib.html**

- **California:** Los Gatos PlaneTree Health Library, **http://planetreesanjose.org/**

- **California:** Sutter Resource Library (Sutter Hospitals Foundation, Sacramento), **http://suttermedicalcenter.org/library/**

- **California:** Health Sciences Libraries (University of California, Davis), **http://www.lib.ucdavis.edu/healthsci/**

- **California:** ValleyCare Health Library & Ryan Comer Cancer Resource Center (ValleyCare Health System, Pleasanton), **http://gaelnet.stmarys-ca.edu/other.libs/gbal/east/vchl.html**

- **California:** Washington Community Health Resource Library (Fremont), **http://www.healthlibrary.org/**

- **Colorado:** William V. Gervasini Memorial Library (Exempla Healthcare), **http://www.saintjosephdenver.org/yourhealth/libraries/**

- **Connecticut:** Hartford Hospital Health Science Libraries (Hartford Hospital), **http://www.harthosp.org/library/**

- **Connecticut:** Healthnet: Connecticut Consumer Health Information Center (University of Connecticut Health Center, Lyman Maynard Stowe Library), **http://library.uchc.edu/departm/hnet/**

- **Connecticut:** Waterbury Hospital Health Center Library (Waterbury Hospital, Waterbury), **http://www.waterburyhospital.com/library/consumer.shtml**

- **Delaware:** Consumer Health Library (Christiana Care Health System, Eugene du Pont Preventive Medicine & Rehabilitation Institute, Wilmington), **http://www.christianacare.org/health_guide/health_guide_pmri_health _info.cfm**

- **Delaware:** Lewis B. Flinn Library (Delaware Academy of Medicine, Wilmington), **http://www.delamed.org/chls.html**

- **Georgia:** Family Resource Library (Medical College of Georgia, Augusta), **http://cmc.mcg.edu/kids_families/fam_resources/fam_res_lib/frl.htm**

- **Georgia:** Health Resource Center (Medical Center of Central Georgia, Macon), **http://www.mccg.org/hrc/hrchome.asp**

- **Hawaii:** Hawaii Medical Library: Consumer Health Information Service (Hawaii Medical Library, Honolulu), **http://hml.org/CHIS/**

- **Idaho:** DeArmond Consumer Health Library (Kootenai Medical Center, Coeur d'Alene), **http://www.nicon.org/DeArmond/index.htm**

- **Illinois:** Health Learning Center of Northwestern Memorial Hospital (Chicago), **http://www.nmh.org/health_info/hlc.html**

- **Illinois:** Medical Library (OSF Saint Francis Medical Center, Peoria), **http://www.osfsaintfrancis.org/general/library/**

- **Kentucky:** Medical Library - Services for Patients, Families, Students & the Public (Central Baptist Hospital, Lexington), **http://www.centralbap.com/education/community/library.cfm**

- **Kentucky:** University of Kentucky - Health Information Library (Chandler Medical Center, Lexington), **http://www.mc.uky.edu/PatientEd/**

- **Louisiana:** Alton Ochsner Medical Foundation Library (Alton Ochsner Medical Foundation, New Orleans), **http://www.ochsner.org/library/**

- **Louisiana:** Louisiana State University Health Sciences Center Medical Library-Shreveport, **http://lib-sh.lsuhsc.edu/**

- **Maine:** Franklin Memorial Hospital Medical Library (Franklin Memorial Hospital, Farmington), **http://www.fchn.org/fmh/lib.htm**

- **Maine:** Gerrish-True Health Sciences Library (Central Maine Medical Center, Lewiston), **http://www.cmmc.org/library/library.html**

- **Maine:** Hadley Parrot Health Science Library (Eastern Maine Healthcare, Bangor), **http://www.emh.org/hll/hpl/guide.htm**

- **Maine:** Maine Medical Center Library (Maine Medical Center, Portland), **http://www.mmc.org/library/**

- **Maine:** Parkview Hospital (Brunswick), **http://www.parkviewhospital.org/**

- **Maine:** Southern Maine Medical Center Health Sciences Library (Southern Maine Medical Center, Biddeford), **http://www.smmc.org/services/service.php3?choice=10**

- **Maine:** Stephens Memorial Hospital's Health Information Library (Western Maine Health, Norway), **http://www.wmhcc.org/Library/**

- **Manitoba, Canada:** Consumer & Patient Health Information Service (University of Manitoba Libraries), **http://www.umanitoba.ca/libraries/units/health/reference/chis.html**

- **Manitoba, Canada:** J.W. Crane Memorial Library (Deer Lodge Centre, Winnipeg), **http://www.deerlodge.mb.ca/crane_library/about.asp**

- **Maryland:** Health Information Center at the Wheaton Regional Library (Montgomery County, Dept. of Public Libraries, Wheaton Regional Library), **http://www.mont.lib.md.us/healthinfo/hic.asp**

- **Massachusetts:** Baystate Medical Center Library (Baystate Health System), **http://www.baystatehealth.com/1024/**

- **Massachusetts:** Boston University Medical Center Alumni Medical Library (Boston University Medical Center), **http://med-libwww.bu.edu/library/lib.html**

- **Massachusetts:** Lowell General Hospital Health Sciences Library (Lowell General Hospital, Lowell), **http://www.lowellgeneral.org/library/HomePageLinks/WWW.htm**

- **Massachusetts:** Paul E. Woodard Health Sciences Library (New England Baptist Hospital, Boston), **http://www.nebh.org/health_lib.asp**

- **Massachusetts:** St. Luke's Hospital Health Sciences Library (St. Luke's Hospital, Southcoast Health System, New Bedford), **http://www.southcoast.org/library/**

- **Massachusetts:** Treadwell Library Consumer Health Reference Center (Massachusetts General Hospital), **http://www.mgh.harvard.edu/library/chrcindex.html**

- **Massachusetts:** UMass HealthNet (University of Massachusetts Medical School, Worchester), **http://healthnet.umassmed.edu/**

- **Michigan:** Botsford General Hospital Library - Consumer Health (Botsford General Hospital, Library & Internet Services), **http://www.botsfordlibrary.org/consumer.htm**

- **Michigan:** Helen DeRoy Medical Library (Providence Hospital and Medical Centers), **http://www.providence-hospital.org/library/**

- **Michigan:** Marquette General Hospital - Consumer Health Library (Marquette General Hospital, Health Information Center), **http://www.mgh.org/center.html**

- **Michigan:** Patient Education Resouce Center - University of Michigan Cancer Center (University of Michigan Comprehensive Cancer Center, Ann Arbor), **http://www.cancer.med.umich.edu/learn/leares.htm**

- **Michigan:** Sladen Library & Center for Health Information Resources - Consumer Health Information (Detroit), **http://www.henryford.com/body.cfm?id=39330**

- **Montana:** Center for Health Information (St. Patrick Hospital and Health Sciences Center, Missoula)

- **National:** Consumer Health Library Directory (Medical Library Association, Consumer and Patient Health Information Section), **http://caphis.mlanet.org/directory/index.html**

- **National:** National Network of Libraries of Medicine (National Library of Medicine) - provides library services for health professionals in the United States who do not have access to a medical library, **http://nnlm.gov/**

- **National:** NN/LM List of Libraries Serving the Public (National Network of Libraries of Medicine), **http://nnlm.gov/members/**

- **Nevada:** Health Science Library, West Charleston Library (Las Vegas-Clark County Library District, Las Vegas), **http://www.lvccld.org/special_collections/medical/index.htm**

- **New Hampshire:** Dartmouth Biomedical Libraries (Dartmouth College Library, Hanover), **http://www.dartmouth.edu/~biomed/resources.htmld/conshealth.htmld**

- **New Jersey:** Consumer Health Library (Rahway Hospital, Rahway), **http://www.rahwayhospital.com/library.htm**

- **New Jersey:** Dr. Walter Phillips Health Sciences Library (Englewood Hospital and Medical Center, Englewood), **http://www.englewoodhospital.com/links/index.htm**

- **New Jersey:** Meland Foundation (Englewood Hospital and Medical Center, Englewood), **http://www.geocities.com/ResearchTriangle/9360/**

- **New York:** Choices in Health Information (New York Public Library) - NLM Consumer Pilot Project participant, **http://www.nypl.org/branch/health/links.html**

- **New York:** Health Information Center (Upstate Medical University, State University of New York, Syracuse), **http://www.upstate.edu/library/hic/**

- **New York:** Health Sciences Library (Long Island Jewish Medical Center, New Hyde Park), **http://www.lij.edu/library/library.html**

- **New York:** ViaHealth Medical Library (Rochester General Hospital), **http://www.nyam.org/library/**

- **Ohio:** Consumer Health Library (Akron General Medical Center, Medical & Consumer Health Library), **http://www.akrongeneral.org/hwlibrary.htm**

- **Oklahoma:** The Health Information Center at Saint Francis Hospital (Saint Francis Health System, Tulsa), **http://www.sfh-tulsa.com/services/healthinfo.asp**

- **Oregon:** Planetree Health Resource Center (Mid-Columbia Medical Center, The Dalles), **http://www.mcmc.net/phrc/**

- **Pennsylvania:** Community Health Information Library (Milton S. Hershey Medical Center, Hershey), **http://www.hmc.psu.edu/commhealth/**

- **Pennsylvania:** Community Health Resource Library (Geisinger Medical Center, Danville), **http://www.geisinger.edu/education/commlib.shtml**

- **Pennsylvania:** HealthInfo Library (Moses Taylor Hospital, Scranton), **http://www.mth.org/healthwellness.html**

- **Pennsylvania:** Hopwood Library (University of Pittsburgh, Health Sciences Library System, Pittsburgh), **http://www.hsls.pitt.edu/guides/chi/hopwood/index_html**

- **Pennsylvania:** Koop Community Health Information Center (College of Physicians of Philadelphia), **http://www.collphyphil.org/kooppg1.shtml**

- **Pennsylvania:** Learning Resources Center - Medical Library (Susquehanna Health System, Williamsport), **http://www.shscares.org/services/lrc/index.asp**

- **Pennsylvania:** Medical Library (UPMC Health System, Pittsburgh), **http://www.upmc.edu/passavant/library.htm**

- **Quebec, Canada:** Medical Library (Montreal General Hospital), **http://www.mghlib.mcgill.ca/**

- **South Dakota:** Rapid City Regional Hospital Medical Library (Rapid City Regional Hospital), **http://www.rcrh.org/Services/Library/Default.asp**

- **Texas:** Houston HealthWays (Houston Academy of Medicine-Texas Medical Center Library), **http://hhw.library.tmc.edu/**

- **Washington:** Community Health Library (Kittitas Valley Community Hospital), **http://www.kvch.com/**

- **Washington:** Southwest Washington Medical Center Library (Southwest Washington Medical Center, Vancouver), **http://www.swmedicalcenter.com/body.cfm?id=72**

# APPENDIX E. NIH CONSENSUS STATEMENT ON MORBIDITY AND MORTALITY OF DIALYSIS

## Overview

NIH Consensus Development Conferences are convened to evaluate available scientific information and resolve safety and efficacy issues related to biomedical technology. The resultant NIH Consensus Statements are intended to advance understanding of the technology or issue in question and to be useful to health professionals and the public.[49] Each NIH consensus statement is the product of an independent, non-Federal panel of experts and is based on the panel's assessment of medical knowledge available at the time the statement was written. Therefore, a consensus statement provides a "snapshot in time" of the state of knowledge of the conference topic.

The NIH makes the following caveat: "When reading or downloading NIH consensus statements, keep in mind that new knowledge is inevitably accumulating through medical research. Nevertheless, each NIH consensus statement is retained on this website in its original form as a record of the NIH Consensus Development Program."[50] The following concensus statement was posted on the NIH site and not indicated as "out of date" in March 2002. It was originally published, however, in November 1993.[51]

---

[49] This paragraph is adapted from the NIH: **http://odp.od.nih.gov/consensus/cons/cons.htm**.
[50] Adapted from the NIH: **http://odp.od.nih.gov/consensus/cons/consdate.htm**.
[51] Morbidity and mortality of dialysis. NIH Consensus Statement Online 1993 Nov 1-3 [cited 2002 February 20]11(2):1-33 **http://consensus.nih.gov/cons/093/093_statement.htm**.

# Abstract

The National Institutes of Health Consensus Development Conference on Morbidity and Mortality of Dialysis brought together experts in general medicine, nephrology, pediatrics, biostatistics, and nutrition as well as the public to address the following questions: (1) How does early medical intervention in predialysis patients influence morbidity and mortality? (2) What is the relationship between delivered dialysis dose and morbidity/mortality? (3) Can co-morbid conditions be altered by nondialytic interventions to improve morbidity/mortality in dialysis patients? (4) How can dialysis-related complications be reduced? and (5) What are the future directions for research in dialysis? Following 1-1/2 days of presentations by experts and discussion by the audience, a consensus panel weighed the evidence and prepared their consensus statement.

Among their findings, the consensus panel concluded that (1) patients including children in the predialysis phase should be referred to a renal team in an effort to reduce the morbidity and mortality incurred during both the predialysis period and when receiving subsequent dialysis therapy; (2) the social and psychological welfare and the quality of life of the dialysis patient are favorably influenced by the early predialytic and continued involvement of a multidisciplinary renal team; (3) attempts should be made by instituting predialytic intervention and the appropriate initiation of dialysis access to avoid a catastrophic onset of dialysis; (4) quantitative methods now available to objectively evaluate the relationship between delivered dose of dialysis and patient morbidity and mortality suggest that the dose of hemodialysis and peritoneal dialysis has been suboptimal for many patients in the United States; (5) factors contributing to underdialysis of some patients include problems with vascular and peritoneal access, nonadherence to dialysis prescription, and underprescription of the dialysis dose; (6) cardiovascular mortality accounts for approximately 50 percent of deaths in dialysis patients, and relative risk factors such as hypertension, smoking, and chronic anemia should be treated as soon as possible after diagnosis of chronic renal failure; (7) early detection and treatment of malnutrition contribute to improved survival of patients on dialysis; and (8) until prospective, randomized, controlled trials have been completed, a delivered hemodialysis dose at least equal to a measured $Kdrt/V$ of 1.2 (single pool) and a delivered peritoneal dialysis dose at least equal to a measured $Kprt/V$ of 1.7 (weekly) are recommended.

The full text of the consensus panel's statement follows.

# What Is Morbidity and Mortality of Dialysis?

Prior to 1960 end-stage renal disease (ESRD) was uniformly fatal. However, with the development by Wayne Quinton and Belding Scribner of an external shunt to provide repeated vascular access coupled with the use of dialysis technology that had evolved some years earlier for the treatment of acute renal failure, chronic intermittent hemodialysis for the management of ESRD was launched in March 1960 at the University of Washington. The application of peritoneal dialysis for the management of ESRD soon followed. A little over a decade elapsed before Congress legislative the provision of Medicare coverage, regardless of the patient's age, for the treatment of ESRD. These as well as subsequent events have made it possible for hundreds of thousands of patients with ESRD to receive life-sustaining renal replacement therapy.

The incidence of treated ESRD in the United States is 180 per million population and continues to rise at a rate of 7.8 percent per year. In 1990, over 45,000 new patients were enrolled in the Medicare ESRD program of which 66 percent were white, 28 percent were African Americans, 2 percent represented Asian/Pacific Islanders, and 1 percent were Native Americans. Forty-three percent were at least 64 years of age and fewer than 2 percent were under 20 years of age. On average, African Americans and Native Americans are younger at the onset of treated ESRD and show dramatically higher incidence rates than whites or Asian/Pacific Islanders. Although clinical experience suggests that the incidence of ESRD in Hispanics is also greater than in whites, data from the United States Renal Data System are not available to confirm this clinical impression. Hypertension and diabetes accounted for 63 percent of the new cases in 1990. The incidence of diabetic ESRD in Native Americans was almost twice that of African-Americans and 6 times that of whites.

Of the more than 195,000 ESRD patients receiving renal replacement therapy during 1990, 70 percent were being treated with either hemodialysis or peritoneal dialysis. Although kidney transplantation is the treatment of choice for many patients with ESRD, the increase in waiting time for cadaveric organs, the presence of disqualifying co-morbid conditions, and the low transplantation rates in an aging ESRD population will likely ensure that dialysis remains the primary method of renal replacement therapy in the foreseeable future.

The cost for care of patients with ESRD from all sources including Federal, State, and private funding was approximately $7.26 billion in 1990, an increase of 21 percent over a similar estimate for the preceding year. Not reflected in this figure are additional expenditures for outpatient drugs and supplies, the cost of disability, and Social Security payments. As the U.S. population continues to grow and a larger proportion of the population at risk attains the age of 65 and beyond, the cost of kidney disease including this end-stage component is projected to increase. According to an analysis conducted by the Health Care Financing Administration, by the turn of the century it is estimated that more than 300,000 patients will be enrolled in the ESRD Program. Furthermore, 85,000 new patients will enter the program in the year 2000 alone. Most of the increase will come from the aged and the diabetic population.

Despite improvements in dialysis technology over the past decade, mortality in the ESRD population remains high. For instance, at age 49 the expected duration of life of an ESRD patient is 7 years compared with approximately 30 years for an individual of the same age from the general population. In addition to increased mortality, patients with ESRD also experience significantly greater morbidity, including a substantial loss in quality of life. In 1986, for example, for all Medicare patients over 65 years of age, hospitalization averaged 2.8 days per year, whereas for those after 1 year on dialysis the median number was 15.0 days per year. The relevant information available to prescribe the appropriate dialysis dose is limited and subject to gross errors. As a consequence, "what is an adequate dialysis dose" remains a controversial question among professionals caring for patients on dialysis.

To resolve questions concerning delivered dialysis dose, as well as co-morbid conditions and dialysis-related complications, all of which appear to cause an increased morbidity and mortality in the United States dialysis population when compared to certain European countries and Japan, the National Institute of Diabetes and Digestive and Kidney Diseases and the Office of Medical Applications of Research of the NIH convened a consensus development conference November 1-3, 1993. Following 1-1/2 days of testimony by experts in the field, a consensus panel representing the professional fields of general medicine, nephrology, pediatrics, biostatistics, nutrition, and nursing, and a representative of the public considered evidence and agreed on answers to the questions that follow.

- How does early medical intervention in predialysis patients influence morbidity and mortality?

- What is the relationship between delivered dialysis dose and morbidity/mortality?

- Can co-morbid conditions be altered by nondialytic interventions to improve morbidity/mortality in dialysis patients?

- How can dialysis-related complications be reduced?
- What are the future directions for research in dialysis?

## Early Medical Intervention in Predialysis Patients

It is clear that factors influencing the morbidity and mortality in dialysis patients are operative for an extended period before ESRD is present and the need for dialysis is imminent. Unfortunately, only a minority of patients (20 to 25 percent) are referred to a renal physician prior to the initiation of dialysis. Managed care programs must recognize the importance of the continued involvement of the renal team in the care of these patients. A number of conditions related to renal failure are present prior to the onset of dialysis including anemia, hypertension, malnutrition, renal osteodystrophy, lipid abnormalities, and metabolic acidosis. In addition, smoking and poor glycemic control in diabetics will influence subsequent morbidity and mortality. The costs of delayed referral include both emergency dialysis, with its higher morbidity and mortality, and excessive utilization of health care dollars. Emergency dialysis jeopardizes the choice for modality of dialysis, endangers the ability to maintain prolonged vascular access, precludes psychological preparation of the patient for ESRD care and necessitates hospitalization for a catastrophic complex illness. The mortality in this crisis situation can be as high as 25 percent.

In the patient with progressing renal insufficiency, early intervention should be aimed at reversal of hypertension and correction of identified nutritional deficiencies and acidosis. While data are limited, the use of erythropoietin will prevent severe anemia and may reverse its associated complications. There is no consensus on the ultimate role of dietary protein restriction in slowing the progression of renal failure. However, an intake level of 0.7 to 0.8 g/kg/day can maintain nutritional status in noncatabolic patients with ESRD without placing an undue burden on the capacity to eliminate potentially toxic metabolites including acid, potassium, sulfate, phosphorus, magnesium, and unidentified uremic toxins. Because of deleterious effects of parathyroid hormone, therapies aimed at prevention or reversal of secondary hyperparathyroidism should be initiated in the predialysis phase.

Referral of a patient to a renal team should occur when the serum creatinine has increased to 1.5 mg/dL in women and 2.0 mg/dL in men. Predialysis referral to a renal team, consisting of a nephrologist, dietitian, nurse, social worker, and mental health professional, allows time to establish a working relationship, to acquaint the patient with the various modes of renal replacement therapy, and to provide information on dialysis access, nutritional modification, avoidance of potentially nephrotoxic drugs, and potential financial support for services. It is essential to initiate the medical interventions, discussed below, to reduce mortality and morbidity as soon as possible.

### Hypertension

Increasing evidence suggests that aggressive therapy of hypertension in the predialysis period delays progression of renal disease and is the most potent intervention to decrease subsequent cardiovascular mortality in dialysis patients. As in patients without renal disease, hypertension is the most important etiologic factor in the development of left ventricular hypertrophy (LVH) and diastolic dysfunction. It has been proposed that delay of adequate therapy or failure to lower blood pressure to normal over several years results in changes that become irreversible or only slowly reversible on dialysis. Hypertension is the highest risk factor for coronary artery disease and cerebral vascular disease. The goal of therapy is a normal systolic and diastolic pressure.

### Anemia

Studies now suggest that aggressive treatment of anemia in the predialysis period is as important as during dialysis. In fact, to reduce cardiovascular morbidity and mortality, predialysis therapy may be critical, since longstanding LVH associated with anemia may be poorly reversible or irreversible if therapy is delayed until the commencement of dialysis. In addition, predialysis correction of anemia appears to improve or maintain functional capacity, nutritional adequacy, sexual function, and psychological health. It also reduces the risk of hepatitis and sensitization to transplant antigens associated with transfusion. As in the dialysis patient, the predialysis patient should be evaluated for other causes of anemia besides the renal failure, and any nutritional deficiencies should be corrected. As the anemia worsens, the physician should initiate therapy with subcutaneous erythropoietin. The target hematocrit has not yet been determined. At present, it is recommended that the hematocrit be maintained above 30 percent, but studies are now being conducted to determine if higher hematocrit levels produce better results.

## Renal Osteodystrophy

It is known that the factors mediating renal osteodystrophy are present early in the course of progressive renal disease. These factors need to be managed throughout the entire predialysis course to prevent the ravages of severe, potentially irreversible hyperparathyroidism. Patients should be instructed early in dietary phosphate restriction, probably before the serum phosphate is elevated. Calcium-containing phosphate binders should be initiated when minimal elevations of phosphate are evident. Metabolic acidosis should be rigorously treated to maintain bicarbonate near or at the normal range because of the effect of acidosis in increasing bone dissolution and inhibiting osteoblastic activity, especially in children and women. Treatment of acidosis may also improve protein metabolism.

## Nutritional Therapy

At an early meeting with the renal team, a nutritional assessment by a trained dietitian should be accomplished and should include as a minimum weight, height, recent weight loss, upper arm anthropometry, and serum proteins (albumin, transferrin, and/or prealbumin). In the absence of obvious malnutrition a modest protein-restricted diet of 0.7 to 0.8 g of protein/kg/day will provide good nutrition. When malnutrition is present, emphasis on adequate caloric intake, greater amounts of dietary protein of up to 1 to 1.2 g/kg are called for in order to allow nutritional repletion or to counter the catabolic effects of stress. Measurement of urinary urea nitrogen to assess net protein catabolic rate (PCR) can be useful for monitoring protein intake. In certain patients in the predialysis period, fluid retentive states will make nutritional assessment more difficult. Newer techniques such as multifrequency bioimpedance analysis and dual-emission x-ray absorptiometry offer promise for ease, reproducibility, and accuracy for assessing states of fluid overload and bone mineral status, respectively.

The dietitian should also design dietary prescriptions for energy, fat and carbohydrate, fluid, sodium, and phosphate, as well as other micronutrients, recognizing that the adequacy of energy intake will be largely monitored by weight change in outpatients. Although modification of the diet to minimize lipid abnormalities is reasonable, such modifications should not be so rigid that they limit energy intake below daily requirements. Lipid abnormalities, particularly hypertriglyceridemia and reduced high-density lipoprotein (HDL) cholesterol along with elevations in lipoprotein(a), are common in ESRD, but there are limited data supporting the efficacy of diet or drug therapy, and there is some evidence that the drugs usually employed have more serious side effects.

## Quality of Life

Quality of life is very important in the predialysis period and should be given strong consideration in the decision to initiate dialysis. Maintenance of physical strength, appetite, and sense of well-being, as well as optimal physiologic functioning promotes interpersonal relationships with family and friends as well as rehabilitation and job retention in the working patient. As the likely need for dialysis approaches, preparation of the patient by introduction to various aspects of the therapy, to members of the renal team, and to the physical site of the therapy as well as to other patients undergoing dialysis will generally facilitate acceptance and compliance. Another potential benefit is the opportunity to discuss the characteristics of the various modes of the therapy in order to involve the patient in this selection and to allow early placement of vascular access if hemodialysis is the method chosen.

## Dialysis Access

The benefits of early establishment of vascular access should be emphasized. Arteriovenous (A-V) fistula surgery must occur weeks to months before the initiation of dialysis to permit maturation of the fistula. Likewise, a peritoneal dialysis catheter should be placed at least 1 month prior to its anticipated use. There may exist advantages to newer catheters in which the external segment is initially buried subcutaneously and exteriorized when needed at a later date. Late referral is clearly associated with increased complications, the need for emergency hemodialysis, and possible long-term access problems.

## Interventions in Renal Failure in Childhood

Chronic renal failure is different in childhood than in adults in that its incidence is low (11 per 106 per year) and its causes are obstructive uropathy, renal dysplasia, and congenital or inherited diseases in a majority of cases. Morbidities associated with childhood chronic renal failure are growth failure, osteodystrophy with bone deformity, salt and water losses due to urologic abnormalities, and neurologic abnormalities, including seizures, deafness, retardation, and learning disabilities. Because of growth requirements, dietary protein intake should be higher than for adults, perhaps as high as 1.3 to 1.5 g/kg/day or even higher for children receiving peritoneal dialysis. The production of erythropoietin and calcitriol and the functions of the growth-hormone-IGF-I axis may be impaired from birth onward. Because of these features, predialysis therapy should be aimed at correcting malnutrition, hormone deficiencies, salt depletion, and neurologic dysfunction.

# Relationship between Delivered Dialysis Dose and Morbidity/Mortality

## Hemodialysis

Indices of hemodialysis adequacy have historically included measurements of serum creatinine and urea, estimates of dialysis delivery (square meter-hour), and assessment of patient well-being.

Recently, an estimate of fractional urea clearance during dialysis has been suggested as a more quantifiable measurement of dialysis efficacy. This estimate uses urea as a marker for uremic toxins cleared during the dialysis procedure. The fractional urea clearance model for hemodialysis is expressed as Kdrt/V, where K[subd]is dialyzer clearance (ml/min), r is residual renal urea clearance (ml/min), t is treatment time (min), and V is total-body urea distribution volume in a single pool (ml). A simpler and more common measurement of fractional urea clearance during a single dialysis treatment is the urea reduction ratio (URR). This ratio is expressed as a percentage and is calculated as [(predialysis BUN minus postdialysis BUN)/predialysis BUN] *100. An approximate relationship between these two means of expressing dialysis dose can be made: Kdrt/V of 1.2 is approximately equal to URR 60 percent. Although urea may be distributed in multiple body pools most current measurements use a single-pool model to calculate urea clearance.

Recent reports demonstrated a direct correlation between dialysis mortality and Kdrt/V (or URR). Several studies have also suggested that the dialysis dose delivered to many hemodialysis patients in the United States was less than that recommended by the National Cooperative Dialysis Study. Although data from controlled, prospective studies are not available, retrospective data presented and opinions expressed at the consensus conference favor a recommendation for a minimum delivered hemodialysis (conventional dialyzer, single urea pool analysis) Kdrt/V of 1.2 in patients with protein intake of approximately 1.0 to1.2 g/kg/day. It is suggested that assessment of dialysis dose, by formal Kdrt/V modeling, be performed on a regular basis. Opinions were expressed that dialysis time may be an independent predictor of mortality irrespective of the dialyzer urea clearance. It is obvious that a prospective, randomized, controlled study relating the dose of delivered dialysis to morbidity and mortality is of great importance.

In the metabolically stable patient, net protein catabolic rate reflects protein intake. As changes in Kdrt/V may be paralleled by corresponding changes in net protein catabolic rate, dietary protein intake may decrease if the dialysis prescription fails to achieve the desired goal and the patient becomes symptomatic.

### Morbidity

Attainment of the recommended Kdrt/V is influenced by a number of factors, modifiable and unmodifiable, which may alter the delivered dose. These include, but are not limited to, the following:

- Vascular access: Obstruction to blood flow in the vascular access may occur and result in recirculation of blood through the dialysis circuit, thereby contributing to decreased dialysis.

- Equipment: Blood flow rate and dialyzer surface area and mass-transfer coefficient must be considered to give optimal delivery to achieve the calculated dialysis dose. Effective dialyzer surface area must be carefully monitored because excessive reuse of dialysis membranes results in loss of dialyzer efficiency and reduction of the delivered dialysis dose.

- Patient factors: Adherence to salt and water intake limitations must be met to avoid unnecessary fluctuations in blood volume during hemodialysis and the associated loss of effective dialysis. Other patient compliance issues include adherence to appointment schedules and time on dialysis. Patients with certain underlying diseases (e.g., diabetes, amyloidosis, drug dependence) have special problems that may interfere with dialysis.

### Dialysis Biocompatibility

The composition of the hemodialyzer membrane may be a factor in establishing urea clearance goals, i.e., biocompatible polymer membranes such as polysulfones, polyacrylonitrile, and polymethylmethacrylate have permeability characteristics different from cellulosic membranes. In addition, the composition of the membrane may be a factor in the nature and intensity of the interaction between the membrane and blood. Generally, cellulosic-based membranes, in contrast to the more biocompatible membranes, have a greater capacity to activate complement and to attenuate the granulocyte response. It has also been suggested that the use of biocompatible membranes may result in lower mortality rates.

## Peritoneal Dialysis

Peritoneal dialysis utilizes a natural membrane to remove nitrogenous products from the body fluids of individuals with impaired renal function. The use of relatively long dwell-time peritoneal exchanges [continuous ambulatory peritoneal dialysis (CAPD)] has enabled individuals to carry on normal daily activities without the use of machines or other appliances. The dose of peritoneal dialysis has been established empirically and depends to some extent on patient acceptance of frequent interruptions for the exchange of peritoneal fluid. Recently, an effort has been made to prescribe for each individual patient the dose of peritoneal dialysis needed to attain target levels of urea clearance. In general, four exchanges of 2 liters each may generate as much as 10 liters of dialysate (allowing for the removal of ultrafiltrate). Assuming nearly complete equilibration of urea between plasma and peritoneal fluid, this equates to a weekly urea clearance of approximately 70 liters. For a 70kg man with a urea "space" of 42 liters, the calculated $K_{pr}t/V$ is 1.7. The weight of current evidence indicates that this value of $K_{pr}t/V$ is a reasonable minimal delivered dose for most functionally anephric CAPD patients who daily eat approximately 0.9 to 1.0 g/kg of protein. The dose of nighttime peritoneal dialysis is usually increased above that of CAPD.

The prescription of dialysis will depend on the volume of urea distribution, the efficiency of peritoneal exchange, and the residual renal urea clearance.

Peritoneal dialysis is a demanding and time-consuming therapy. Omission of exchanges or shortening exchange times by the patient will reduce urea clearance and lead to increased morbidity and mortality. The use of urea as an index of peritoneal dialysis efficiency is complicated because the peritoneal membrane is more permeable to large molecules than are dialyzer membranes.

Peritoneal dialysis efficiency can be increased by more frequent exchange (5/day), increased volume per exchange (2.5 to 3.0 liters), and the coupling of CAPD with nighttime cycler dialysis in large individuals or those with relatively low peritoneal clearances.

### Children

Children undergoing chronic dialysis therapy are more likely to receive peritoneal dialysis than adults. This preference is based on technical factors including problems maintaining chronic hemodialysis access. Because of the serious problems of growth failure and neurologic dysfunction, children require appropriate hormone therapy (erythropoietin, calcitriol, and growth hormone), nutrition support services, and neurologic evaluation. A qualified pediatric nephrologist is an essential member of the renal team. Data exist that intervention with specified nutrition, growth hormone, erythropoietin and calcitrol therapy, and avoidance of aluminum can clearly improve growth velocity. Because of the serious problems of growth failure and neurologic dysfunction, children with renal insufficiency should be referred to centers with specialized pediatric nephrologic care. Children also require educational and play facilities at the dialysis center.

Children of all ages with ESRD benefit from treatment with peritoneal and hemodialysis. The principles of dialysis outlined for adults generally hold for children, although no retrospective or prospective studies have been performed that indicate reasonable targets of $Kprt/V$ or $Kdrt/V$ to maximally allay morbidity and mortality.

Children with chronic renal failure suffer from a cycle of depression, anxiety and loss of self-esteem. The difficulties encountered often result in family stress with a high divorce rate among the parents of a child undergoing dialysis. For these reasons, a mental health professional is an essential component of the pediatric renal disease center.

Finally, dialysis should be a temporary therapy, since renal transplantation is considered the treatment of choice for children.

# Can Comorbid Conditions Be Altered by Nondialytic Interventions?

## Cardiovascular Abnormalities

Cardiovascular events (principally systolic and diastolic dysfunction, myocardial infarction, and stroke) account for 50 percent of the mortality in dialysis patients, and also contribute importantly to mortality after renal transplantation.

Studies of patients entering dialysis treatment demonstrate a high prevalence of established cardiovascular abnormalities including hypertension, LVH, coronary artery disease, and cardiac failure. For example, two-dimensional echocardiograms are abnormal in 70 percent of such patients. The rising mean age of dialysis patients likely will further increase this cardiovascular pathology.

We believe that optimum reduction of dialysis morbidity and mortality begins with predialysis intervention. The patient with chronic renal failure is at high risk for cardiovascular events. It is likely, but not yet proven, that prevention of severe anemia by erythropoietin will also prevent, diminish, or partially reverse left ventricular overload.

Cessation of smoking, correction of obesity, and regular aerobic exercise may also contribute to reducing mortality from cardiovascular disease. Normotension and non-smoking have been two characteristics of 20-year-plus survivors on chronic dialysis.

It is not yet known whether modifications of the common lipid abnormalities in chronic renal failure and ESRD patients can be safely achieved in the long term by currently available lipid-lowering agents or whether this would be beneficial.

Because myocardial calcification and fibrosis may contribute especially to diastolic dysfunction (which accounts for 50 percent of cardiac failure in dialysis patients) control of calcium, phosphorus, and parathyroid hormone levels may help to prevent cardiovascular disease as well as bone disease.

Two-thirds of ESRD is due to two primary diseases--diabetes mellitus and essential hypertension--that themselves contribute importantly to cardiovascular disease. Not infrequently such patients have had erratic treatment and followup programs prior to the onset of chronic renal disease.

The identification of a diabetic patient has not routinely led to inclusion of that patient in a program of strict glycemic control and followup of potential microvascular and renal complications, such as micro or gross albuminuria. We also now understand that careful control of blood pressure upon diagnosis of diabetes mellitus is crucial.

Current studies suggest that blood pressure is not being adequately controlled in many dialysis patients. Blood pressure at the initiation of each dialysis treatment should be in the normal range or as near as possible to it. Adequate ultrafiltration and restriction of interdialytic intake of sodium chloride should establish normotension in up to 80 percent of dialysis patients. Mechanisms of hypertension in the remainder include an inappropriately hyperactive renin-angiotensin system, nephrogenic activation of the sympathetic nervous system and, possibly, an altered balance of endothelial factors (nitric oxide and endothelin) influencing arteriolar smooth muscle tone.

### Nutritional Deficiency

The nutritional status of the patient is a major factor in the outcome of hemodialysis treatment and may be maintained in the predialysis period by the use of low-protein diets, in the range of 0.7 to 0.8 g/kg/day together with adequate calorie intake of 35 kcal/kg/day. It is essential that during this period, malnutrition, as evidenced by a decrease in albumin and body weight, is not allowed to develop in renal patients. Serum albumin levels above 3.5 g/dL are associated with little mortality, while mortality rises dramatically with lower values for serum albumin.

Once the patient is on hemodialysis, dietary protein should be liberalized to equal 1.0 g/kg/day, with appropriate calorie supplementation, to sustain nutrition at a normal level. The complexity of nutritional intervention for the renal patient is of such degree and, at the same time, of such importance as to require the expert guidance of a well-trained renal dietitian. High cholesterol is indicative of increased risk of morbidity and mortality, but values below 100 mg/dL are also associated with increased mortality. The reasons why hypoalbuminemia and hypocholesterolemia are indexes of high mortality are not known.

Educational programs instituted by the renal center and by organizations concerned with the welfare of all kidney patients should explain the need for adequate dialysis time and correction of malnutrition, because these factors contribute to longer life of higher quality and correction of many co-morbid conditions. Patient participation, as an integral part of the renal team, is of the essence if success in improving quality of life is to be achieved.

Current concerns about morbidity and mortality raise issues regarding the present uniform reimbursement system for dialysis, especially in the area of nutritional and psychosocial support systems. Linking direct reimbursement for such care to important outcomes such as levels of serum albumin, mean blood pressure, and measurements of fractional urea clearance during dialysis should be explored.

# How Can Dialysis-Related Complications Be Reduced?

Although dialysis allows effective and productive lives for many patients with ESRD, a variety of complications can occur. Problems with dialysis access, infections, atherosclerosis and cardiovascular disease, malnutrition, and metabolic abnormalities, as well as persisting uremic symptoms and acute symptoms related to the dialysis procedure itself, may limit a patient's health and quality of life. Disorders of calcium, phosphorus, vitamin D, and parathyroid hormone are common and may be disabling.

### Hemodialysis

Perhaps the major complication limiting continued effective hemodialysis involves vascular access. The most effective, durable access is the A-V fistula. Unfortunately a satisfactory fistula cannot be established in many patients, because of inadequate vessels (especially in diabetic patients). The chances of a successful fistula are enhanced by early planning and placement well before dialysis becomes necessary. When early planning is not possible, the use of a tunnelled subcutaneous catheter may make dialysis possible while an A-V fistula is maturing, but repeated use of temporary subclavian catheters is often accompanied by infection or thrombosis with ultimate impairment of subclavian flow and loss of the whole arm for dialysis access purposes. Use of temporary catheters should be avoided when possible.

When a fistula is unsuccessful or not feasible, a synthetic graft is ordinarily placed. Current experience indicates that 60 percent of these grafts fail each year due to thrombosis. Anatomic stenosis is responsible for four-fifths of these clots (almost all are on the venous side of the anastomosis) while the rest result from other causes such as excessive post-venipuncture pressure by manual compression or clamp or sleeping on the graft. Medical thrombolysis may remove the clot and restore flow, but often surgical thrombectomy is required. The stenosis, usually formed by endothelial proliferation, sometimes responds to percutaneous angioplasty but may require surgical intervention. The present life of a synthetic graft is about 2 years with loss due to thrombosis in 80 percent and infection in 20 percent of patients.

Consistently elevated venous dialysis pressure may provide a warning of developing stenosis and hence of impending thrombosis and may indicate the need for a fistulogram. An increase in recirculation may also indicate an incipient problem. Attention to these signs may allow for intervention prior to clotting of the graft and prevent its loss.

The need for meticulous, experienced surgical skill in establishing satisfactory fistulas and shunts must be emphasized. Although the procedure may not be dramatic, a dialysis patient's life often depends on the presence of a reliable access. Nursing skill in access use has a major influence on dialysis success.

### Infection

Infection remains the major cause of death in 15 to 30 percent of all dialysis patients; a figure that has not changed significantly over the years. Infections are usually due to common organisms and often appear to be access-related. About 60 percent of bacteremic infections are Gram-positive, especially Staphylococcus aureus. Perhaps 50 to 60 percent of dialysis patients are carriers of this organism (compared to 10 to 30 percent of the general population), and the carrier rate among diabetic patients is still higher. It is possible to reduce the carrier rate with prophylactic antibiotic treatment, but this may encourage the emergence of resistant organisms.

Uremia itself causes an impairment in cell-mediated immunity that is not totally corrected by dialysis. In addition, granulocyte phagocytosis and killing functions appear to be impaired by cellulosic dialysis membranes. Biocompatible membranes may have less deleterious effects on white cell function and other defense mechanisms. Some studies suggest a 50 percent fall in incidence of infection accompanying a switch to more biocompatible dialyzers.

### Peritoneal Dialysis

The overwhelming cause of unsuccessful peritoneal dialysis is peritonitis. Although improvement has followed recent changes in tubing and connection systems, recurrent peritonitis is a continuing problem for many patients. Catheter tunnel infection often underlies this peritonitis, and changes in catheter design (e.g., U shape), placement (with both peritoneal and skin ends directed caudad and a cuff placed in the rectus muscle), and the use of prophylactic antibiotics at the time of placement or thereafter have been proposed as deterrents to infection. The use of vaccine against Staphylococcus organisms and of bacteriostatics such as silver-coated catheters are under investigation.

## Calcium, Phosphorus, and Parathyroid Hormone

The disturbances in body calcium, phosphorus, vitamin D, parathyroid hormone, and bone disease that usually start prior to the initiation of dialysis continue to demand consistent attention so long as dialysis is required. Mainstays in therapy include control of dietary phosphorus, minimization of its absorption by use of phosphate-binders, and the use of calcitriol. Control of dietary intake of phosphorus requires patient education by the renal team and adherence by the patient to the recommended diet. Previous reliance on aluminum hydroxide to prevent absorption of phosphorus has been largely discontinued because of accumulation of aluminum in the brain and bone, leading to severe neurological disorders and osteomalacia. Ingestion of calcium carbonate or calcium acetate with meals is currently recommended for most patients to prevent absorption of phosphorus. Use of these calcium salts may require adjustments in the concentration of calcium in the dialysate fluid to prevent hypercalcemia and consequent deposition of calcium phosphate salts with damage to the heart, blood vessels, and other tissues. Careful titration of the calcitriol dosage is required to obtain its benefits without causing hyperphosphatemia or hypercalcemia. Careful attention to dietary phosphorus, calcium salts, and calcitriol often enable parathyroid hormone concentrations to be maintained at or near normal. Of serious concern is the emergence of "adynamic bone disease," a condition diagnosed by bone biopsy in which the normal correction of bone wear and tear by "remodeling" fails to occur. The exact cause(s) and consequences of adynamic bone disease are not yet known.

## Amyloid

Amyloidosis in dialysis patients is associated with long-term (greater than 6 years) dialysis, and is increased in frequency in older patients. The deposition of beta-2-microglobulin protein as amyloid causes carpal tunnel syndrome, destructive arthropathy in medium- and large-sized joints, and cystic bone disease. The disorder may be due both to increased release of beta-2-microglobulin from macrophages and, significantly, to reduction in the destruction of beta-2-microglobulin that normally occurs in functioning kidneys. Some evidence indicates that amyloidosis is a lesser problem in patients dialyzed with high-flux membranes than in those with cellulosic membranes, perhaps because of both decreased release of the protein from macrophages and from partial removal of the protein during dialysis by filtration or binding with some synthetic polymer membranes. Serious consideration should be given to the use of these membranes for dialysis of patients in whom amyloidosis is a problem or may become a clinical concern.

### Anemia

Attention to the management of anemia, begun in the predialysis phase of care, must be continued into dialysis.

### Intradialytic Complications

Acute complications related to the dialysis procedure itself may severely compromise the quality of life in chronic dialysis patients. A mild degree of hypotension is "normal" in dialysis, but severe degrees may be disabling. Muscle cramps, chest or back pain, hypoxemia, fever, nausea, seizures, or cardiac arrhythmias may occur. In addition, mechanical problems related to dialysis machines, cartridges, and water purifiers may occur.

Some of these problems have been lessened by the use of bicarbonate rather than acetate dialysis solutions, by longer dialysis periods with lower rates of ultrafiltration, with the use of synthetic polymer dialysis membranes that are more biocompatible, and perhaps by reuse of these membranes. Reuse brings the potential for problems as well as benefits; however, additional research will be necessary to define the optimum mix of membranes, reuse, solutions, and time and intensity of dialysis to ensure maximum safety and minimum complications of dialysis.

### Psychosocial Concerns

Early predialysis assessment and continuous, active intervention by the renal team, including mental health professionals, in the care of a patient beginning dialysis are more likely to be effective than efforts initiated later in treatment. This assessment should include measures of quality of life and social role function in addition to lack of mental acuity and depression. Ensuring patients' understanding and positive participation in their care is a primary goal of this intervention in addition to optimizing the relationship between patient and physician and patient with staff. The earlier this assessment is accomplished the greater will be the potential for a positive impact on physical and social rehabilitation. Exercise and physical training can add to physical well-being and should also be initiated at the beginning of dialysis, or in the predialysis period.

## Future Directions for Research

- Studies should be conducted to evaluate the effect of aggressive nutritional support in malnourished predialysis patients, and to determine the mechanisms by which malnutrition increases mortality and morbidity rates, and to develop sensitive and specific methodology to detect the early stages of malnutrition.

- Studies should be instituted to determine the benefits and risks of early control of renal osteodystrophy on morbidity and to explore the causes and therapy of disturbances in calcium, phosphorus, and vitamin D, both at the basic level on regulation of bone metabolism and at the clinical level on the importance of soft tissue calcium deposition. Studies should include development of new phosphate-binding agents and noncalcemic analogues of vitamin D, and determination of the optimal degree of suppression of parathyroid hormone.

- Basic and clinical studies should be initiated to evaluate the effect of chronic uremia on neurologic function.

- Basic and clinical studies should be conducted to evaluate the effect of uremia on growth in children.

- Studies should be initiated to determine the impact of early treatment of anemia on mortality, morbidity, and rehabilitation. Studies to determine when to initiate treatment of anemia and what the target hematocrit should be are needed in both the predialysis and dialysis patient.

- A prospective, randomized, controlled clinical trial should be initiated to examine the differences in patient morbidity and mortality at to examine the differences in patient morbidity and mortality at Kdrt/V levels of 1.2 (single pool) and 1.6 for hemodialysis patients.

- A prospective, randomized, controlled clinical trial should be initiated to examine the differences in patient morbidity and mortality at delivered weekly Kprt/V levels of 1.47 and 2.10 in peritoneal dialysis patients.

- A prospective, randomized, controlled clinical trial should be initiated to determine the differences in the effects of biocompatible, high-flux versus cellulosic membranes in studies which include, but are not limited to, patient survival, incidence of infection, and incidence and course of beta-2-microglobulin amyloidosis.

- Additional studies to establish the effect of reuse of dialysis membranes on hemodialysis effectiveness and morbidity and mortality are recommended.

- A prospective study of the feasibility and effectiveness of modification of cardiovascular risk factors in chronic renal failure patients both before and after initiation of dialysis should be undertaken. Risk factors to be evaluated would include hypertension (mechanism of development and regression of left ventricular hypertrophy and characterization of the best pharmacological approaches to antihypertensive treatment), smoking, obesity, and uremic dyslipidemia. The role of metabolic factors such as hyperinsulinemia and parathyroid hormone and calcium phosphorous relationships including tissue calcium burden in the myocardium and methods of its detection should be examined. Finally, development of noninvasive testing for coronary artery disease in this patient population should be explored.

- Studies to determine the mechanisms of interdialytic hypertension should be initiated and should include the respective roles of abnormal renin-angiotensin responses, abnormal thirst and salt craving, vascular endothelial factors (endothelin, nitric oxide production, and inhibitors), the renal-sympathetic axis, the relationship to erythropoietin administration, and the role for continuous blood pressure monitoring.

- Studies of the mechanisms by which malnutrition increases mortality and morbidity rates due to infections, anorexia, hypogusia, and related problems in the dialysis patient should be undertaken.

- Improved methods for detecting stenosis and thrombosis of access grafts and understanding the mechanism of endothelial proliferation leading to vascular graft stenosis are needed. Improved material and techniques should be developed to diminish access clotting and infection and new methods identified for cost-effective thrombolysis in clotted grafts.

- Study of the immunodeficiency of uremia and evaluation of antibacterial vaccines, antibiotic prophylaxis, and dialyzer membrane characteristics in the prevention of infection in dialysis patients should be initiated.

- Evaluating and standardizing methods for measurement of psychological well-being and quality of life in dialysis patients, and applying these instruments in studies on the effectiveness of interventions should be undertaken.

## Conclusions

- Patients, including children, in the predialysis phase should be referred to a renal team consisting of a nephrologist, dietitian, nurse, social worker, and mental health professional in an effort to reduce the morbidity and mortality incurred during both the predialysis period and when receiving the subsequent dialysis therapy.

- The social and psychological welfare and the quality of life of the dialysis patient are favorably influenced by early predialytic and continued involvement of a multidisciplinary renal team.

- Attempts should be made through predialytic intervention and the appropriate initiation of dialysis access to avoid a catastrophic onset of dialysis.

- Quantitative methods to measure the delivered dose of hemodialysis and peritoneal dialysis have now been developed. These methods permit an objective evaluation of the relationship between the delivered dose of dialysis and patient morbidity and mortality. These methods suggest that the dose of hemodialysis and peritoneal dialysis has been suboptimal for many patients in the United States.

- Factors contributing to underdialysis of some patients include problems with vascular and peritoneal access, nonadherence to the dialysis prescription, and underprescription of the dialysis dose.

- Until prospective, randomized, controlled trials have been completed, a delivered hemodialysis dose at least equal to a measured Kdrt/V of 1.2 (single pool) and a delivered peritoneal dialysis dose at least equal to a measured Kprt/V of 1.7 (weekly) are recommended.

- Cardiovascular mortality accounts for approximately 50 percent of deaths in dialysis patients. Relevant risk factors should be treated as soon as possible after diagnosis of chronic renal failure. These factors include hypertension, smoking, and chronic anemia.

- Patients with diabetes mellitus face especially severe cardiovascular risk, which contributes to reduced survival on dialysis.

- Malnutrition is another important co-morbid condition contributing to mortality. A serum albumin of less than 3.5 g/dL is clearly associated with increased relative risk. Early detection and treatment of malnutrition should substantially improve survival.

- Control of renal osteodystrophy requires patient adherence to the prescribed regimen and careful attention by the renal team to calcium and phosphorus intake and to the use of phosphate binders and calcitriol.

- Early creation of an A-V fistula is preferable to placement of a synthetic graft for vascular access. Both require an experienced, meticulous surgeon.

- Skilled management by nursing and other clinical personnel will help prolong the life of the vascular access.

- Attention to catheter design, placement, and care, and to exchange procedures can minimize infection in patients on peritoneal dialysis.

- Biocompatible dialysis membranes may reduce infection and amyloid deposition in hemodialysis patients, but evidence is inconclusive at present.

- Financial support to conduct clinical investigation, including outcomes and health services delivery research, should be incorporated into the budgets of the Medicare End-Stage Renal Disease program, Health Care Financing Administration, Agency for Health Care Policy Research, and the Food and Drug Administration. This support will enable the conduct of studies that promise to improve morbidity and mortality, enhance cost-effective care, and create long-term financial savings in the Medicare ESRD program.

# Appendix F. Your Rights and Insurance

## Overview

Any patient with kidney failure faces a series of issues related more to the healthcare industry than to the medical condition itself. This appendix covers two important topics in this regard: your rights and responsibilities as a patient, and how to get the most out of your medical insurance plan.

## Your Rights as a Patient

The President's Advisory Commission on Consumer Protection and Quality in the Healthcare Industry has created the following summary of your rights as a patient.[52]

### Information Disclosure

Consumers have the right to receive accurate, easily understood information. Some consumers require assistance in making informed decisions about health plans, health professionals, and healthcare facilities. Such information includes:

- *Health plans.* Covered benefits, cost-sharing, and procedures for resolving complaints, licensure, certification, and accreditation status, comparable measures of quality and consumer satisfaction, provider network composition, the procedures that govern access to specialists and emergency services, and care management information.

---

[52]Adapted from Consumer Bill of Rights and Responsibilities:
**http://www.hcqualitycommission.gov/press/cbor.html#head1.**

- *Health professionals.* Education, board certification, and recertification, years of practice, experience performing certain procedures, and comparable measures of quality and consumer satisfaction.

- *Healthcare facilities.* Experience in performing certain procedures and services, accreditation status, comparable measures of quality, worker, and consumer satisfaction, and procedures for resolving complaints.

- *Consumer assistance programs.* Programs must be carefully structured to promote consumer confidence and to work cooperatively with health plans, providers, payers, and regulators. Desirable characteristics of such programs are sponsorship that ensures accountability to the interests of consumers and stable, adequate funding.

### Choice of Providers and Plans

Consumers have the right to a choice of healthcare providers that is sufficient to ensure access to appropriate high-quality healthcare. To ensure such choice, the Commission recommends the following:

- *Provider network adequacy.* All health plan networks should provide access to sufficient numbers and types of providers to assure that all covered services will be accessible without unreasonable delay -- including access to emergency services 24 hours a day and 7 days a week. If a health plan has an insufficient number or type of providers to provide a covered benefit with the appropriate degree of specialization, the plan should ensure that the consumer obtains the benefit outside the network at no greater cost than if the benefit were obtained from participating providers.

- *Women's health services.* Women should be able to choose a qualified provider offered by a plan -- such as gynecologists, certified nurse midwives, and other qualified healthcare providers -- for the provision of covered care necessary to provide routine and preventative women's healthcare services.

- *Access to specialists.* Consumers with complex or serious medical conditions who require frequent specialty care should have direct access to a qualified specialist of their choice within a plan's network of providers. Authorizations, when required, should be for an adequate number of direct access visits under an approved treatment plan.

- *Transitional care.* Consumers who are undergoing a course of treatment for a chronic or disabling condition (or who are in the second or third trimester of a pregnancy) at the time they involuntarily change health plans or at a time when a provider is terminated by a plan for other than cause should be able to continue seeing their current specialty providers for up to 90 days (or through completion of postpartum care) to allow for transition of care.

- *Choice of health plans.* Public and private group purchasers should, wherever feasible, offer consumers a choice of high-quality health insurance plans.

### Access to Emergency Services

Consumers have the right to access emergency healthcare services when and where the need arises. Health plans should provide payment when a consumer presents to an emergency department with acute symptoms of sufficient severity--including severe pain--such that a "prudent layperson" could reasonably expect the absence of medical attention to result in placing that consumer's health in serious jeopardy, serious impairment to bodily functions, or serious dysfunction of any bodily organ or part.

### Participation in Treatment Decisions

Consumers have the right and responsibility to fully participate in all decisions related to their healthcare. Consumers who are unable to fully participate in treatment decisions have the right to be represented by parents, guardians, family members, or other conservators. Physicians and other health professionals should:

- Provide patients with sufficient information and opportunity to decide among treatment options consistent with the informed consent process.

- Discuss all treatment options with a patient in a culturally competent manner, including the option of no treatment at all.

- Ensure that persons with disabilities have effective communications with members of the health system in making such decisions.

- Discuss all current treatments a consumer may be undergoing.

- Discuss all risks, benefits, and consequences to treatment or nontreatment.

- Give patients the opportunity to refuse treatment and to express preferences about future treatment decisions.

- Discuss the use of advance directives -- both living wills and durable powers of attorney for healthcare -- with patients and their designated family members.

- Abide by the decisions made by their patients and/or their designated representatives consistent with the informed consent process.

Health plans, health providers, and healthcare facilities should:

- Disclose to consumers factors -- such as methods of compensation, ownership of or interest in healthcare facilities, or matters of conscience -- that could influence advice or treatment decisions.

- Assure that provider contracts do not contain any so-called "gag clauses" or other contractual mechanisms that restrict healthcare providers' ability to communicate with and advise patients about medically necessary treatment options.

- Be prohibited from penalizing or seeking retribution against healthcare professionals or other health workers for advocating on behalf of their patients.

### Respect and Nondiscrimination

Consumers have the right to considerate, respectful care from all members of the healthcare industry at all times and under all circumstances. An environment of mutual respect is essential to maintain a quality healthcare system. To assure that right, the Commission recommends the following:

- Consumers must not be discriminated against in the delivery of healthcare services consistent with the benefits covered in their policy, or as required by law, based on race, ethnicity, national origin, religion, sex, age, mental or physical disability, sexual orientation, genetic information, or source of payment.

- Consumers eligible for coverage under the terms and conditions of a health plan or program, or as required by law, must not be discriminated against in marketing and enrollment practices based on race, ethnicity, national origin, religion, sex, age, mental or physical disability, sexual orientation, genetic information, or source of payment.

### Confidentiality of Health Information

Consumers have the right to communicate with healthcare providers in confidence and to have the confidentiality of their individually identifiable healthcare information protected. Consumers also have the right to review and copy their own medical records and request amendments to their records.

### Complaints and Appeals

Consumers have the right to a fair and efficient process for resolving differences with their health plans, healthcare providers, and the institutions that serve them, including a rigorous system of internal review and an independent system of external review. A free copy of the Patient's Bill of Rights is available from the American Hospital Association.[53]

## Patient Responsibilities

Treatment is a two-way street between you and your healthcare providers. To underscore the importance of finance in modern healthcare as well as your responsibility for the financial aspects of your care, the President's Advisory Commission on Consumer Protection and Quality in the Healthcare Industry has proposed that patients understand the following "Consumer Responsibilities."[54] In a healthcare system that protects consumers' rights, it is reasonable to expect and encourage consumers to assume certain responsibilities. Greater individual involvement by the consumer in his or her care increases the likelihood of achieving the best outcome and helps support a quality-oriented, cost-conscious environment. Such responsibilities include:

- Take responsibility for maximizing healthy habits such as exercising, not smoking, and eating a healthy diet.

- Work collaboratively with healthcare providers in developing and carrying out agreed-upon treatment plans.

- Disclose relevant information and clearly communicate wants and needs.

- Use your health insurance plan's internal complaint and appeal processes to address your concerns.

- Avoid knowingly spreading disease.

---

[53] To order your free copy of the Patient's Bill of Rights, telephone 312-422-3000 or visit the American Hospital Association's Web site: **http://www.aha.org**. Click on "Resource Center," go to "Search" at bottom of page, and then type in "Patient's Bill of Rights." The Patient's Bill of Rights is also available from Fax on Demand, at 312-422-2020, document number 471124.

[54] Adapted from **http://www.hcqualitycommission.gov/press/cbor.html#head1**.

- Recognize the reality of risks, the limits of the medical science, and the human fallibility of the healthcare professional.

- Be aware of a healthcare provider's obligation to be reasonably efficient and equitable in providing care to other patients and the community.

- Become knowledgeable about your health plan's coverage and options (when available) including all covered benefits, limitations, and exclusions, rules regarding use of network providers, coverage and referral rules, appropriate processes to secure additional information, and the process to appeal coverage decisions.

- Show respect for other patients and health workers.

- Make a good-faith effort to meet financial obligations.

- Abide by administrative and operational procedures of health plans, healthcare providers, and Government health benefit programs.

## Choosing an Insurance Plan

There are a number of official government agencies that help consumers understand their healthcare insurance choices.[55] The U.S. Department of Labor, in particular, recommends ten ways to make your health benefits choices work best for you.[56]

**1. Your options are important.** There are many different types of health benefit plans. Find out which one your employer offers, then check out the plan, or plans, offered. Your employer's human resource office, the health plan administrator, or your union can provide information to help you match your needs and preferences with the available plans. The more information you have, the better your healthcare decisions will be.

**2. Reviewing the benefits available.** Do the plans offered cover preventive care, well-baby care, vision or dental care? Are there deductibles? Answers to these questions can help determine the out-of-pocket expenses you may face. Matching your needs and those of your family members will result in the best possible benefits. Cheapest may not always be best. Your goal is high quality health benefits.

---

[55] More information about quality across programs is provided at the following AHRQ Web site:
http://www.ahrq.gov/consumer/qntascii/qnthplan.htm.
[56] Adapted from the Department of Labor:
http://www.dol.gov/dol/pwba/public/pubs/health/top10-text.html.

**3. Look for quality.** The quality of healthcare services varies, but quality can be measured. You should consider the quality of healthcare in deciding among the healthcare plans or options available to you. Not all health plans, doctors, hospitals and other providers give the highest quality care. Fortunately, there is quality information you can use right now to help you compare your healthcare choices. Find out how you can measure quality. Consult the U.S. Department of Health and Human Services publication "Your Guide to Choosing Quality Health Care" on the Internet at **www.ahcpr.gov/consumer**.

**4. Your plan's summary plan description (SPD) provides a wealth of information.** Your health plan administrator can provide you with a copy of your plan's SPD. It outlines your benefits and your legal rights under the Employee Retirement Income Security Act (ERISA), the federal law that protects your health benefits. It should contain information about the coverage of dependents, what services will require a co-pay, and the circumstances under which your employer can change or terminate a health benefits plan. Save the SPD and all other health plan brochures and documents, along with memos or correspondence from your employer relating to health benefits.

**5. Assess your benefit coverage as your family status changes.** Marriage, divorce, childbirth or adoption, and the death of a spouse are all life events that may signal a need to change your health benefits. You, your spouse and dependent children may be eligible for a special enrollment period under provisions of the Health Insurance Portability and Accountability Act (HIPAA). Even without life-changing events, the information provided by your employer should tell you how you can change benefits or switch plans, if more than one plan is offered. If your spouse's employer also offers a health benefits package, consider coordinating both plans for maximum coverage.

**6. Changing jobs and other life events can affect your health benefits.** Under the Consolidated Omnibus Budget Reconciliation Act (COBRA), you, your covered spouse, and your dependent children may be eligible to purchase extended health coverage under your employer's plan if you lose your job, change employers, get divorced, or upon occurrence of certain other events. Coverage can range from 18 to 36 months depending on your situation. COBRA applies to most employers with 20 or more workers and requires your plan to notify you of your rights. Most plans require eligible individuals to make their COBRA election within 60 days of the plan's notice. Be sure to follow up with your plan sponsor if you don't receive notice, and make sure you respond within the allotted time.

**7. HIPAA can also help if you are changing jobs, particularly if you have a medical condition.** HIPAA generally limits pre-existing condition exclusions to a maximum of 12 months (18 months for late enrollees). HIPAA also requires this maximum period to be reduced by the length of time you had prior "creditable coverage." You should receive a certificate documenting your prior creditable coverage from your old plan when coverage ends.

**8. Plan for retirement.** Before you retire, find out what health benefits, if any, extend to you and your spouse during your retirement years. Consult with your employer's human resources office, your union, the plan administrator, and check your SPD. Make sure there is no conflicting information among these sources about the benefits you will receive or the circumstances under which they can change or be eliminated. With this information in hand, you can make other important choices, like finding out if you are eligible for Medicare and Medigap insurance coverage.

**9. Know how to file an appeal if your health benefits claim is denied.** Understand how your plan handles grievances and where to make appeals of the plan's decisions. Keep records and copies of correspondence. Check your health benefits package and your SPD to determine who is responsible for handling problems with benefit claims. Contact PWBA for customer service assistance if you are unable to obtain a response to your complaint.

**10. You can take steps to improve the quality of the healthcare and the health benefits you receive.** Look for and use things like Quality Reports and Accreditation Reports whenever you can. Quality reports may contain consumer ratings -- how satisfied consumers are with the doctors in their plan, for instance-- and clinical performance measures -- how well a healthcare organization prevents and treats illness. Accreditation reports provide information on how accredited organizations meet national standards, and often include clinical performance measures. Look for these quality measures whenever possible. Consult "Your Guide to Choosing Quality Health Care" on the Internet at **www.ahcpr.gov/consumer**.

## Medicare and Medicaid

Illness strikes both rich and poor families. For low-income families, Medicaid is available to defer the costs of treatment. The Health Care Financing Administration (HCFA) administers Medicare, the nation's largest health insurance program, which covers 39 million Americans. In the following pages, you will learn the basics about Medicare insurance as well as useful contact information on how to find more in-depth information about Medicaid.[57]

## Who Is Eligible for Medicare?

Generally, you are eligible for Medicare if you or your spouse worked for at least 10 years in Medicare-covered employment and you are 65 years old and a citizen or permanent resident of the United States. You might also qualify for coverage if you are under age 65 but have a disability or End-Stage Renal disease (permanent kidney failure requiring dialysis or transplant). Here are some simple guidelines:

You can get Part A at age 65 without having to pay premiums if:

- You are already receiving retirement benefits from Social Security or the Railroad Retirement Board.

- You are eligible to receive Social Security or Railroad benefits but have not yet filed for them.

- You or your spouse had Medicare-covered government employment.

If you are under 65, you can get Part A without having to pay premiums if:

- You have received Social Security or Railroad Retirement Board disability benefit for 24 months.

- You are a kidney dialysis or kidney transplant patient.

Medicare has two parts:

- Part A (Hospital Insurance). Most people do not have to pay for Part A.

- Part B (Medical Insurance). Most people pay monthly for Part B.

## Part A (Hospital Insurance)

**Helps Pay For:** Inpatient hospital care, care in critical access hospitals (small facilities that give limited outpatient and inpatient services to people in rural areas) and skilled nursing facilities, hospice care, and some home healthcare.

---

[57] This section has been adapted from the Official U.S. Site for Medicare Information: http://www.medicare.gov/Basics/Overview.asp.

**Cost:** Most people get Part A automatically when they turn age 65. You do not have to pay a monthly payment called a premium for Part A because you or a spouse paid Medicare taxes while you were working.

If you (or your spouse) did not pay Medicare taxes while you were working and you are age 65 or older, you still may be able to buy Part A. If you are not sure you have Part A, look on your red, white, and blue Medicare card. It will show "Hospital Part A" on the lower left corner of the card. You can also call the Social Security Administration toll free at 1-800-772-1213 or call your local Social Security office for more information about buying Part A. If you get benefits from the Railroad Retirement Board, call your local RRB office or 1-800-808-0772. For more information, call your Fiscal Intermediary about Part A bills and services. The phone number for the Fiscal Intermediary office in your area can be obtained from the following Web site: **http://www.medicare.gov/Contacts/home.asp**.

### Part B (Medical Insurance)

**Helps Pay For:** Doctors, services, outpatient hospital care, and some other medical services that Part A does not cover, such as the services of physical and occupational therapists, and some home healthcare. Part B helps pay for covered services and supplies when they are medically necessary.

**Cost:** As of 2001, you pay the Medicare Part B premium of $50.00 per month. In some cases this amount may be higher if you did not choose Part B when you first became eligible at age 65. The cost of Part B may go up 10% for each 12-month period that you were eligible for Part B but declined coverage, except in special cases. You will have to pay the extra 10% cost for the rest of your life.

Enrolling in Part B is your choice. You can sign up for Part B anytime during a 7-month period that begins 3 months before you turn 65. Visit your local Social Security office, or call the Social Security Administration at 1-800-772-1213 to sign up. If you choose to enroll in Part B, the premium is usually taken out of your monthly Social Security, Railroad Retirement, or Civil Service Retirement payment. If you do not receive any of the above payments, Medicare sends you a bill for your part B premium every 3 months. You should receive your Medicare premium bill in the mail by the 10th of the month. If you do not, call the Social Security Administration at 1-800-772-1213, or your local Social Security office. If you get benefits from the Railroad Retirement Board, call your local RRB office or 1-800-808-0772. For more information, call your Medicare carrier about bills and services. The phone number for the Medicare carrier in your area can be found at the following Web site: **http://www.medicare.gov/Contacts/home.asp**. You may have choices in how you get your healthcare including the Original Medicare Plan, Medicare Managed Care Plans (like HMOs), and Medicare Private Fee-for-Service Plans.

### Medicaid

Medicaid is a joint federal and state program that helps pay medical costs for some people with low incomes and limited resources. Medicaid programs vary from state to state. People on Medicaid may also get coverage for nursing home care and outpatient prescription drugs which are not covered by Medicare. You can find more information about Medicaid on the HCFA.gov Web site at **http://www.hcfa.gov/medicaid/medicaid.htm**.

States also have programs that pay some or all of Medicare's premiums and may also pay Medicare deductibles and coinsurance for certain people who have Medicare and a low income. To qualify, you must have:

- Part A (Hospital Insurance),

- Assets, such as bank accounts, stocks, and bonds that are not more than $4,000 for a single person, or $6,000 for a couple, and

- A monthly income that is below certain limits.

For more information, look at the Medicare Savings Programs brochure, **http://www.medicare.gov/Library/PDFNavigation/PDFInterim.asp?Langua ge=English&Type=Pub&PubID=10126**. There are also Prescription Drug Assistance Programs available. Find information on these programs which offer discounts or free medications to individuals in need at **http://www.medicare.gov/Prescription/Home.asp**.

## NORD's Medication Assistance Programs

Finally, the National Organization for Rare Disorders, Inc. (NORD) administers medication programs sponsored by humanitarian-minded pharmaceutical and biotechnology companies to help uninsured or under-insured individuals secure life-saving or life-sustaining drugs.[58] NORD programs ensure that certain vital drugs are available "to those individuals whose income is too high to qualify for Medicaid but too low to pay for their

---

[58] Adapted from NORD: **http://www.rarediseases.org/programs/medication**.

prescribed medications." The program has standards for fairness, equity, and unbiased eligibility. It currently covers some 14 programs for nine pharmaceutical companies. NORD also offers early access programs for investigational new drugs (IND) under the approved "Treatment INDs" programs of the Food and Drug Administration (FDA). In these programs, a limited number of individuals can receive investigational drugs that have yet to be approved by the FDA. These programs are generally designed for rare diseases or disorders. For more information, visit **www.rarediseases.org**.

## Additional Resources

In addition to the references already listed in this chapter, you may need more information on health insurance, hospitals, or the healthcare system in general. The NIH has set up an excellent guidance Web site that addresses these and other issues. Topics include:[59]

- Health Insurance:
  **http://www.nlm.nih.gov/medlineplus/healthinsurance.html**
- Health Statistics:
  **http://www.nlm.nih.gov/medlineplus/healthstatistics.html**
- HMO and Managed Care:
  **http://www.nlm.nih.gov/medlineplus/managedcare.html**
- Hospice Care: **http://www.nlm.nih.gov/medlineplus/hospicecare.html**
- Medicaid: **http://www.nlm.nih.gov/medlineplus/medicaid.html**
- Medicare: **http://www.nlm.nih.gov/medlineplus/medicare.html**
- Nursing Homes and Long-Term Care:
  **http://www.nlm.nih.gov/medlineplus/nursinghomes.html**
- Patient's Rights, Confidentiality, Informed Consent, Ombudsman Programs, Privacy and Patient Issues:
  **http://www.nlm.nih.gov/medlineplus/patientissues.html**
- Veteran's Health, Persian Gulf War, Gulf War Syndrome, Agent Orange:
  **http://www.nlm.nih.gov/medlineplus/veteranshealth.html**

---

[59] You can access this information at
**http://www.nlm.nih.gov/medlineplus/healthsystem.html**.

## Vocabulary Builder

The following vocabulary builder provides definitions of words used in this chapter that have not been defined in previous chapters:

**Belding:** An expression based on the ratio of the sweat evaporation rate necessary to maintain thermal equilibrium at the maximum evaporative capacity of the environment. Generally used in the form E sub eq/E sub max x 1000, where E denotes evaporation. [NIH]

**Fistulas:** An abnormal passage from one hollow structure of the body to another, or from a hollow structure to the surface, formed by an abscess, disease process, incomplete closure of a wound, or by a congenital anomaly. [NIH]

**Modeling:** A treatment procedure whereby the therapist presents the target behavior which the learner is to imitate and make part of his repertoire. [NIH]

**Subclavian:** The direct continuation of the axillary vein at the lateral border of the first rib. It passes medially to join the internal jugular vein and form the brachiocephalic vein on each side. [NIH]

# ONLINE GLOSSARIES

The Internet provides access to a number of free-to-use medical dictionaries and glossaries. The National Library of Medicine has compiled the following list of online dictionaries:

- ADAM Medical Encyclopedia (A.D.A.M., Inc.), comprehensive medical reference: **http://www.nlm.nih.gov/medlineplus/encyclopedia.html**

- MedicineNet.com Medical Dictionary (MedicineNet, Inc.): **http://www.medterms.com/Script/Main/hp.asp**

- Merriam-Webster Medical Dictionary (Inteli-Health, Inc.): **http://www.intelihealth.com/IH/**

- Multilingual Glossary of Technical and Popular Medical Terms in Eight European Languages (European Commission) - Danish, Dutch, English, French, German, Italian, Portuguese, and Spanish: **http://allserv.rug.ac.be/~rvdstich/eugloss/welcome.html**

- On-line Medical Dictionary (CancerWEB): **http://www.graylab.ac.uk/omd/**

- Technology Glossary (National Library of Medicine) - Health Care Technology: **http://www.nlm.nih.gov/nichsr/ta101/ta10108.htm**

- Terms and Definitions (Office of Rare Diseases): **http://rarediseases.info.nih.gov/ord/glossary_a-e.html**

Beyond these, MEDLINEplus contains a very user-friendly encyclopedia covering every aspect of medicine (licensed from A.D.A.M., Inc.). The ADAM Medical Encyclopedia can be accessed via the following Web site address: **http://www.nlm.nih.gov/medlineplus/encyclopedia.html**. ADAM is also available on commercial Web sites such as Web MD (**http://my.webmd.com/adam/asset/adam_disease_articles/a_to_z/a**) and drkoop.com (**http://www.drkoop.com/**). Topics of interest can be researched by using keywords before continuing elsewhere, as these basic definitions and concepts will be useful in more advanced areas of research. You may choose to print various pages specifically relating to kidney failure and keep them on file. The NIH, in particular, suggests that patients with kidney failure visit the following Web sites in the ADAM Medical Encyclopedia:

- **Basic Guidelines for Kidney Failure**

  **End-stage renal disease**
  Web site:
  http://www.nlm.nih.gov/medlineplus/ency/article/000500.htm

- **Signs & Symptoms for Kidney Failure**

**Anemia**
Web site:
http://www.nlm.nih.gov/medlineplus/ency/article/000560.htm

**Blood in the vomit**
Web site:
http://www.nlm.nih.gov/medlineplus/ency/article/003118.htm

**Bruising**
Web site:
http://www.nlm.nih.gov/medlineplus/ency/article/003235.htm

**Coma**
Web site:
http://www.nlm.nih.gov/medlineplus/ency/article/003202.htm

**Confusion**
Web site:
http://www.nlm.nih.gov/medlineplus/ency/article/003205.htm

**Decreased alertness**
Web site:
http://www.nlm.nih.gov/medlineplus/ency/article/003202.htm

**Decreased sensation**
Web site:
http://www.nlm.nih.gov/medlineplus/ency/article/003206.htm

**Decreased urine output**
Web site:
http://www.nlm.nih.gov/medlineplus/ency/article/003147.htm

**Drowsiness**
Web site:
http://www.nlm.nih.gov/medlineplus/ency/article/003208.htm

**Fatigue**
Web site:
http://www.nlm.nih.gov/medlineplus/ency/article/003088.htm

**General ill feeling**
Web site:
http://www.nlm.nih.gov/medlineplus/ency/article/003089.htm

**Headache**
Web site:
http://www.nlm.nih.gov/medlineplus/ency/article/003024.htm

**Hiccups**
Web site:
http://www.nlm.nih.gov/medlineplus/ency/article/003068.htm

**Impotence**
Web site:
http://www.nlm.nih.gov/medlineplus/ency/article/003164.htm

**Itching**
Web site:
http://www.nlm.nih.gov/medlineplus/ency/article/003217.htm

**Lethargy**
Web site:
http://www.nlm.nih.gov/medlineplus/ency/article/003088.htm

**Menstrual irregularities**
Web site:
http://www.nlm.nih.gov/medlineplus/ency/article/003263.htm

**Muscle twitching**
Web site:
http://www.nlm.nih.gov/medlineplus/ency/article/003296.htm

**Nail abnormalities**
Web site:
http://www.nlm.nih.gov/medlineplus/ency/article/003247.htm

**Nausea**
Web site:
http://www.nlm.nih.gov/medlineplus/ency/article/003117.htm

**Nausea and vomiting**
Web site:
http://www.nlm.nih.gov/medlineplus/ency/article/003117.htm

### No urine output
Web site:
http://www.nlm.nih.gov/medlineplus/ency/article/003147.htm

### Pruritus
Web site:
http://www.nlm.nih.gov/medlineplus/ency/article/003217.htm

### Seizures
Web site:
http://www.nlm.nih.gov/medlineplus/ency/article/003200.htm

### Somnolence
Web site:
http://www.nlm.nih.gov/medlineplus/ency/article/003208.htm

### Stress
Web site:
http://www.nlm.nih.gov/medlineplus/ency/article/003211.htm

### Vomiting
Web site:
http://www.nlm.nih.gov/medlineplus/ency/article/003117.htm

### Weight loss
Web site:
http://www.nlm.nih.gov/medlineplus/ency/article/003107.htm

- **Diagnostics and Tests for Kidney Failure**

### BUN
Web site:
http://www.nlm.nih.gov/medlineplus/ency/article/003474.htm

### Creatinine
Web site:
http://www.nlm.nih.gov/medlineplus/ency/article/003475.htm

### Creatinine clearance
Web site:
http://www.nlm.nih.gov/medlineplus/ency/article/003611.htm

**Dialysis**
Web site:
http://www.nlm.nih.gov/medlineplus/ency/article/003421.htm

**Erythropoietin**
Web site:
http://www.nlm.nih.gov/medlineplus/ency/article/003683.htm

**Urine volume**
Web site:
http://www.nlm.nih.gov/medlineplus/ency/article/003425.htm

- **Nutrition for Kidney Failure**

**Carbohydrate**
Web site:
http://www.nlm.nih.gov/medlineplus/ency/article/002469.htm

**Protein in diet**
Web site:
http://www.nlm.nih.gov/medlineplus/ency/article/002467.htm

- **Background Topics for Kidney Failure**

**Acute**
Web site:
http://www.nlm.nih.gov/medlineplus/ency/article/002215.htm

**Chronic**
Web site:
http://www.nlm.nih.gov/medlineplus/ency/article/002312.htm

**Electrolyte**
Web site:
http://www.nlm.nih.gov/medlineplus/ency/article/002350.htm

**Electrolytes**
Web site:
http://www.nlm.nih.gov/medlineplus/ency/article/002350.htm

**Fractures**
Web site:
http://www.nlm.nih.gov/medlineplus/ency/article/000001.htm

**Kidney disease - support group**
Web site:
http://www.nlm.nih.gov/medlineplus/ency/article/002172.htm

**Metabolism**
Web site:
http://www.nlm.nih.gov/medlineplus/ency/article/002257.htm

**Support group**
Web site:
http://www.nlm.nih.gov/medlineplus/ency/article/002150.htm

## Online Dictionary Directories

The following are additional online directories compiled by the National Library of Medicine, including a number of specialized medical dictionaries and glossaries:

- Medical Dictionaries: Medical & Biological (World Health Organization):
  **http://www.who.int/hlt/virtuallibrary/English/diction.htm#Medical**

- MEL-Michigan Electronic Library List of Online Health and Medical Dictionaries (Michigan Electronic Library):
  **http://mel.lib.mi.us/health/health-dictionaries.html**

- Patient Education: Glossaries (DMOZ Open Directory Project):
  **http://dmoz.org/Health/Education/Patient_Education/Glossaries/**

- Web of Online Dictionaries (Bucknell University):
  **http://www.yourdictionary.com/diction5.html#medicine**

# KIDNEY FAILURE GLOSSARY

The following is a complete glossary of terms used in this sourcebook. The definitions are derived from official public sources including the National Institutes of Health [NIH] and the European Union [EU]. After this glossary, we list a number of additional hardbound and electronic glossaries and dictionaries that you may wish to consult.

**Ablation:** The removal of an organ by surgery. [NIH]

**Adjustment:** The dynamic process wherein the thoughts, feelings, behavior, and biophysiological mechanisms of the individual continually change to adjust to the environment. [NIH]

**Airway:** A device for securing unobstructed passage of air into and out of the lungs during general anesthesia. [NIH]

**Allografts:** A graft of tissue obtained from the body of another animal of the same species but with genotype differing from that of the recipient; tissue graft from a donor of one genotype to a host of another genotype with host and donor being members of the same species. [NIH]

**Ameliorating:** A changeable condition which prevents the consequence of a failure or accident from becoming as bad as it otherwise would. [NIH]

**Anorexia:** Lack or loss of appetite for food. Appetite is psychologic, dependent on memory and associations. Anorexia can be brought about by unattractive food, surroundings, or company. [NIH]

**Antibiotic:** A substance usually produced by vegetal micro-organisms capable of inhibiting the growth of or killing bacteria. [NIH]

**Aspartate:** A synthetic amino acid. [NIH]

**ATP:** ATP an abbreviation for adenosine triphosphate, a compound which serves as a carrier of energy for cells. [NIH]

**Belding:** An expression based on the ratio of the sweat evaporation rate necessary to maintain thermal equilibrium at the maximum evaporative capacity of the environment. Generally used in the form E sub eq/E sub max x 1000, where E denotes evaporation. [NIH]

**Benson:** Snowball-like bodies of calcium soaps occurring in a structurally intact vitreous body. [NIH]

**Bernstein:** A sensitive means of determining whether acid reflux is the cause of pain, but may be falsely negative in the patient receiving treatment. [NIH]

**Biophysics:** The science of physical phenomena and processes in living organisms. [NIH]

**Blot:** To transfer DNA, RNA, or proteins to an immobilizing matrix such as nitrocellulose. [NIH]

**Cataracts:** In medicine, an opacity of the crystalline lens of the eye obstructing partially or totally its transmission of light. [NIH]

**Catheters:** A small, flexible tube that may be inserted into various parts of the body to inject or remove liquids. [NIH]

**CDNA:** Synthetic DNA reverse transcribed from a specific RNA through the action of the enzyme reverse transcriptase. DNA synthesized by reverse transcriptase using RNA as a template. [NIH]

**Chickenpox:** A mild, highly contagious virus characterized by itchy blisters all over the body. [NIH]

**Clamp:** A u-shaped steel rod used with a pin or wire for skeletal traction in the treatment of certain fractures. [NIH]

**Cloning:** The production of a number of genetically identical individuals; in genetic engineering, a process for the efficient replication of a great number of identical DNA molecules. [NIH]

**Communis:** Common tendon of the rectus group of muscles that surrounds the optic foramen and a portion of the superior orbital fissure, to the anterior margin of which it is attached at the spina recti lateralis. [NIH]

**Compassionate:** A process for providing experimental drugs to very sick patients who have no treatment options. [NIH]

**Consultation:** A deliberation between two or more physicians concerning the diagnosis and the proper method of treatment in a case. [NIH]

**Contraindications:** Any factor or sign that it is unwise to pursue a certain kind of action or treatment, e. g. giving a general anesthetic to a person with pneumonia. [NIH]

**Cyclin:** Molecule that regulates the cell cycle. [NIH]

**Cytokine:** Small but highly potent protein that modulates the activity of many cell types, including T and B cells. [NIH]

**Deletion:** A genetic rearrangement through loss of segments of DNA (chromosomes), bringing sequences, which are normally separated, into close proximity. [NIH]

**Density:** The logarithm to the base 10 of the opacity of an exposed and processed film. [NIH]

**Diaphragm:** Contraceptive intra-uterine device. [NIH]

**Dilution:** A diluted or attenuated medicine; in homeopathy, the diffusion of a given quantity of a medicinal agent in ten or one hundred times the same quantity of water. [NIH]

**Dissection:** Cutting up of an organism for study. [NIH]

**Effector:** It is often an enzyme that converts an inactive precursor molecule into an active second messenger. [NIH]

**Efferent:** Nerve fibers which conduct impulses from the central nervous system to muscles and glands. [NIH]

**Electrode:** Component of the pacing system which is at the distal end of the lead. It is the interface with living cardiac tissue across which the stimulus is transmitted. [NIH]

**Emboli:** Bit of foreign matter which enters the blood stream at one point and is carried until it is lodged or impacted in an artery and obstructs it. It may be a blood clot, an air bubble, fat or other tissue, or clumps of bacteria. [NIH]

**Embryogenesis:** The process of embryo or embryoid formation, whether by sexual (zygotic) or asexual means. In asexual embryogenesis embryoids arise directly from the explant or on intermediary callus tissue. In some cases they arise from individual cells (somatic cell embryoge). [NIH]

**Enamel:** A very hard whitish substance which covers the dentine of the anatomical crown of a tooth. [NIH]

**Endoscopic:** A technique where a lateral-view endoscope is passed orally to the duodenum for visualization of the ampulla of Vater. [NIH]

**Enkephalin:** A natural opiate painkiller, in the hypothalamus. [NIH]

**Enzymatic:** Phase where enzyme cuts the precursor protein. [NIH]

**Exhaustion:** The feeling of weariness of mind and body. [NIH]

**Fatigue:** The feeling of weariness of mind and body. [NIH]

**Fistulas:** An abnormal passage from one hollow structure of the body to another, or from a hollow structure to the surface, formed by an abscess, disease process, incomplete closure of a wound, or by a congenital anomaly. [NIH]

**Fold:** A plication or doubling of various parts of the body. [NIH]

**Forearm:** The part between the elbow and the wrist. [NIH]

**FRC:** The functional residual capacity is the volume of gas remaining in the lungs at the end-expiratory level; the FRC has to be measured indirectly because the residual volume, RV, which is a subdivision of the FRC, cannot be removed from the lung; the techniques. [NIH]

**Gallate:** Antioxidant present in tea. [NIH]

**Generator:** Any system incorporating a fixed parent radionuclide from which is produced a daughter radionuclide which is to be removed by elution or by any other method and used in a radiopharmaceutical. [NIH]

**Hemodialyzer:** Apparatus for hemodialysis performing the functions of human kidneys in place of the damaged organs; highly specialized medical equipment used for treating kidney failure by passing the body's toxic substances through an external artificial kidney. [NIH]

**Hepatitis:** Infectious disease of the liver. [NIH]

**Heterogeneity:** The property of one or more samples or populations which implies that they are not identical in respect of some or all of their parameters, e. g. heterogeneity of variance. [NIH]

**HLA:** A glycoprotein found on the surface of all human leucocytes. The HLA region of chromosome 6 produces four such glycoproteins-A, B, C and D. [NIH]

**Hospice:** Institution dedicated to caring for the terminally ill. [NIH]

**Imidazole:** C3H4N2. The ring is present in polybenzimidazoles. [NIH]

**Immunologic:** The ability of the antibody-forming system to recall a previous experience with an antigen and to respond to a second exposure with the prompt production of large amounts of antibody. [NIH]

**Impairment:** In the context of health experience, an impairment is any loss or abnormality of psychological, physiological, or anatomical structure or function. [NIH]

**Infections:** The illnesses caused by an organism that usually does not cause disease in a person with a normal immune system. [NIH]

**Initiation:** Mutation induced by a chemical reactive substance causing cell changes; being a step in a carcinogenic process. [NIH]

**Insight:** The capacity to understand one's own motives, to be aware of one's own psychodynamics, to appreciate the meaning of symbolic behavior. [NIH]

**Islet:** Cell producing insulin in pancreas. [NIH]

**Kb:** A measure of the length of DNA fragments, 1 Kb = 1000 base pairs. The largest DNA fragments are up to 50 kilobases long. [NIH]

**Lactulose:** A mild laxative. [NIH]

**Linkage:** The tendency of two or more genes in the same chromosome to remain together from one generation to the next more frequently than expected according to the law of independent assortment. [NIH]

**Lod:** The lowest analyte content which, if actually present, will be detected with reasonable statistical certainty and can be identified according to the identification criteria of the method. If both accuracy and precision are constant over a concentration range. [NIH]

**Lymphoma:** Tumor of lymphatic tissue. [NIH]

**Migration:** The systematic movement of genes between populations of the same species, geographic race, or variety. [NIH]

**Modeling:** A treatment procedure whereby the therapist presents the target behavior which the learner is to imitate and make part of his repertoire. [NIH]

**Modification:** A change in an organism, or in a process in an organism, that is acquired from its own activity or environment. [NIH]

**Monitor:** An apparatus which automatically records such physiological signs as respiration, pulse, and blood pressure in an anesthetized patient or one undergoing surgical or other procedures. [NIH]

**MRNA:** The RNA molecule that conveys from the DNA the information that is to be translated into the structure of a particular polypeptide molecule. [NIH]

**Nerve:** A cordlike structure of nervous tissue that connects parts of the nervous system with other tissues of the body and conveys nervous impulses to, or away from, these tissues. [NIH]

**Networks:** Pertaining to a nerve or to the nerves, a meshlike structure of interlocking fibers or strands. [NIH]

**Neutrophil:** A motile, short-lived polymorphonuclear leucocyte with a multilobed nucleus and a cytoplasm filled with numerous minute granules, which is primarily responsible for maintaining normal host defenses against invading microorganisms. [NIH]

**Orf:** A specific disease of sheep and goats caused by a pox-virus that is transmissible to man and characterized by vesiculation and ulceration of the lips. [NIH]

**Outpatient:** A patient who is not an inmate of a hospital but receives diagnosis or treatment in a clinic or dispensary connected with the hospital. [NIH]

**Patch:** A piece of material used to cover or protect a wound, an injured part, etc.: a patch over the eye. [NIH]

**Pediatrics:** The branch of medical science concerned with children and their diseases. [NIH]

**Pharmacodynamic:** Is concerned with the response of living tissues to chemical stimuli, that is, the action of drugs on the living organism in the absence of disease. [NIH]

**Pharmacokinetic:** The mathematical analysis of the time courses of absorption, distribution, and elimination of drugs. [NIH]

**Phosphorylated:** Attached to a phosphate group. [NIH]

**Phosphorylating:** Attached to a phosphate group. [NIH]

**Physiology:** The science that deals with the life processes and functions of organismus, their cells, tissues, and organs. [NIH]

**Plaque:** A clear zone in a bacterial culture grown on an agar plate caused by localized destruction of bacterial cells by a bacteriophage. The concentration of infective virus in a fluid can be estimated by applying the fluid to a culture and counting the number of. [NIH]

**Plasticity:** In an individual or a population, the capacity for adaptation: a) through gene changes (genetic plasticity) or b) through internal physiological modifications in response to changes of environment (physiological plasticity). [NIH]

**Pneumology:** The study of disease of the air passages. [NIH]

**Polymorphism:** The occurrence together of two or more distinct forms in the same population. [NIH]

**Potassium:** It is essential to the ability of muscle cells to contract. [NIH]

**Promoter:** A chemical substance that increases the activity of a carcinogenic process. [NIH]

**Protocol:** The detailed plan for a clinical trial that states the trial's rationale, purpose, drug or vaccine dosages, length of study, routes of administration, who may participate, and other aspects of trial design. [NIH]

**Race:** A population within a species which exhibits general similarities within itself, but is both discontinuous and distinct from other populations of that species, though not sufficiently so as to achieve the status of a taxon. [NIH]

**Recombination:** The formation of new combinations of genes as a result of segregation in crosses between genetically different parents; also the rearrangement of linked genes due to crossing-over. [NIH]

**Rehabilitative:** Instruction of incapacitated individuals or of those affected with some mental disorder, so that some or all of their lost ability may be regained. [NIH]

**Salivary:** The duct that convey saliva to the mouth. [NIH]

**Sarcoma:** A malignant tumor of connective tissue or its derivatives. [NIH]

**Schematic:** Representative or schematic eye computed from the average of a large number of human eye measurements by Allvar Gullstrand. [NIH]

**Sebaceous:** Gland that secretes sebum. [NIH]

**Segal:** The alternate presentation of two visual stimuli consisting of concentric circular spots of light of different size. [NIH]

**Segmental:** Describing or pertaining to a structure which is repeated in similar form in successive segments of an organism, or which is undergoing segmentation. [NIH]

**Sendai:** A virus that causes an important and widespread infection of laboratory mice; it belongs to the parainfluenza group of mixoviruses. The virus is widely used in cell fusion studies. [NIH]

**Specialist:** In medicine, one who concentrates on 1 special branch of medical science. [NIH]

**Sperm:** The fecundating fluid of the male. [NIH]

**Stimulants:** Any drug or agent which causes stimulation. [NIH]

**Stimulus:** That which can elicit or evoke action (response) in a muscle, nerve, gland or other excitable issue, or cause an augmenting action upon any function or metabolic process. [NIH]

**Streptococcal:** Caused by infection due to any species of streptococcus. [NIH]

**Subclavian:** The direct continuation of the axillary vein at the lateral border of the first rib. It passes medially to join the internal jugular vein and form the brachiocephalic vein on each side. [NIH]

**Therapeutics:** The branch of medicine which is concerned with the treatment of diseases, palliative or curative. [NIH]

**Threshold:** For a specified sensory modality (e. g. light, sound, vibration), the lowest level (absolute threshold) or smallest difference (difference threshold, difference limen) or intensity of the stimulus discernible in prescribed conditions of stimulation. [NIH]

**Translation:** The process whereby the genetic information present in the linear sequence of ribonucleotides in mRNA is converted into a corresponding sequence of amino acids in a protein. It occurs on the ribosome and is unidirectional. [NIH]

**Trauma:** Any injury, wound, or shock, must frequently physical or structural shock, producing a disturbance. [NIH]

**Ulcer:** A localized necrotic lesion of the skin or a mucous surface. [NIH]

**Vasodilators:** Any nerve or agent which induces dilatation of the blood vessels. [NIH]

**Vector:** Plasmid or other self-replicating DNA molecule that transfers DNA between cells in nature or in recombinant DNA technology. [NIH]

**Vitro:** Descriptive of an event or enzyme reaction under experimental investigation occurring outside a living organism. Parts of an organism or microorganism are used together with artificial substrates and/or conditions. [NIH]

**Zestril:** A heart drug. [NIH]

**Zoster:** A virus infection of the Gasserian ganglion and its nerve branches, characterized by discrete areas of vesiculation of the epithelium of the forehead, the nose, the eyelids, and the cornea together with subepithelial infiltration. [NIH]

## General Dictionaries and Glossaries

While the above glossary is essentially complete, the dictionaries listed here cover virtually all aspects of medicine, from basic words and phrases to more advanced terms (sorted alphabetically by title; hyperlinks provide rankings, information and reviews at Amazon.com):

- **Dictionary of Medical Acronymns & Abbreviations** by Stanley Jablonski (Editor), Paperback, 4th edition (2001), Lippincott Williams & Wilkins Publishers, ISBN: 1560534605,
  **http://www.amazon.com/exec/obidos/ASIN/1560534605/icongroupinterna**

- **Dictionary of Medical Terms: For the Nonmedical Person (Dictionary of Medical Terms for the Nonmedical Person, Ed 4)** by Mikel A. Rothenberg, M.D, et al, Paperback - 544 pages, 4th edition (2000), Barrons Educational Series, ISBN: 0764112015,
  **http://www.amazon.com/exec/obidos/ASIN/0764112015/icongroupinterna**

- **A Dictionary of the History of Medicine** by A. Sebastian, CD-Rom edition (2001), CRC Press-Parthenon Publishers, ISBN: 185070368X,
  **http://www.amazon.com/exec/obidos/ASIN/185070368X/icongroupinterna**

- **Dorland's Illustrated Medical Dictionary (Standard Version)** by Dorland, et al, Hardcover - 2088 pages, 29th edition (2000), W B Saunders Co, ISBN: 0721662544,
  **http://www.amazon.com/exec/obidos/ASIN/0721662544/icongroupinterna**

- **Dorland's Electronic Medical Dictionary** by Dorland, et al, Software, 29th Book & CD-Rom edition (2000), Harcourt Health Sciences, ISBN: 0721694934,
  **http://www.amazon.com/exec/obidos/ASIN/0721694934/icongroupinterna**

- **Dorland's Pocket Medical Dictionary (Dorland's Pocket Medical Dictionary, 26th Ed)** Hardcover - 912 pages, 26th edition (2001), W B Saunders Co, ISBN: 0721682812,
  **http://www.amazon.com/exec/obidos/ASIN/0721682812/icongroupinterna/103-4193558-7304618**

- **Melloni's Illustrated Medical Dictionary (Melloni's Illustrated Medical Dictionary, 4th Ed)** by Melloni, Hardcover, 4th edition (2001), CRC Press-Parthenon Publishers, ISBN: 85070094X,

http://www.amazon.com/exec/obidos/ASIN/85070094X/icongroupintern
a

- **Stedman's Electronic Medical Dictionary Version 5.0 (CD-ROM for Windows and Macintosh, Individual)** by Stedmans, CD-ROM edition (2000), Lippincott Williams & Wilkins Publishers, ISBN: 0781726328, http://www.amazon.com/exec/obidos/ASIN/0781726328/icongroupinter na

- **Stedman's Medical Dictionary** by Thomas Lathrop Stedman, Hardcover - 2098 pages, 27th edition (2000), Lippincott, Williams & Wilkins, ISBN: 068340007X, http://www.amazon.com/exec/obidos/ASIN/068340007X/icongroupinter na

- **Tabers Cyclopedic Medical Dictionary (Thumb Index)** by Donald Venes (Editor), et al, Hardcover - 2439 pages, 19th edition (2001), F A Davis Co, ISBN: 0803606540, http://www.amazon.com/exec/obidos/ASIN/0803606540/icongroupinter na

# INDEX

Printed in the United States
46767LVS00004B/202

9 780497 009892